Handbook of Diabetes

Rudy Bilous, MD, FRCP
Professor Emeritus of Clinical Medicine, Newcastle University;
Consultant in Medical Education, South Tees NHS Foundation Trust
Middlesbrough, UK

Richard Donnelly, MD, PhD, FRCP, FRACP
Professor Emeritus and Consultant Physician
School of Medicine, University of Nottingham
Nottingham, UK

Iskandar Idris, DM, FRCP
Clinical Associate Professor in Diabetes and Vascular Medicine
Division of Graduate Entry Medicine and Medical Sciences
School of Medicine, University of Nottingham, Nottingham, UK;
Honorary Consultant Endocrinologist and General Physician
University Hospitals of Derby and Burton Foundation Trust, Derby, UK

5th edition

WILEY Blackwell

Registered Office(s)
John Wiley & Sons, Inc., 111 River Street, Hoboken, NJ 07030, USA
John Wiley & Sons Ltd, The Atrium, Southern Gate, Chichester, West Sussex, PO19 8SQ, UK

Editorial Office
9600 Garsington Road, Oxford, OX4 2DQ, UK

For details of our global editorial offices, customer services, and more information about Wiley products visit us at www.wiley.com.

Wiley also publishes its books in a variety of electronic formats and by print-on-demand. Some content that appears in standard print versions of this book may not be available in other formats.

Library of Congress Cataloging-in-Publication Data

Names: Bilous, Rudy W., author. | Donnelly, Richard, 1960- author. | Idris,
   Iskandar, author.
Title: Handbook of diabetes / Rudy Bilous, Richard Donnelly, Iskandar
   Idris.
Description: Fifth edition. | Hoboken, NJ : Wiley-Blackwell, [2021] |
   Includes bibliographical references and index.
Identifiers: LCCN 2020051205 (print) | LCCN 2020051206 (ebook) |
   ISBN 9781118976043 (paperback) | ISBN 9781118975992 (adobe pdf) |
   ISBN 9781118975978 (epub)
Subjects: MESH: Diabetes Mellitus | Diabetes Complications
Classification: LCC RC660.4 (print) | LCC RC660.4 (ebook) | NLM WK 810 |
   DDC 616.4/62–dc23
LC record available at https://lccn.loc.gov/2020051205
LC ebook record available at https://lccn.loc.gov/2020051206

Cover Design: Wiley
Cover Images: (top, left to right) © BSIP/Getty Images, © artursfoto/Getty Images, © Click_and_Photo/Getty Images, © Goffkein / Adobe Stock Photo, (main) © vgajic/Getty Images

Set in 9/12pt Meridien by Spi Global, Pondicherry, India
Printed and bound by CPI Group (UK) Ltd, Croydon, CR0 4YY

C9781118976043_250321

Handbook of
Diabetes

Contents

Preface

It is more than 10 years since the last edition and much has changed in diabetes understanding and therapy. Advances in diabetes technologies such as continuous glucose monitoring have made the use of closed-loop insulin infusion devices commonplace in many countries. New therapies for type 2 diabetes have led to the concept of personalised management algorithms for patients based upon individual circumstances such as age, weight and presence of complications or comorbidities. Large randomised trials of these treatments have shown benefit in terms of reduction of cardiovascular and renal risk. Diabetic retinopathy is no longer the leading cause of blindness in the working age population in the UK. Bariatric surgery and very low calorie diets have demonstrated the reversibility of type 2 diabetes.

Some things are sadly the same, however, such as the seemingly inexorable rise in prevalence, with the 2019 global figures already exceeding the 2025 predictions of the last edition. Others have fallen short of initial promise, such as islet cell transplantation, and while genetic research into the causes of diabetes has increased our understanding it has not yet been translated into new treatments.

This latest version of the Handbook has been revised and updated incorporating all of these developments and more, and there are new chapters on Cancer and Liver disease. We have tried to maintain the standards and ethos of previous editions. References are again selective but focus on reviews that are freely available wherever possible; key guidance from NICE, SIGN, ADA and other specialist bodies is also included.

Iskandar Idris is a new member of the editorial team and we would like to thank Alistair Lumb for his contribution to the chapters on type 1 diabetes treatment and psychological problems.

The team at Wiley have been notable for their patience. We would like to thank Priyanka Gibbons, Anupama Srikanth, and Jennifer Seward. Their forbearance during the long gestation of this edition is much appreciated. Any errors of commission or omission are, of course, the responsibility of the editors.

The goal with this latest edition is to continue to provide a useful desktop reference for all involved in providing care to people with diabetes.

Rudy Bilous
Richard Donnelly
Iskandar Idris

Key to the boxes

KEY POINTS

These points summarise important learning topics, things to remember and/or areas that are sometimes misunderstood by healthcare professionals.

CASE HISTORY

This is a typical case summary that illustrates a number of learning topics from the chapter.

LANDMARK CLINICAL TRIALS

These are often major trials underpinning the evidence base for clinical practice and decision-making in the area.

KEY WEBSITES

Websites that contain further information, practice guidelines and/or learning topics to supplement the information in the chapter.

FURTHER READING

Published reviews, original research or meta-analyses relevant to the chapter.

List of abbreviations

ABPI	Ankle Brachial Pressure Index	DCCT	Diabetes Control and Complications Trial
ABPM	ambulatory blood pressure measurement	DESMOND	Diabetes Education and Self-Management Ongoing and Newly Diagnosed
ACCORD	Action to Control Cardiovascular Risk in Diabetes	DIDMOAD	diabetes insipidus diabetes mellitus optic atrophy deafness
ACE	angiotensin-converting enzyme	DKA	diabetic ketoacidosis
ACEI	angiotensin-converting enzyme inhibitors	DME	diabetes-related macular oedema
ACR	albumin creatinine ratio	DPP-4	dipeptidyl peptidase-4 (IV)
ADA	American Diabetes Association	DSN	diabetes specialist nurse
ADVANCE	Action in Diabetes and Vascular Disease: Preterax and Diamicron MR Controlled Evaluation	DVA	Driving and Vehicle Agency
		DVLA	Driving and Vehicle Licensing Authority
AGE	advanced glycation endproduct	eAG	estimated average glucose
AKI	acute kidney injury	ED	erectile dysfunction
ALT	alanine aminotransferase	EDIC	Epidemiology of Diabetes Complications
AMI	acute myocardial infarction	eGFR	estimated glomerular filtration rate
ARB	angiotensin type 1 receptor blocker	eNOS	endothelial nitric oxide synthase
AST	aspartate aminotransferase	EPO	erythropoietin
ATP	adenosine triphosphate	ESRD	end-stage renal disease
BB	BioBreeding	ETDRS	Early Treatment Diabetic Retinopathy Study
BMI	Body Mass Index	EURODIAB	European Diabetes complications study group
BP	blood pressure	FATP	fatty acid transporter protein
CABG	coronary artery bypass grafting		
CBT	cognitive behavioural therapy	FDA	Food and Drug Administration
CCB	calcium channel blockers	FFA	free fatty acids
CETP	cholesterol ester transfer protein	FPG	fasting plasma glucose
CF	cystic fibrosis	FSD	female sexual dysfunction
CGM	continuous glucose monitoring	GAD	glutamic acid decarboxylase
CHD	coronary heart disease	GBM	glomerular basement membrane
CI	confidence interval	GCK	glucokinase
CIDP	chronic inflammatory demyelinating polyneuropathy	GDM	gestational diabetes mellitus
		GFAT	glutamine:fructose-6-phosphate amidotransferase
CKD	chronic kidney disease		
CSF	cerebrospinal fluid	GFR	glomerular filtration rate
CSII	continuous subcutaneous insulin infusion	GI	gastrointestinal
CT	computed tomography	GIP	gastric inhibitory polypeptide
CVD	cardiovascular disease	GIR	glucose infusion rate
DAFNE	Dose Adjustment for Normal Eating	GKI	glucose potassium insulin infusion
DAG	diacylglycerol	GLP-1	glucagon-like peptide-1

GLUT	glucose transporter		NOD	non-obese diabetic
GWAS	genome wide association study		NPH	neutral protamine Hagedorn
HBPM	home blood pressure measurement		NPY	neuropeptide Y
HDL	high-density lipoprotein		NVD	new vessels on the disc
HHS	hyperosmolar hyperglycaemic state		NVE	new vessels elsewhere
HL	hepatic lipase		OCT	optical coherence tomography
HLA	human leukocyte antigen		OGTT	oral glucose tolerance test
HOMA	Homeostasis Model Assessment		OR	odds ratio
HPLC	high-pressure liquid chromatography		PAD	peripheral arterial disease
HR	hazard ratio		PAI-1	plasminogen activator inhibitor-1
hsCRP	high-sensitivity C-reactive protein		PCI	percutaneous coronary intervention
IAA	insulin autoantibody		PCOS	polycystic ovary syndrome
IAPP	islet amyloid polypeptide		PG	plasma glucose
ICA	islet cell antibody		PI	phospatidylinositol
	insulin-dependent diabetes mellitus		PKC	Protein kinase C
IFG	impaired fasting glycaemia		PNDM	permanent neonatal diabetes mellitus
IGF	Insulin-like growth factor		PP	pancreatic polypeptide
IGT	impaired glucose tolerance		PPARγ	peroxisome proliferator-activated receptor-γ
IM	intramuscular		PRP	panretinal laser photocoagulation
IPPV	intermittent positive pressure ventilation		PTDM	post-transplant diabetes mellitus
IQR	interquartile range		QALY	quality-adjusted life-year
IRMA	intraretinal microvascular abnormality		RAGE	receptor for AGE
IRS	insulin receptor substrate		RAS	renin-angiotensin system
ITU	intensive therapy unit		RCT	randomised controlled trial
IV	intravenous		ROS	reactive oxygen species
KATP	ATP-sensitive potassium channel		RRR	relative risk reduction
LADA	latent autoimmune diabetes of adults		RRT	renal replacement therapy
LDL	low-density lipoprotein		RXR	retinoid X receptor
LH	luteinising hormone		SC	subcutaneous
MAP	mitogen-activated protein		SGLT2	sodium-glucose transporter 2
MAPK	mitogen-activated protein kinase		SMI	severe mental illness
MDI	multiple daily injection		SPK	simultaneous pancreas and kidney transplantation
MHC	major histocompatibility complex			
MI	myocardial infarction		SU	sulfonylurea
MODY	maturity-onset diabetes of the young		TCC	total contact casting
mTOR	mammalian target of rapamycin		TCF7L2	transcription factor 7-like 2 gene
NADH	nicotinamide adenine dinucleotide plus hydrogen		TG	triglyceride
			TGF	transforming growth factor
NADPH	nicotinamide adenine dinucleotide		TIA	transient ischaemic attack
NDIP	phospate hydrogen		TNF	tumour necrosis factor
	National Diabetes in Pregnancy audit		TZD	Thiazolidinediones
NEFA	non-esterified fatty acid		UKPDS	UK Prospective Diabetes Study
NDIP	National Diabetes in Pregnancy audit		UTI	urinary tract infections
NFκB	nuclear factor kappa-light-chain-enhancer of activated B cells		VCAM	vascular cell adhesion molecule
			VDT	vibration detection threshold
NGT	normal glucose tolerance		VEGF	vascular endothelium-derived growth factor
NICE	National Institute of Health and Clinical Excellence		VIP	vasoactive intestinal peptide
			VLDL	very low-density lipoprotein
NK	natural killer		VRIII	variable rate intravenous insulin infusion
NKCF	natural killer cell factor		WESDR	Wisconsin epidemiologic study of diabetic retinopathy
NLD	necrobiosis lipoidica diabeticorum			
NO	nitric oxide		WHO	World Health Organization

Part 1

Introduction to diabetes

Chapter 1

Introduction to diabetes

KEY POINTS

- Diabetes is common, and its incidence is rising.
- Type 2 diabetes is by far the most common accounting for 85–95% of cases.
- Complications in the microvasculature (eye, kidney and nerve) and the macrovasculature are responsible for considerable morbidity and excess mortality.

- Mortality from some complications is decreasing but absolute numbers for many are still rising.

Diabetes mellitus is a condition of chronically elevated blood glucose concentrations which give rise to its main symptom of passing large quantities of sweet–tasting urine (*diabetes* from the Greek word meaning 'a siphon', as the body acts as a conduit for the excess fluid, and *mellitus* from the Greek and Latin for honey). The fundamental underlying abnormality is a net (relative or absolute) deficiency of the hormone insulin. Insulin is essentially the only hormone that can lower blood glucose.

There are two main types of diabetes: type 1 is caused by an autoimmune destruction of the insulin-producing β cell of the islets of Langerhans in the pancreas (absolute deficiency); and type 2 is a result of both impaired insulin secretion and resistance to its action – often secondary to obesity (relative deficiency).

The precise level of blood glucose that defines diabetes has been revised several times and is covered in more detail in Chapter 3. Diabetes is common and is becoming more common. In absolute numbers, globally there are 463 million people aged 20–79 with known diabetes in 2019, projected to rise to 700 million in 2045. Alarmingly it is thought that there are almost as many again with undiagnosed diabetes. World-wide, age-adjusted prevalence is set to rise from 9.3 to 10.9% in 2045. The numbers of those with impaired glucose tolerance are equally startling with a prevalence of 7.5% in 2019, projected to rise to 8.6% in 2045 (Figure 1.1). The relative proportions of type 1 to type 2 vary from 15 : 85% for Western populations to 5 : 95% in developing countries.

It is the short- and long-term complications of diabetes which make it a major public health problem. Absolute deficiency of insulin leads to ketoacidosis and coma with an appreciable mortality even in the UK and other Western countries. Hyperglycaemic hyperosmolar state is less common but remains an equally serious problem for people with type 2 diabetes (see Chapter 12).

Long-term hyperglycaemia affects the microvasculature of the eye, kidney, and nerve as well as the larger arteries, leading to accelerated atherosclerosis. Diabetes is the most common cause of blindness in those of working age, the most common single cause of end-stage renal failure worldwide, and the consequences of neuropathy and peripheral vascular disease make it the most common cause of non-traumatic lower limb amputation. Diabetes and its complications are estimated to account for 11.3% of all cause mortality in adults aged 20–79 years in 2019 and nearly 50% of these are in people of working age (< 60 years).

Handbook of Diabetes, Fifth Edition. Rudy Bilous, Richard Donnelly, and Iskandar Idris.

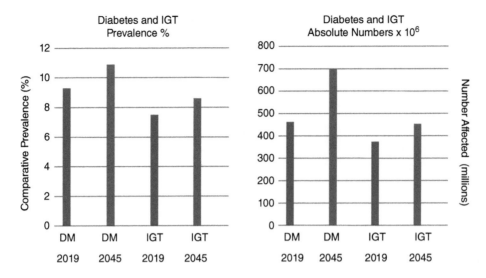

Figure 1.1 Estimated comparative raw prevalence of diabetes and impaired glucose tolerance (IGT) together with numbers affected for the global population age 20–79 years for 2019 (BLUE) and 2045 (RED). Data from *Diabetes Atlas*, 9th edn, International Diabetes Federation.

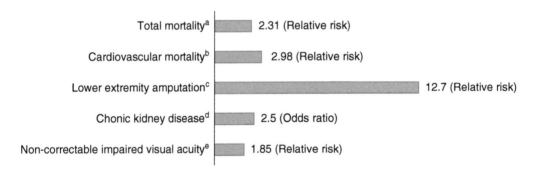

Figure 1.2 Rates of major complications of diabetes for the US population derived from NHANES or Medicare data. [a]NHANES data 1988–2000; [b]Medicare population Minnesota 1993–5; [c]NHANES data, 1999–2006 (chronic kidney disease defined as estimated GFR <60 mL/min/1.73 m[2].); [d]NHANES data, 1999–2002.

Mortality from ischaemic heart disease and stroke is 2–4-fold higher than in the age- and sex-matched non-diabetic population (Figure 1.2). These relative rates have not substantially changed since the last edition, although, encouragingly, mortality rates from acute myocardial infarction and hyperglycaemic crises have reduced, at least in the USA and Sweden (Figure 1.3). Because of the increasing numbers of people with diabetes, however, absolute numbers experiencing stroke, amputation, and end stage renal disease are increasing with massive associated financial costs. In 2019

the IDF estimates total diabetes healthcare expenditure will be US$760 billion and predicts that this will rise to US$ 825 billion in 2030 and US$ 845 billion by 2045 (Figure 1.4).

This handbook sets out to cover the essentials of diagnosis, epidemiology and management of diabetes and its' distressingly many complications. By using case vignettes and summaries of key trials together with web links and suggestions for further reading, it will hopefully serve as a useful desktop reference for all healthcare professionals who provide diabetes care.

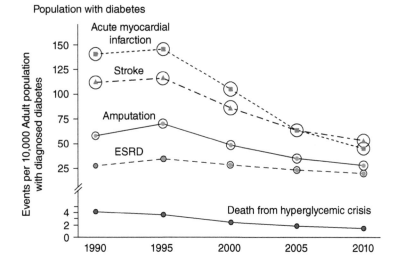

Mortality rates per 10,000 adults with diabetes	1990	1995	2000	2005	2010
AMI	8.5	10.1	9.6	7.3	5.7
Stroke	7.6	8.9	9.0	8.0	7.9
Amputation	3.0	4.2	4.0	3.2	3.0
ESRD	1.1	1.6	2.1	2.2	2.1
Hypergly - caemia	0.17	0.15	0.12	0.10	0.10

Figure 1.3 Age standardised mortality rates from diabetes-related complications in the US population with known diabetes 1990–2010. Circle size is proportional to the absolute number of cases. The table shows the rate per 10,000 population with or without diabetes. AMI = acute myocardial infarction, ESRD = End Stage Renal Disease. Figure and data from Gregg, E.W. et al. *NEJM* 2014; 370:1514–23 with permission.

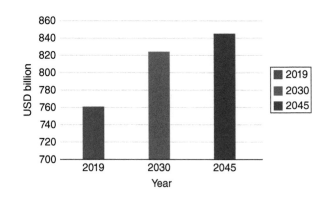

Figure 1.4 Estimated global diabetes-related healthcare costs for adults aged 20–79 years in 2019, 2030 and 2045. Source: IDF Diabetes Atlas 9th Edition 2019.

Chapter 2

History of diabetes

Diseases with the clinical features of diabetes have been recognised since antiquity. The Ebers papyrus (Figure 2.1), dating from 1550 BC, describes a polyuric state that resembles diabetes.

The word 'diabetes' was first used by Aretaeus of Cappadocia in the second century CE. Aretaeus gave a clinical description of the disease (Box 2.1), noting the increased urine flow, thirst, and weight loss, features that are instantly recognisable today.

The sweet, honey-like taste of urine in polyuric states, which attracted ants and other insects, was reported by Hindu physicians such as Sushrut (Susruta) during the fifth and sixth centuries CE. These descriptions even mention two forms of diabetes, the more common occurring in older, overweight, and indolent people, and the other in lean people who did not survive for long. This empirical subdivision predicted the modern classification into type 1 and type 2 diabetes.

Diabetes was largely neglected in Europe until a seventeenth-century English physician, Thomas Willis (1621–75) (Figure 2.2), rediscovered the sweetness of diabetic urine. Willis, who was physician to King Charles II, thought that the disease had been rare in ancient times, but that its frequency was increasing in his age 'given to good fellowship'. Nearly a century later, the Liverpool physician Matthew

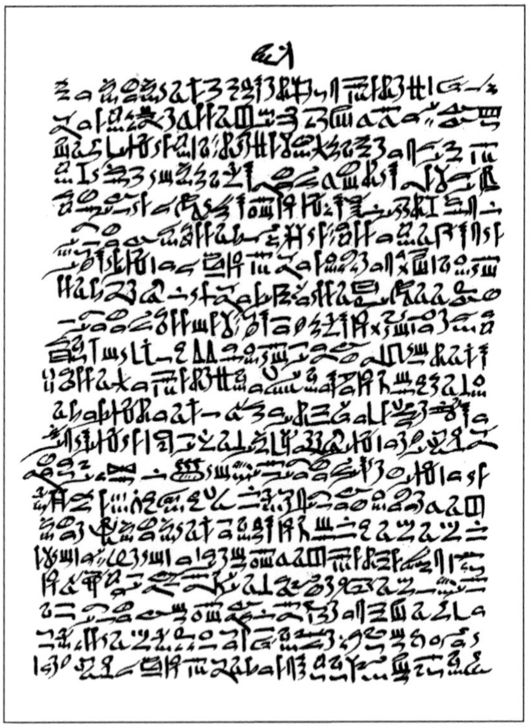

Figure 2.1 The Ebers papyrus. The Wellcome Institute Library, London, UK.

Handbook of Diabetes, Fifth Edition. Rudy Bilous, Richard Donnelly, and Iskandar Idris.
© 2021 John Wiley & Sons Ltd. Published 2021 by John Wiley & Sons Ltd.

Box 2.1 Description of diabetes by Aretaeus.

Diabetes is a dreadful affliction, not very frequent among men, being a melting down of the flesh and limbs into urine. The patients never stop making water and the flow is incessant, like the opening of aqueducts. Life is short, unpleasant and painful, thirst unquenchable, drinking excessive, and disproportionate to the large quantity of urine, for yet more urine is passed. One cannot stop them either from drinking or making water. If for a while they abstain from drinking, their mouths become parched and their bodies dry; the viscera seem scorched up, the patients are affected by nausea, restlessness and a burning thirst, and within a short time, they expire.

Adapted from Papaspyros S. *The History of Diabetes Mellitus*, 2nd edn. Stuttgart: Thieme, 1964.

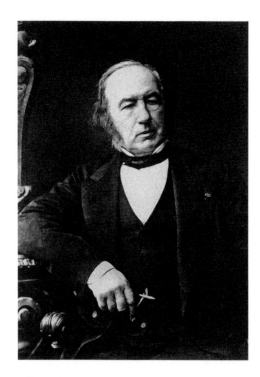

Figure 2.3 Claude Bernard. The Wellcome Institute Library, London, UK.

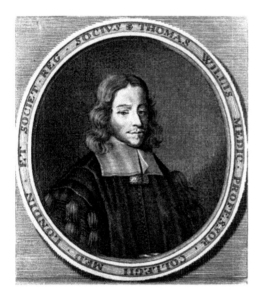

Figure 2.2 Thomas Willis. The Wellcome Institute Library, London, UK.

Dobson (1735–84) showed that the sweetness of urine and serum was caused by sugar. John Rollo (d. 1809) was the first to apply the adjective 'mellitus' to the disease.

In the 19th century, the French physiologist Claude Bernard (1813–78) (Figure 2.3) made many discoveries relating to diabetes. Among these was the finding that the sugar that appears in the urine was stored in the liver as glycogen. Bernard also demonstrated links between the central nervous system and diabetes when he observed temporary hyperglycaemia (piqûre diabetes) when the medulla of conscious rabbits was transfixed with a needle.

In 1889, Oskar Minkowski (1858–1931) and Joseph von Mering (1849–1908) from Strasbourg removed the pancreas

from a dog to see if the organ was essential for life. The animal displayed typical signs of diabetes, with thirst, polyuria, and wasting, which were associated with glycosuria and hyperglycaemia. This experiment showed that a pancreatic disorder causes diabetes, but they did not follow up on their observation.

Paul Langerhans (1847–88) (Figure 2.4) from Berlin, in his doctoral thesis of 1869, was the first to describe small clusters of cells in teased preparations of the pancreas. He did not speculate on the function of the cells, and it was Edouard Laguesse in France who later (1893) named the cells 'islets of Langerhans' and suggested that they were endocrine tissue of the pancreas that produced a glucose-lowering hormone.

In the early twentieth century, several workers isolated impure hypoglycaemic extracts from the pancreas, including the Berlin physician Georg Zuelzer (1840–1949), the Romanian Nicolas Paulesco (1869–1931), and the Americans Ernest Scott (1877–1966) and Israel Kleiner (1885–1966).

Insulin was discovered in 1921 at the University of Toronto, Canada, through a collaboration between the surgeon Frederick G Banting (1891–1941), his student assistant Charles H Best (1899–1978), the biochemist James B Collip (1892–1965) and the physiologist JJR Macleod (1876–1935). Banting and Best made chilled extracts of dog pancreas, injected them into pancreatectomised diabetic dogs, and showed a fall in blood glucose concentrations (Figure 2.5).

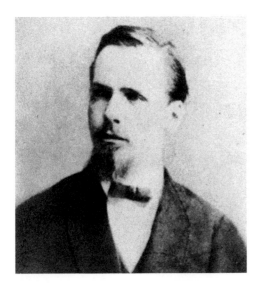

Figure 2.4 Paul Langerhans. The Wellcome Institute Library, London, UK.

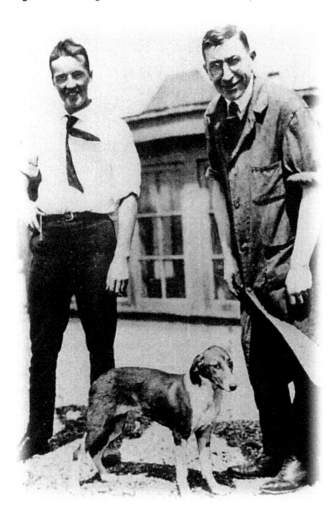

Figure 2.5 Charles Best and Frederick Banting in Toronto in 1922 (the dog is thought to have been called Marjorie). The Wellcome Institute Library, London, UK.

Banting and Best's notes of the dog experiments refer to the administration of 'isletin', later called insulin at the suggestion of Macleod. They were unaware that the Belgian Jean de Meyer had already coined the term 'insuline' in 1909. (All these names ultimately derive from the Latin for 'island'.)

Collip improved the methods for the extraction and purification of insulin from the pancreas, and the first person with diabetes, a 14-year-old boy called Leonard Thompson, was treated on 11 January 1922. A commercially viable extraction procedure was then developed in collaboration with chemists from Eli Lilly and Co. in the USA, and insulin became widely available in North America and Europe from 1923. The 1923 Nobel Prize for Physiology or Medicine was awarded to Banting and Macleod, who decided to share their prizes with Best and Collip.

The American physician Elliot P Joslin (1869–1962) was one of the first doctors to gain experience with insulin. Working in Boston, he treated 293 patients in the first year after August 1922. Joslin also introduced systematic education for his diabetic patients.

In the UK, the discovery of insulin saved the life of the London physician Robin D Lawrence (1892–1968), who had recently developed type 1 diabetes. He subsequently played a leading part in the founding of the British Diabetic Association now Diabetes UK.

Among the many major advances since the introduction of insulin into clinical practice was the elucidation in 1955 of its primary structure (amino acid sequence) (Figure 2.6) by the Cambridge UK scientist Frederick Sanger (b. 1918), who received the Nobel Prize for this work in 1958.

Oxford-based Dorothy Hodgkin (1910–1994), another Nobel Prize winner, and her colleagues described the three-dimensional structure of insulin using X-ray crystallography (1969). In total, there have been five Nobel Prizes awarded for scientific discoveries related to diabetes and carbohydrate metabolism.

By the 1950s, it was accepted that tissue complications, such as those that occur in the eye and kidney, continued to develop in long-standing diabetes, in spite of insulin treatment. The definitive proof that normalisation of glycaemia could prevent or delay the development of diabetic complications had to wait until 1993 for type 1 diabetes (the Diabetes Control and Complications Trial in North America) and 1998 for type 2 diabetes (the UK Prospective Diabetes Study – UKPDS).

Until the 1980s, insulin was derived only from animal pancreata, in increasingly more refined preparations. Using additives such as protamine or zinc, the subcutaneous absorption could be delayed, thus providing 24-hour availability using 2–4 injections a day of different preparations.

With the development of genetic engineering, it became possible to produce human insulin and subsequent further

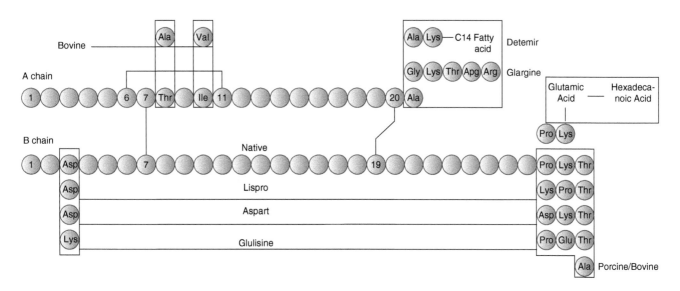

Figure 2.6 Schematic amino acid sequence of human insulin; porcine and bovine insulin; the short-acting insulin analogues aspart, lispro, and glulisine; and the long-acting analogues glargine, detemir, and degludec.

manipulations of the molecule have led to a wide range of preparations (Figure 2.6) with different absorption profiles (Chapter 10). There has been extensive research into an orally effective form of insulin but a continuing dependence upon subcutaneous injection as the main route of administration is likely for the foreseeable future.

In the 1980s, capillary blood glucose testing was a major breakthrough for patients allowing them to precisely assess their blood glucose levels and check for hypoglycaemia. Modern meters allow downloading of results enabling better informed modification of insulin regimens.

The rapid evolution of insulin delivery devices and continuous subcutaneous glucose sensing over the last decade has led to the production of closed loop systems which are effectively acting as an artificial pancreas. These systems are revolutionising the management of type 1 diabetes, although

their cost poses significant challenges for health care funders and has inevitably limited their use.

In type 2 diabetes oral agents have been available since the 1950s, bur the last few decades have seen the production of many different classes of compound that affect insulin secretion, its efficacy and sensitivity, as well as whole body glucose dispersal and excretion. This has led to the development of personalised diabetes therapy based upon the likely defect in the individual patient. This concept of personalised medicine forms the basis of recent guidelines for type 2 diabetes (Chapter 11).

FURTHER READING

Bliss, M. *The Discovery of Insulin*. Toronto: McLelland and Stewart, 1982.

Diagnosis and classification of diabetes

Diabetes mellitus is diagnosed by identifying chronic hyperglycaemia. The World Health Organisation (WHO) and the American Diabetes Association (ADA) use a fasting plasma glucose (FPG) of 7 mmol/L or higher to define diabetes (Table 3.1). This originates from epidemiological studies in the 1990s which appeared to show that the risk of microvascular complications (e.g retinopathy) increases sharply at a FPG threshold of 7 mmol/L (Figure 3.1). Lately, the notion of a clear glycaemic threshold separating people at high and low risk of diabetic microvascular complications has been called into question. The relationship between plasma glucose and microangiopathy is likely to be continuous, thus a FPG of 7 mmol/L is an arbitrary cut-off for defining diabetes which may be lowered in the future.

There are currently 34.2 million people in the USA with diabetes (10.5% of the population). Approximately 7 million of these are not yet aware that they have diabetes. The total number of people with diabetes worldwide is projected to increase from 171 million in 2000 to 366 million in 2030. A key demographic change to the rising prevalence of diabetes worldwide is an increasing proportion of people >65 years of age.

FPG, 2-h PG after 75-g OGTT, and A1C are equally appropriate for diagnostic testing. It should be noted that the tests do not necessarily detect diabetes in the same individuals. The concordance between the FPG and 2-h PG tests is imperfect. The overlap depends on the ethnic and geographical population, and on other characteristics such as age and body mass index. Some individuals have asymptomatic, isolated post-challenge hyperglycaemia, while others

Table 3.1 Diagnostic criteria for Type 2 diabetes.

Diabetes may be diagnosed based on plasma glucose criteria, either the fasting plasma glucose (FPG) or the 2-h plasma glucose (2-h PG) value after a 75-g oral glucose tolerance test (OGTT) or A1C criteria.

Criteria for the diagnosis of diabetes.
- FPG ≥126 mg/dL (7.0 mmol/L). Fasting is defined as no caloric intake for at least 8 h.*
- 2-h PG ≥200 mg/dL (11.1 mmol/L) during an OGTT. The test should be performed as described by the WHO, using a glucose load containing the equivalent of 75 g anhydrous glucose dissolved in water.*
- A1C ≥6.5% (48 mmol/mol). The test should be performed in a laboratory using a method that is NGSP certified and standardized to the DCCT assay.*

In a patient with classic symptoms of hyperglycemia or hyperglycemic crisis, a random plasma glucose ≥200 mg/dL (11.1 mmol/L).

* In the absence of unequivocal hyperglycemia, results should be confirmed by repeat testing.

Table 3.2 Use of HbA1c >6.5% (48 mmol/mol) as a cut-off for making the diagnosis of diabetes offers some advantages but there are several disadvantages.

Advantages	Disadvantages

• Avoids the need for a fasting blood sample, and the pre-analytical instability of glucose measurements.
• HbA1c reflects glycaemia over several weeks.
• Lower biological variability of HbA1c compared with FPG or 2 h glucose.
• Virtual absence of significant retinopathy among people with HbA1c < 6.5%.
	• HbA1c measurements can give spurious results in:
	  ○ anaemia (Fe-deficiency)
	  ○ haemoglobinopathies
	  ○ renal failure
	  ○ different ethnic groups.
	• Diagnosis by HbA1c will identify a different population to that diagnosed by FPG.
	• Distribution of HbA1c values varies in different ethnic groups.
	• HbA1c increases with age
	• Some patients and ethnic groups may be diagnosed with diabetes by some criteria but not others.

Handbook of Diabetes, Fifth Edition. Rudy Bilous, Richard Donnelly, and Iskandar Idris.
© 2021 John Wiley & Sons Ltd. Published 2021 by John Wiley & Sons Ltd.

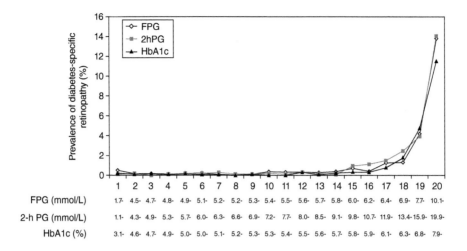

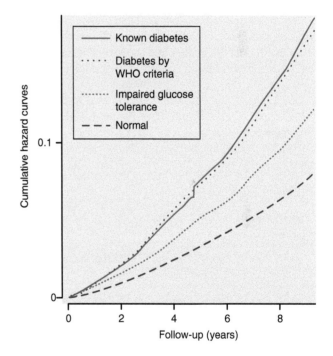

Figure 3.1 Prevalence of diabetes-specific retinopathy (moderate or more severe retinopathy) by vigintiles of the distribution of FPG, 2-h PG, and A1C. Adapted from Colaguiri et al. Diabetes Care *2011; 34: 145-150.*

have fasting hyperglycaemia but normal post-load glycaemic responses. The fasting criteria for diabetes tend to pick out younger and more obese subjects.

Numerous studies have confirmed that, compared with FPG and A1C cut points, the 2-h PG value diagnoses more people with diabetes. When using A1C to diagnose diabetes, it is important to recognize that A1C is an indirect measure of average blood glucose levels and to take other factors into consideration that may impact haemoglobin glycation independently of glycaemia including age, race/ethnicity, and anaemia/haemoglobinopathies.

Intermediate categories of hyperglycaemia: Pre-diabetes

During the natural history of all forms of diabetes, the disease passes through a stage of impaired glucose tolerance (IGT), defined as a plasma glucose of 7.8–11.0 mmol/L (140–200 mg/dL) 2 hours after an OGTT (Figure 3.2). Impaired fasting glucose (IFG) is an analogous category based on fasting glucose levels, and is defined as a FPG of 6.1–6.9 mmol/L (110–126 mg/dL).

IGT and IFG are intermediate metabolic stages between normal glucose homeostasis and diabetes. They are both risk factors for future diabetes and cardiovascular disease, but the 2-hour plasma glucose concentration is a particularly strong predictor of cardiovascular risk and mortality.

As with the glucose measures, several prospective studies that used A1C to predict the progression to diabetes as defined by A1C criteria demonstrated a strong, continuous

Figure 3.2 The relationship between 2-hour plasma glucose and survival in patients with normal glucose tolerance, patients with IGT, those with newly-diagnosed diabetes by OGTT, and those with known diabetes, as shown by the DECODE study (combining data from 13 European cohort studies). From Glucose tolerance and mortality: comparison of WHO and American Diabetic Association diagnostic criteria. *The Lancet* 354(9179), 617–621.

association between A1C and subsequent diabetes. Based on numerous studies and meta-analysis, it is now considered that A1C range of 5.7–6.4% (39–47 mmol/mol) as identifying individuals with prediabetes or with impaired glucose regulation IGR).

A proportion of patients with IFG, IGT and/or IGR (5-10% per annum) will deteriorate metabolically into overt diabetes. Lifestyle modification (diet, exercise and weight loss) is the best approach to diabetes prevention for these patients.

For an OGTT, the subject is tested in the morning after an overnight fast, in the seated position. After taking a fasting blood sample, 75 g of glucose is given by mouth, often in the form of a glucose drink such as Lucozade (843 mL based on the new formulation of 8.9g/100ml of glucose). For children, the glucose dose is calculated as 1.75 g/kg. A further blood sample is taken at 2 hours, and the fasting and 2 hour glucose values are interpreted as in Figure 3.3.

Glycosuria (the presence of glucose in the urine) is responsible for the classic diabetic symptoms and was previously regarded as a diagnostic hallmark of the disease. Nowadays, it indicates the need to test blood glucose, but cannot be used to diagnose diabetes because of the poor relationship between blood and urine glucose (Figure 3.6). This is for several reasons: the renal threshold for glucose reabsorption varies considerably within and between individuals, the urine glucose concentration is affected by the subject's state of hydration and the result reflects the average blood glucose during the period that urine has accumulated in the bladder. The average renal threshold is 10 mmol/L (i.e. blood glucose concentration above this level will 'spill over' into the urine), but a negative urine test can be associated with marked hyperglycaemia.

Longer term indices of hyperglycaemia include the HbA1c, a measure of integrated blood glucose control over the preceding few weeks. HbA1c is used primarily to assess glycaemic control among people with diabetes on treatment. HbA1c analyses are now being calibrated to the IFCC assay. Thus the units of HbA1c in many countries have changed from percent to mmol/mol (Table 3.3).

Table 3.3 Historically, HbA1c has been reported in percentage values describing the proportion of haemoglobin that is glycated. The assay was aligned to that used in the Diabetes Control and Complications (DCCT) trial. The International Federation of Clinical Chemistry (IFCC) has now established a new reference system, and values will be reported in mmol HbA1c per mol haemoglobin without glucose attached. Conversion for HbA1c is shown below.

DCCT (%)	IFCC (mmol/mol)	DCCT (%)	IFCC (mmol/mol)
6.0	42	9.0	75
6.2	44	9.2	77
6.4	46	9.4	79
6.5	48	9.5	80
6.6	49	9.6	81
6.8	51	9.8	84
7.0	53	10.0	86
7.2	55	10.2	88
7.4	57	10.4	90
7.5	58	10.5	91
7.6	60	10.6	92
7.8	62	10.8	95
8.0	64	11.0	97
8.2	66	11.2	99
8.4	68	11.4	101
8.5	69	11.5	102
8.6	70	11.6	103
8.8	73	11.8	105

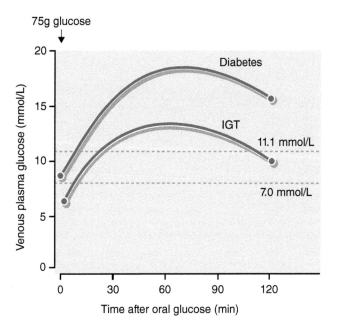

Figure 3.3 *Diagnosis of diabetes and IGT by the oral glucose tolerance test.*

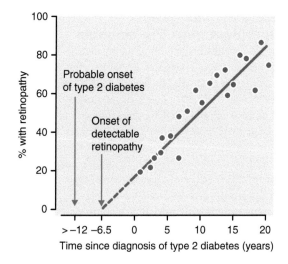

Figure 3.4 *The prevalence of retinopathy in type 2 diabetes relative to the time of clinical diagnosis. Note the presence of retinopathy at diagnosis and the likely onset of retinopathy and diabetes some years before diagnosis.* From Paisey. Diabetologia 1980; 19: 31 – 34.

The potential value of screening for diabetes is to facilitate early diagnosis and treatment. About 20% of newly diagnosed type 2 diabetic subjects already have evidence of vascular complications, such as retinopathy, the prevalence of which increases with diabetes duration. This suggests that complications begin about 5–6 years before a diagnosis is made, and that the actual onset of (type 2) diabetes may be several years before the clinical diagnosis.

In most countries, there is no systematic screening policy for diabetes, yet there are estimates that up to 50% of patients with diabetes are undiagnosed. Ad-hoc screening of high-risk groups is becoming more common. The fasting

---

High-risk patients who should be screened annually for type 2 diabetes

- Metabolic syndrome
- Patients >45 years of age, especially the obese
- Those with parents or siblings with type 2 diabetes
- Ethnic minorities, e.g. South Indians, even if non-obese
- Patients with cardiovascular risk factors, e.g. hypertension or dyslipidaemia, and those with established atherosclerotic disease
- Women with previous gestational diabetes
- Women with polycystic ovary syndrome
- Patients with IFG/IGT

Figure 3.5 *High-risk patients who should be screened annually for type 2 diabetes.*

Classification of diabetes

- Type 1 (β cell destruction, usually leading to absolute insulin deficiency)
  - Autoimmune
  - Idiopathic
- Type 2
  - Ranges from predominantly insulin resistant, with relative insulin deficiency, to a predominantly insulin-secretory defect, with or without insulin resistance
- Other specific types
  - Genetic defects of β cell function
  - Genetic defects of insulin action
  - Diseases of exocrine pancreas
  - Endocrinopathies
  - Drug induced or chemical induced, e.g. steroids
  - Infections
  - Uncommon forms of immune-mediated diabetes
  - Other genetic syndromes sometimes associated with diabetes
- Gestational diabetes

Figure 3.6 *Classification of diabetes.*

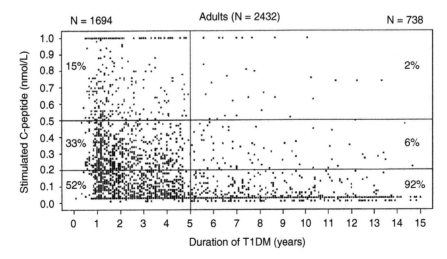

Peak C-peptide during MMTT (2-h) in patients 18 years of age at onset of diabetes and with type 1 diabetes (TIDM) of 1-15 years' duration when screened for entry into the DCCT.

Figure 3.7 Using C-peptide to confirm type 1 diabetes based on residual beta cell function. MMT-mixed meal tolerance test – i.e. patients ingested a standardized breakfast ingested over 10 min based on the total caloric need of the patient (25–30% of their daily caloric intake; 50% of the calories as carbohydrates). In routine practice this is utilised as a random 'c-peptide' level.

plasma glucose is simple, quick, acceptable to patients and of low cost, but can miss those with isolated post-challenge hyperglycaemia and requires patient to be fasted. The OGTT is more difficult to perform, impractical for large numbers and expensive, but is the only way to identify post-load hyperglycaemia. Screening should focus on high-risk groups. HbA1c is widely used to screen individuals at high risk of developing diabetes.

1 Severe Autoimmune Diabetes (SAID)
2 Severe Insulin Deficient Diabetes (SIDD)
3 Severe Insulin Resistance Diabetes (SIRD)
4 Moderate Obesity Diabetes (MOD)
5 Moderate Age Related Diabetes (MARD)

Figure 3.8 Five replicable clusters of patients with diabetes.
Source: Adapted from Ahlqvist et al. Lancet Diabetes & Endocrinology, 1 March 2018.

Clinical features of type 1 and type 2 diabetes

Type 1 diabetes
- Sudden onset with severe symptoms of thirst and ketoacidosis (vomiting, hyperventilation, dehydration)
- Recent, marked weight loss. Usually lean
- Spontaneous ketosis
- Life-threatening; needs urgent insulin replacement
- Absent C-peptide
- Markers of autoimmunity present (e.g. islet cell antibodies)

Type 2 diabetes
- Usually insidious onset of tiredness, thirst, polyuria, nocturia
- No ketoacidosis
- Usually overweight or obese; often no recent weight loss
- Frequent infections, e.g. urine, skin, chest
- Symptoms may be minimal and/or ignored by patient
- Often other features of 'metabolic syndrome' , e.g. hypertension
- C- peptide detectable

Figure 3.9 Clinical features of type 1 and type 2 diabetes.

Other specific types of diabetes

Genetic defects of β cell function
- Chromosome 12, HNF-1a (formerly MODY-3)
- Chromosome 7, glucokinase (formerly MODY-2)
- Chromosome 20, HNF-4a (formerly MODY-1)
- Mitochondrial DNA
- Insulinopathies

Genetic defects in insulin action
- Type A insulin resistance
- Leprechaunism
- Rabson–Mendenhall syndrome
- Lipoatrophic diabetes

Diseases of the exocrine pancreas
- Pancreatitis
- Trauma/pancreatectomy
- Neoplasia
- Cystic fibrosis
- Haemochromatosis
- Fibrocalculous pancreatopathy

Endocrinopathies
- Acromegaly
- Cushing's syndrome
- Glucagonoma
- Phaeochromocytoma
- Hyperthyroidism
- Somatostatinoma
- Aldosteronoma

Drug induced or chemical induced
- Glucocorticoids
- Thiazides
- Pentamidine
- Nicotinic acid
- Thyroid hormone
- β- adrenergic agonists
- Interferon-α

Infections
- Congenital rubella
- Cytomegalovirus
- Others
- Uncommon forms of immune-mediated diabetes
- 'Stiff man' syndrome
- Anti-insulin receptor antibodies

Other genetic syndromes sometimes a ssociated with diabetes
- Down's syndrome
- Klinefelter' s syndrome
- Turner's syndrome
- Wolfram' s syndrome
- Friedreich' s ataxia
- Huntington' s chorea
- Lawrence–Moon–Biedl syndrome
- Myotonic dystrophy
- Porphyria
- Prader–Willi syndrome

Figure 3.10 Other specific types of diabetes.

Classification of diabetes

The current classification of diabetes is based on the aetiology of the disease. There are four categories:

- Type 1 diabetes (caused by pancreatic islet cell destruction);
- Type 2 diabetes (caused by a combination of insulin resistance and β-cell insulin secretory dysfunction);
- Other specific types of diabetes (caused by conditions such as endocrinopathies, diseases of the exocrine pancreas, genetic syndromes, steroid induced etc., see below);
- Gestational diabetes (defined as diabetes that occurs for the first time in pregnancy).

Type 1 diabetes is subdivided into two main types: 1a or autoimmune (about 90% of type 1 patients in Europe and North America, in which immune markers, such as circulating islet cell antibodies, suggest autoimmune destruction of the β-cells) and 1b or idiopathic (where there is no evidence of autoimmunity).

A steady increase (2.5–3% per annum) in the incidence of type 1 diabetes has been reported worldwide, especially among young children <4 years old. There are large differences between countries in the incidence of type 1 diabetes, e.g up to 10-fold differences among European countries.

This classification has now replaced the earlier, clinical classification into 'insulin-dependent diabetes mellitus' (IDDM) and 'non-insulin-dependent diabetes mellitus' (NIDDM), which was based on the need for insulin treatment at diagnosis. IDDM is broadly equivalent to type 1 diabetes and NIDDM to type 2 diabetes. One of the disadvantages of the old classification according to treatment was that subjects could change their type of diabetes – for example, some type 1a patients diagnosed after the age of 40 years masquerade as NIDDM, before eventually becoming truly insulin-dependent (this is now classified as latent autoimmune diabetes in adults, LADA). Where diagnostic uncertainty exists between type 1 versus non type 1 diabetes, c-peptide assessments can determine residual function beta cells (and insulin dependency to prevent ketoacidosis).

Various clinical and biochemical features can be used to decide whether the patient has type 1 or type 2 diabetes. The distinction may be difficult in individual cases.

A recent study have suggested a novel classification of adult onset diabetes according to patient characteristics (glutamate decarboxylase antibodies, age at diagnosis, BMI, HbA1c and homoeostatic model assessment 2 estimates of beta cell function and insulin resistance) and risk of diabetic complications.

1. Severe Autoimmune Diabetes (SAID)
2. Severe Insulin Deficient Diabetes (SIDD)
3. Severe Insulin Resistance Diabetes (SIRD)
4. Moderate Obesity Diabetes (MOD)
5. Moderate Age Related Diabetes (MARD)

Their study showed that individuals in cluster 3 (Most resistant to insulin) had significantly higher risk of diabetic kidney disease than individuals in cluster 4 and 5. Cluster 2 (insulin deficient) had the highest risk of diabetic eye disease. The largest cluster is cluster 5.

The category of 'other specific types of diabetes' is a large group of conditions, which includes genetic defects in insulin secretion [such as in maturity-onset diabetes of the young (MODY) and insulinopathies], genetic defects in insulin action (e.g. syndromes of severe insulin resistance), pancreatitis, steroid induced and other exocrine disorders, hormone-secreting tumours such as acromegaly (growth hormone) and Cushing's syndrome (cortisol). Some cases are caused by the administration of drugs such as glucocorticoids. Some genetic syndromes are sometimes associated with diabetes (e.g. Down syndrome, Klinefelter's syndrome and many more).

CASE HISTORY

A 66-year-old retired policeman attends his family doctor for a routine BP check. He has had hypertension for 4 years. He reports incidentally that he has been feeling generally tired and lethargic. On further questioning, he admits to nocturia x3 and volunteers that in recent months he has been taking a glass of water to bed since he often wakes feeling thirsty. The GP notices that he had a cutaneous boil lanced 6 weeks ago. Apart from hypertension, there is no other significant past medical history, but his body weight has gradually risen (95kg, BMI 32). He takes an ACE inhibitor, lisinopril 10mg, for hypertension. His mother had type 2 diabetes, he is a non-smoker and drinks 15 units of alcohol per week. His only exercise is golf, twice per week. The doctor takes a random venous blood sample, which shows a plasma glucose level of 13 mmol/L. Further blood tests show a normal haematology profile, normal electrolytes and renal function, HbA1c 8.3%, and fasting lipids show total cholesterol 6.6mmol/L, LDL-cholesterol 4.3mmol/L, triglycerides 3.9mmol/L and HDL-cholesterol 0.6mmol/L. Minor abnormalities of liver function are also noted (AST & ALT 2-3x upper limit).

Comment: This man presents with typical symptoms of type 2 diabetes and several risk factors (age, obesity, hypertension, family history). The random plasma glucose and HbA1c in the context of symptoms, is diagnostic. He has features of the metabolic syndrome, including hypertension, dyslipidaemia (high triglycerides and low HDL-cholesterol) and central obesity, and fatty infiltration of the liver is common in this scenario. Susceptibility to infections is typical.

LANDMARK TRIALS

DECODE Study Group. Glucose tolerance and mortality: comparison of WHO and American Diabetes Association diagnostic criteria. *Lancet* 1999; 354: 617–621.

Wong TY, et al. Relation between fasting glucose and retinopathy for diagnosis of diabetes: three population-based cross-sectional studies. *Lancet* 2008; 371: 736–743.

Wild S, et al. Global Prevalence of Diabetes: Estimates for the year 2000 and projections for 2030. *Diabetes Care* 2004; 27: 1047–1053.

Diabetes Prevention Program Research Group. The prevalence of retinopathy in impaired glucose tolerance and recent-onset diabetes in the Diabetes Prevention Program. *Diabet. Med.* 2007; 24: 137–144.

Li G, et al. The long-term effect of lifestyle interventions to prevent diabetes in the China Da Qing Diabetes Prevention Study: a 20-year follow-up study. *Lancet* 2008; 371: 1783–1789.

Tabak AG, et al. Trajectories of glycaemia, insulin sensitivity, and insulin secretion before diagnosis of type 2 diabetes: an analysis from the Whitehall II study. *Lancet* 2009; 373: 2215–2221.

Dabelea D et al SEARCH for Diabetes in Youth Study Group. Trends in the prevalence of ketoacidosis at diabetes diagnosis: the Search for Diabetes in Youth Study. *Pediatrics* 2014;133:e938–e945

Herman WH, et al. Early detection and treatment of type 2 diabetes reduce cardiovascular morbidity and mortality: a simulation of the results of the Anglo-Danish-Dutch study of intensive treatment in people with screen-detected diabetes in primary care (ADDITION-Europe). *Diabetes Care* 2015;38:1449–1455

WEBSITES

- http://www.who.int/diabetes/publications/en/
- http://www.diabetes.org/about-diabetes.jsp
- http://www.idf.org/home/index.cfm?node=4

FURTHER READING

International Expert Committee International Expert Committee report on the role of the A1C assay in the diagnosis of diabetes. *Diabetes Care* 2009;32:1327–1334

Florez JC, et al. TCF7L2 Polymorphisms and progression to diabetes in the Diabetes Prevention Program. *N. Engl. J. Med.* 2006; 355: 241–250.

Gillies CL, et al. Different strategies for screening and prevention of type 2 diabetes in adults: cost effectiveness analysis. *Br. Med. J.* 2008; 336: 1180–1184.

Classification and diagnosis of diabetes American Diabetes Association Diabetes Care 2017 *Jan*; 40(Supplement 1): S11–S24. https://doi.org/10.2337/dc17-S005

Harris MI, et al. Onset of NIDDM occurs at least 4-7 years before clinical diagnosis. *Diabetes Care* 1992; 15: 815–819.

Ahlqvist et al. Novel subgroups of adult-onset diabetes and their association with outcomes: a data-driven cluster analysis of six variables. *Lancet Diabetes & Endocrinology*, 2018; 6:361–369

Public health aspects of diabetes

KEY POINTS

- The annual economic burden of diabetes in the USA is estimated at $450 billion in 2016.
- The cost-effectiveness of healthcare interventions in diabetes is a topic of importance.
- There are currently circa 425m patients with diabetes worldwide (2017).
- Providing structured education for all patients with diabetes, and implementation of a targeted screening and diabetes prevention programme are public health priorities.

Diabetes has become a major public health challenge in the 21st century (Figures 4.1 and 4.2). Over 26m people (8% of the population) now have diabetes in the USA and 7 million of these are not even aware of their diagnosis (Figure 4.3). The prevalence has increased 5- to 7-fold in recent years, and diabetes is responsible for significant reductions in life-expectancy as well as longterm disabling complications such as blindness, renal failure, lower limb amputation, and premature cardiovascular disease (Figures 4.4 and 4.5).

Overweight and obesity are major factors driving this trend. A recent report from Public Health England suggests that 90% of adults with type 2 diabetes are overweight or obese and there is a direct linear relationship between BMI and mortality among type 2 diabetes patients who have never smoked. In those with a smoking history, the relationship is J-shaped because smoking off-sets any benefits of a lower BMI. The relationship between HbA1c and any diabetes-related endpoint is also linear.

Aside from the human costs of diabetes, there is a huge economic impact on the healthcare budget (Figures 4.6 and 4.7). About 75% of the direct costs are attributable to managing the long-term vascular complications of diabetes, only a relatively small fraction is spent on diabetes treatments and surveillance. Furthermore, 90% of resources are spent on patients with type 2 diabetes. In the USA, the total direct costs of diabetes in 2012 were estimated to be $176b.

For an individual patient, the lifetime healthcare costs of diabetes were estimated at $85 200. In the UK, expenditure on diabetes accounts for 9% of the entire NHS budget (approximately £8.8b per year) and is forecast to reach 17% of NHS spending by 2035.

Given that hyperglycaemia has cumulative adverse effects, it makes good clinical and economic sense to maximise glycaemic control and weight reduction in the early years after diagnosis. The UK National Diabetes Audit reported data on 1.9m patients with diabetes and showed that, in the period 2009–2015, 90–95% of patients with type 2 diabetes had 6-monthly HbA1c monitoring performed and two-thirds of them achieved the NICE treatment target (applicable at the time) of HbA1c <7.5% (58 mmol/mol). However, there were significant regional variations in achievement of HbA1c targets, and the lowest rates of attainment were among younger age groups (those <40 years and in the 40–64 yr age band).

Declining mortality rates for patients with diabetes, combined with aging population demographics and the increasing prevalence of diabetes risk factors, will likely fuel the continuation of a diabetes epidemic (Figure 4.8). Clinical management is becoming more complex and more intensive, and therefore more expensive. In particular there has been a shift towards using more expensive analogue insulins (Figure 4.9)

Handbook of Diabetes, Fifth Edition. Rudy Bilous, Richard Donnelly, and Iskandar Idris.
© 2021 John Wiley & Sons Ltd. Published 2021 by John Wiley & Sons Ltd.

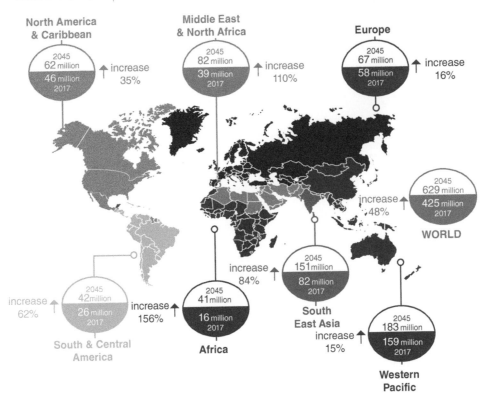

Figure 4.1 Rising numbers of people with diabetes worldwide. IDF Atlas, 2017.

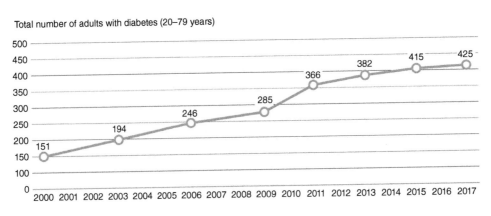

Figure 4.2 There are estimated to be 425m patients with diabetes worldwide in 2017. IDF Atlas, 2017.

Public health strategies are focused in several key areas:

Primary prevention of Type 2 Diabetes

Primary prevention of diabetes is a public health priority for a number of good reasons: (i) the overall burden of diabetes justifies strategies at a population level: (ii) current treatments are costly, confer risks of serious adverse events (e.g. hypoglycaemia) and often have limited efficacy on key clinical outcomes; (iii) access to, and adherence to, diabetes treatments is still a challenge for many patients; and (iv)

prevention of type 2 diabetes through lifestyle modification is likely to confer added benefits in terms of reducing the risks of hypertension, hyperlipidaemia, heart disease, and certain cancers.

Thus, assessing an individual's diabetes risk status, discussing the risk and, referring the patient to a proven community-based diabetes prevention program is an important role for the primary care practitioner. RCTs of structured lifestyle modification have consistently demonstrated that caloric reduction plus increased physical activity leading to

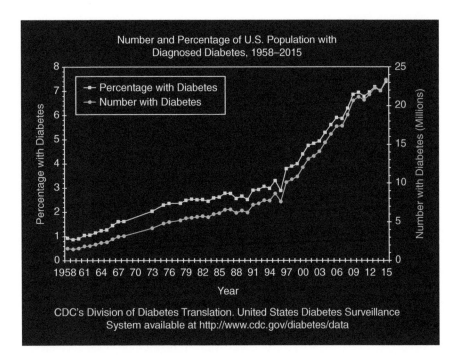

Figure 4.3 An alarming trend in the USA with increasing numbers of patients. CDC's Division of Diabetes Translation. United States Diabetes Surveillance System.

Number of deaths due to diabetes (20–79 years) in 2017 in millions

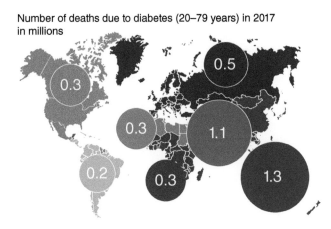

Figure 4.4 Mortality rates due to diabetes-related complications. IDF Atlas, 2017.

modest weight loss reduces the risk of incident type 2 diabetes in adults at high risk by 50–70%.

The Diabetes Prevention program (DPP) recruited 3234 middle-aged overweight or obese adults with impaired glucose tolerance, who were then randomised to one of three treatment groups: (i) a lifestyle intervention that employed behavioural counselling to promote caloric reduction and physical activity; (ii) metformin therapy; or (iii) placebo metformin therapy. The lifestyle intervention group achieved an initial weight loss of ~6% of body weight after 12 months, reducing to ~4% after 3 years, and an increase in self-reported physical activity (equivalent to brisk walking) from 100 to 190 minutes per week. Compared to their counterparts in the control group, participants in the lifestyle intervention group showed a 58% reduction in incident diabetes over 4 years. This benefit was evident in men and women across different ethnic groups and it was even greater among older age participants (Figure 4.10).

The intensive and quite costly lifestyle intervention used in the DPP trial was designed to give maximum efficacy with limited consideration for the ease or sustainability of delivering the program in a real world community setting. Thus, two barriers have hampered the widespread implementation of the DPP findings to the growing population of people who might benefit: (i) the cost of the one-to-one lifestyle coaching and intervention format; and (ii) limitations in the practicalities of identifying suitable patients, optimising referral pathways and maintaining patient participation.

In the UK, the ambition is to achieve a country-wide, evidence-based type 2 diabetes prevention program, known as *'The Healthier You'* programme, to prevent or delay diabetes in those identified to be at high risk. The scheme was rolled out in 2016, and participants undergo an intensive 9-month programme that includes at least 13 face-to-face interactions and at least 16 hours of contact time. So far, >50,000 referrals have been made with attendance rates over 40% across diverse socio-economic groups (Figure 4.11).

Providing access to structured diabetes education

Diabetes education is key to successful day-to-day diabetes management, yet few patients are offered high quality education, in part because of myths that it doesn't really work.

Deaths attributable to diabetes by age (20–79 years)

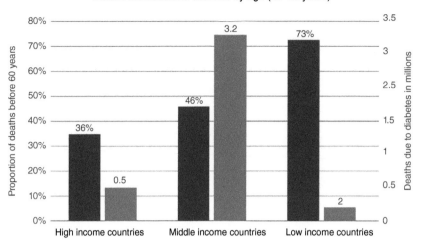

"Half of the 4 million people who die from diabetes are under the age of 60"

Figure 4.5 Premature mortality affects low-, medium- and high-income countries. IDF Atlas, 2017.

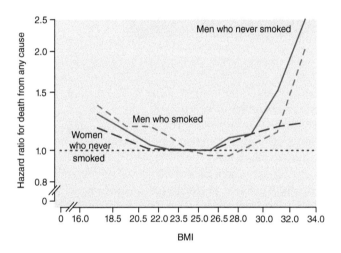

Figure 4.6 The relationship between Body Mass Index and the hazard ratio for death from any cause. Data for men according to smoking status, relative to females who never smoked, in a large Asian cohort study. Obesity carries an increased risk of several unwanted health outcomes, including diabetes, cardiovascular disease and certain forms of cancer. Adapted from Jee et al. N Engl J Med 2006; 355: 779–787.

However, randomised trials, and a meta-analysis, have shown that group-based diabetes self-management education results in statistically significant improvements in key clinical (HbA1c, fasting glucose), lifestyle (diabetes knowledge and self-management skills), and psycho-social

A shift to new and more expensive insulins

Since 2000, prescriptions for newer, pricier analog insulins have increased, while those for older human insulins have sharply decreased.

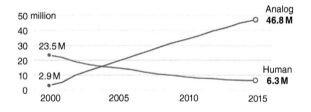

Figure 4.7 Healthcare expenditure on diabetes is rising steeply. IDF Atlas, 2017.

U.S. Diabetes Forecast: Total Annual Cost (2015 Dollars)

Total Health Care Spending in Billions

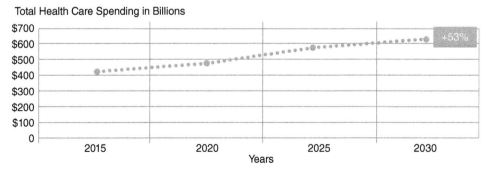

Figure 4.8 In the USA the costs of providing diabetes care are enormous. Based on Rowley et.al. 2016. Diabetes 2030: Insights from Yesterday, Today, and Future Trends.

Factors that affect prevalence of type 2 diabetes

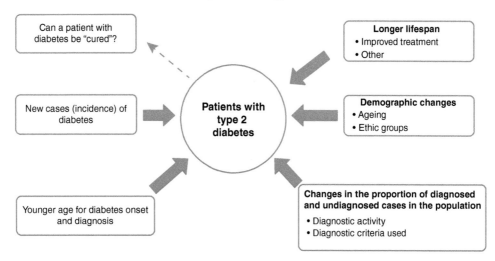

Figure 4.9 Factors affecting the numbers of patients with type 2 diabetes.

outcomes. As a result, diabetes education is recommended by NICE and SIGN (Table 4.1).

The definition of structured patient education is: 'A planned and graded programme that is comprehensive in scope, flexible in content, responsive to an individual's clinical and psychological needs and adaptable to his or her educational and cultural background'. Work initially undertaken to support people with type 1 diabetes identified three different levels of patient education:

- Level 1:   Basic skills at diagnosis
- Level 2:   Content on living with diabetes
- Level 3:   Content on managing diabetes

A systematic review of group-based education for people with type 2 diabetes assessed 21 RCTs and concluded that education achieved reductions in HbA1c of 0.46% at 1 year, reduced body weight at 1 year and significant improvements in self-empowerment, knowledge and satisfaction.

In the UK, audits of two major education programmes for type 2 diabetes, the X-PERT and DESMOND diabetes programmes, have shown clinical benefits that are highly cost effective. The cost of delivering these courses is circa £70, which means that diabetes education could be provided to everyone in the UK with type 2 diabetes for £40m per year over 5 years (i.e <0.6% of what the NHS currently spends

Table 4.1 Criteria that define structured patient education in the NICE guidance.

- A philosophy of education
- An evidence-based curriculum meeting the needs of an individual
- Aims and learning outcomes that support self management
- Delivered by a trained educator with an understanding of educational theory
- Quality assured and audited

on diabetes). Lay educators, partnering healthcare professionals, can also deliver effective education to patients with type 2 diabetes.

In type 1 diabetes the evidence for group-based education is extremely strong. The DAFNE programme – which costs £308 per person for a 5-day course – achieves long-term improvements in glycaemic control, less hypoglycaemia and improved quality of life. The UK Department of Health estimates that in the long run the DAFNE course could save the NHS £48m per year if it was made accessible to everyone in the UK with type 1 diabetes.

Improving diabetes treatment and care

A key public health strategy is to implement a systematic approach to evaluate the quality of care provided to patients with diabetes. In the UK, since 2004, disease-specific indicators for both the processes of diabetes care and the attainment of treatment targets have been assessed through the pay-for-performance Quality and Outcomes Framework (QoF).

In the UK in 2017, NHS England has allocated £36m to target four clinical areas where intervention is likely to result in improved outcomes, better quality care and longer term cost savings (Table 4.2).

The number of diabetes treatments has increased sharply in the last 10 years. The global market for products used in the management of diabetes is in excess of $100b annually. Spending on insulin has increased faster than other diabetes drugs, and there has been a big shift towards analog insulins (Figure 4.10).

Digital health interventions are likely to play an important role in improving the quality of diabetes care in the next 5–10 years. Digital and E-health initiatives will include:

- Wearable technologies that monitor levels of exercise.
- Apps which allow users to access health coaches.

- Online peer support groups.
- Provide the ability to set and monitor goals electronically.

Table 4.2 Transformation Funding in the UK in 2017 is targeting 4 key areas to improve quality of care, outcomes and to achieve longer term cost savings.

Work stream	Approx funding
Improving Attainment of NICE recommended Targets (HbA1c, BP, Lipids)	£14m
Increased Access to Structured Education For T1 and T2 DM	£11m
Reducing the No of Amputations by Improving Access to Multidisciplinary Foot Teams	£6m
Improving Access to in-patient Diabetes specialist nurses	£4m

A shift to new and more expensive insulins

Since 2000, prescriptions for newer, pricier analog insulins have increased, while those for older human insulins have sharply decreased.

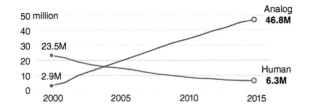

Figure 4.10 The shift towards using new, expensive analogue insulins. IMS Health.

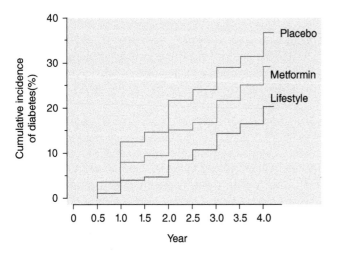

Figure 4.11 A structured lifestyle modification program (aimed at delivering >7% weight loss and 150 minutes of physical activity per week) is superior to drug treatment with metformin and placebo in diabetes prevention. Lifestyle intervention reduced the risk of type 2 diabetes by 58%. Adapted from Diabetes Prevention Study. N Engl J Med 2002; 346: 393–403.

Commissioning diabetes services

Improving population metrics for the quality of diabetes care as well as clinical outcomes hinges on effective local and national commissioning of diabetes services. Public Health England uses a Diabetes Outcomes versus Expenditure (DOVE) scoring tool to judge how cost-effective local Clinical Commissioning Groups (CCGs) are in procuring services for their population. Guidance has been produced (Table 4.3).

Table 4.3 Top Tips For Commissioning Diabetes Services.

1. Involve Patients
2. Use Data: to Identify local & national variations and to identify areas for intervention
3. Strong Leadership: Especially from GP's
4. Identify Diabetes Champions: Both in Primary & Secondary Care
5. Develop Partnerships: For example with industry to support implementation
6. Outcome-Based Approached: Collaborate with healthcare providers to move from activity to outcomes-based approaches

Adapted From: NHS Clinical Commissioners: Excellence in Commissioning Diabetes Care, April 2017.

LANDMARK CLINICAL TRIALS

Diabetes Prevention Program Research Group. Reduction in the incidence of type 2 diabetes with lifestyle intervention or metformin. N Engl J Med 2002; 346: 393–403.

Huxley R, Barzi F, Woodward M. Excess risk of fatal coronary heart disease associated with diabetes in men and women: meta-analysis of 37 prospective cohort studies. BMJ 2006; 332: 73–76.

Li G, Zhang P, Wang J, et al. The long-term effect of lifestyle interventions to prevent diabetes in the China Da Qing Diabetes Prevention study: a 20-year follow-up study. Lancet 2008; 371: 1783–1789.

Patterson CC, Dahlquist G, Gyurus E, et al. Incidence trends for childhood type 1 diabetes in Europe during 1989–2003 and predicted new cases 2005–2020: a multicentre prospective registration study. Lancet 2009; 373: 2027–2033.

FURTHER READING

Alexander GC, Sehgal N, Moloney R, Stafford R. National trends in treatment of type 2 diabetes mellitus, 1994–2007. *Arch Intern Med* 2008; 168: 2088–2094.

Bain SC, Feher M, Russell-Jones D, et al. Management of type 2 diabetes: the current situation and key opportunities to improve care in the UK. *Diab. Obes. Metab.* 2016;18:1157–1166.

Currie CJ, Peters JR, Tynan A, et al. Survival as a function of HbA$_{1c}$ in people with type 2 diabetes: a retrospective cohort study. *Lancet* 2010; 375: 481–489.

Goyder EC. Screening for and prevention of type 2 diabetes. *BMJ* 2008; 336: 1140–1141.

Jee SH, Sull J, Park J, et al. Body–mass index and mortality in Korean men and women. *N Engl J Med* 2006; 355: 779–787.

Rosella LC, Lebenbaum M, Fitzpatrick T, et al. Impact of Diabetes on healthcare costs in a population-based cohort: a cost analysis. *Diabet. Med* 2016; DOI: 10.1111/dme.12858.

Selvin E, Steffes MW, Zhu H, et al. Glycated haemoglobin, diabetes and cardiovascular risk in nondiabetic adults. *N Engl J Med* 2010; 362: 800–811.

Zghebi SS, Steinke DT, Carr MJ, et al. Examining trends in type 2 diabetes incidence, prevalence and mortality in the UK between 2004 and 2014. *Diab. Obes. Metab.* 2017; doi: 10.1111/dom.12964.

Normal physiology of insulin secretion and action, and the incretin effect

Islet structure and function

Insulin is synthesised in and secreted from the β cells within the islets of Langerhans in the pancreas. The normal pancreas has about 1 million islets, which are derived embryologically from endodermal outgrowths of the foetal gut. The islets can be identified easily with various histological stains with which the cells react less intensely than does the surrounding exocrine tissue (Figure 5.1). Pancreatic islets vary in size from having a few dozen to several thousands of cells and they are scattered irregularly throughout the exocrine pancreas.

The main cell types of the pancreatic islets are β-cells that produce insulin, α-cells that secrete glucagon, δ-cells that produce somatostatin and PP-cells that produce pancreatic polypeptide. Different islet cell types can be identified by various immunostaining techniques. β-cells are the most numerous cell type and are located mainly in the core of the islet, while α and δ cells are located in the periphery (Figure 5.2).

Islet cells interact with each other through direct physical contact and through paracrine effects of their hormone products (e.g. glucagon stimulates insulin secretion and somatostatin inhibits insulin and glucagon secretion) (Figure 5.3).

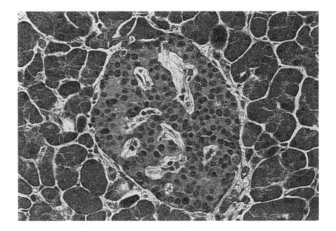

Figure 5.1 A section of normal pancreas stained with haematoxylin and eosin. As observed by Paul Langerhans, the islet in the centre is identified easily by its distinct morphology and lighter staining than that of the surrounding exocrine tissue (original magnification ×350).

The blood flow within the islets is organised centrifugally so that the different cell types are supplied in the sequence β → α → δ. Insulin also has an 'autocrine' (self-regulating) effect

Handbook of Diabetes, Fifth Edition. Rudy Bilous, Richard Donnelly, and Iskandar Idris.
© 2021 John Wiley & Sons Ltd. Published 2021 by John Wiley & Sons Ltd.

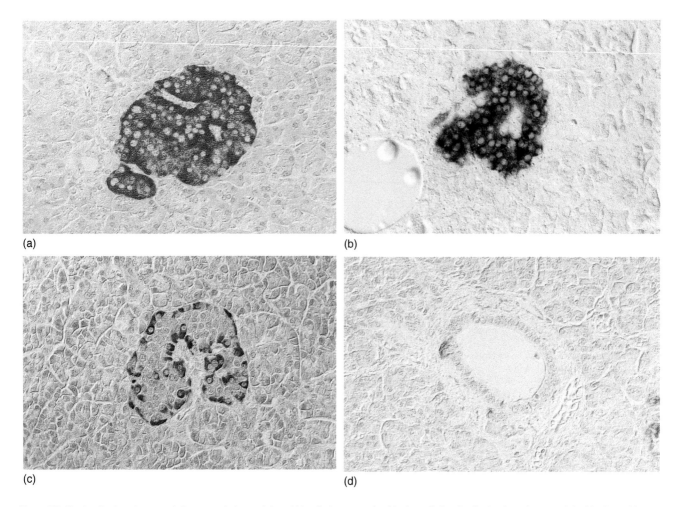

(a)

(b)

(c)

(d)

Figure 5.2 The localisation of pancreatic hormones in human islets. (a) Insulin immunostained in the majority of cells that form the core of the islet (peroxidase–antiperoxidase immunostain with haematoxylin counterstain). (b) Insulin mRNA localised by *in situ* hybridization with a digoxigenin-labelled sequence of rat insulin cRNA (which cross-reacts fully with human insulin mRNA). (c) Peripherally located α cells immunostained with antibodies to pancreatic glucagon using the same method as for (a). (d) Weakly immunoreactive PP cells in the epithelium of a duct in the ventral portion of the pancreatic head. Magnifications approximately ×150.

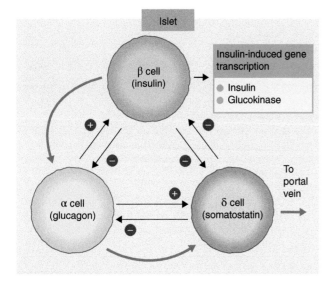

Figure 5.3 Potential interactions between the secretory products of the major islet cell types. Black arrows indicate paracrine stimulation or inhibition. The direction of blood flow within the islet is indicated by the red arrows.

that alters the transcription of insulin and glucokinase genes in the β cell.

Pancreatic islets are densely innervated with autonomic and peptidergic nerve fibres (Figure 5.4). Parasympathetic innervation from the vagus stimulates insulin release, while adrenergic sympathetic nerves inhibit insulin and stimulate glucagon secretion. Other nerve fibres that supply the pancreas release peptides which also regulate pancreatic function, e.g vasoactive intestinal peptide (VIP) stimulates the release of all islet hormones and neuropeptide Y (NPY) inhibits insulin secretion. Neural pathways are important in the regulation of pancreatic function.

Pancreatic β-cells may change in size, number, and function during normal aging and development (Figure 5.5). β cell mass is determined by the net effect of four independent mechanisms: (i) β cell replication (i.e. division of existing β cells), (ii) β cell size, (iii) β cell neogenesis (i.e. emergence of new β cells from pancreatic ductal epithelial cells), and (iv) β cell apoptosis. The contribution made by each of these processes is variable and may change at different stages of life.

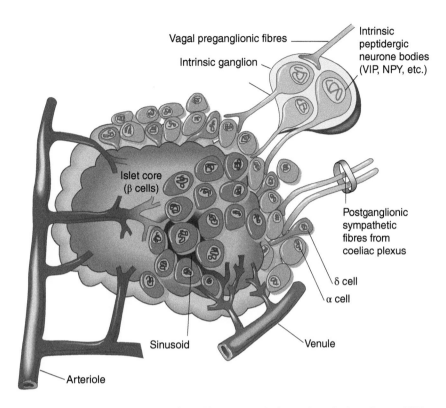

Figure 5.4 Structure of a pancreatic islet, showing the anatomical relationships between the four major endocrine cell types. NPY, neuropeptide Y; VIP, vasoactive intestinal polypeptide.

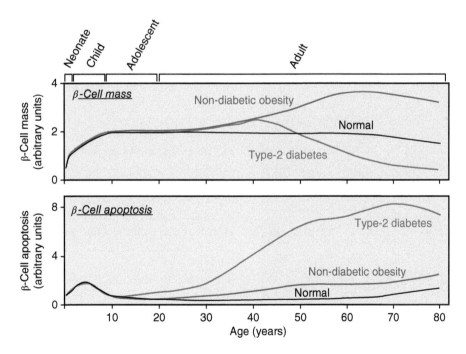

Figure 5.5 A hypothetical model for postnatal pancreatic β cell growth in humans. Adapted from Rhodes et al. Science 2005; 307: 380–384.

Insulin synthesis and insulin polypeptide structure

Insulin consists of two polypeptide chains linked by disulphide bridges; the A-chain contains 21 amino acids and the B-chain contains 30 amino acids (Figure 5.6). In the circulation, insulin exists as a monomer of 6000 Da molecular weight. The tertiary (three-dimensional) structure of monomeric insulin consists of a hydrophobic core buried beneath

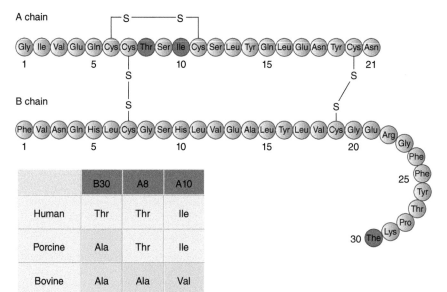

	B30	A8	A10
Human	Thr	Thr	Ile
Porcine	Ala	Thr	Ile
Bovine	Ala	Ala	Val

Figure 5.6 The primary structure (amino acid sequence) of human insulin. The highlighted residues are those that differ in porcine and bovine insulins, as shown in the inset.

a surface that is hydrophilic, except for two non-polar regions involved in the aggregation of the monomers into dimers and hexamers.

In concentrated solution (such as in the insulin vial supplied by the pharmaceutical company for injection) and in crystals (such as in the insulin secretory granule), six monomers self-associate with two zinc ions to form a hexamer (Figure 5.7). This is of therapeutic importance because the slow absorption of native insulin from the subcutaneous

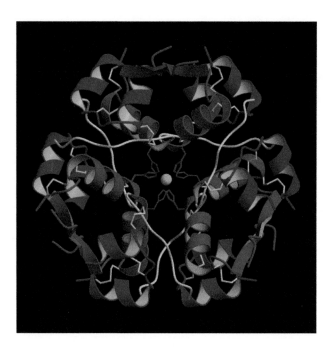

Figure 5.7 The double zinc insulin hexamer composed of three insulin dimers in a threefold symmetrical pattern.

tissue partly results from the time taken for the hexameric insulin to dissociate into the smaller, more easily absorbed monomeric form.

Insulin is synthesised in the β cells from a single amino acid precursor called proinsulin (Figure 5.8). Synthesis begins with the formation of an even larger precursor, preproinsulin, which is cleaved by protease activity to proinsulin. The gene for preproinsulin (and therefore the 'gene for insulin') is located on chromosome 11. Proinsulin is packaged into vesicles in the Golgi apparatus of the β cell; in the maturing secretory granules that bud off it, proinsulin is converted by enzymes into insulin and connecting peptide (C-peptide).

Insulin and C-peptide are released from the β cell when the secretory granules are transported ('translocated') to the cell surface and fuse with the plasma membrane (exocytosis) (Figure 5.9). Microtubules, formed of polymerised tubulin, probably provide the mechanical framework for granule transport, and microfilaments of actin, interacting with myosin and other motor proteins such as kinesin, may provide the mechanical force that propels the granules along the tubules. Although the actin cytoskeleton is a key mediator of biphasic insulin release, cyclic GTPases are involved in F-actin reorganization in the islet β cell and play a crucial role in stimulus-secretion coupling.

The 'regulated pathway', with almost complete cleavage of proinsulin to insulin, normally accounts for about 95% of the β cell insulin production. In certain conditions, however, e.g insulinoma and type 2 diabetes, an alternative 'constitutive' pathway operates, in which large amounts of unprocessed proinsulin and intermediate insulin precursors ('split proinsulins') are released directly from vesicles that originate in the endoplasmic reticulum (Figure 5.10).

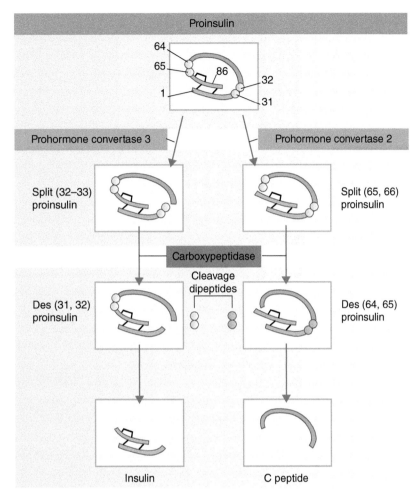

Figure 5.8 Insulin biosynthesis and processing. Proinsulin is cleaved on the C-terminal side of two dipeptides. The cleavage dipeptides are liberated, so yielding the 'split' proinsulin products and ultimately insulin and C-peptide.

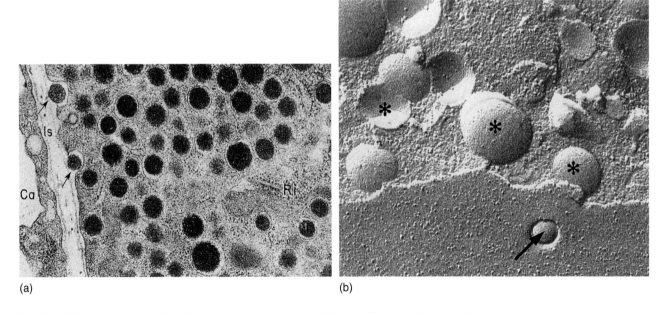

(a)

(b)

Figure 5.9 (a) Electron micrograph of insulin secretory granules in a pancreatic β cell and their secretion by exocytosis. Arrows show exocytosis occurring. Ca, capillary lumen; Is, interstitial space. (b) Freeze-fracture views of β cells that reveal the secretory granules in the cytoplasm (*asterisks*) and the granule content released by exocytosis at the cell membrane (*arrows*). Magnification: ×52,000. From Orci. Diabetologia 1974; 10: 163–187.

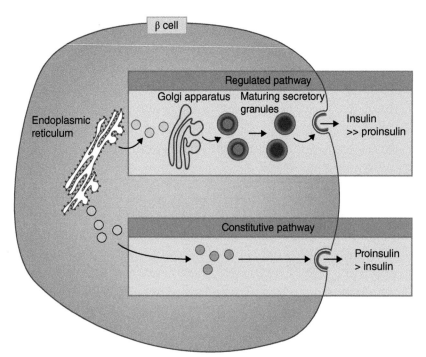

Figure 5.10 The regulated (normal) and constitutive (active in type 2 diabetes) pathways of insulin processing.

Insulin secretion

Glucose is the main stimulator of insulin release from the β cells, and insulin secretion occurs in a characteristic biphasic pattern – an immediate 'first phase' response that lasts only a few minutes, followed by a more gradual sustained 'second phase' (Figure 5.11). The first phase of insulin release involves a small, readily releasable pool of granules fusing with the plasma membrane. Of particular importance is the observation that first-phase insulin secretion is lost in patients with type 2 diabetes.

Various types of fuels, hormones, and neurotransmitters regulate insulin secretion. Glucose is the most important regulator and glucose stimulates insulin secretion by mechanisms that depend upon the metabolism of glucose and other nutrients in the β cells. A triggering pathway involves closure of ATP-sensitive potassium channels (K_{ATP} channels), cellular depolarisation, an influx of calcium through voltage-dependent calcium channels and an increase in intracellular calcium concentration. Simultaneously, a metabolic amplifying pathway augments the stimulatory effect of calcium on the exocytosis of insulin-containing granules. The second messenger cAMP is an important amplifier of insulin secretion triggered by Ca^{2+} elevation in the β cells.

Glucose enters the β cell by facilitated diffusion via GLUT-2 transporters. It is then phosphorylated by the enzyme glucokinase, which acts as the 'glucose sensor' that couples insulin secretion to the prevailing glucose concentration (Figure 5.12). Glycolysis and mitochondrial metabolism of glucose produce adenosine triphosphate (ATP), which leads to the closure of the K_{ATP} channels. This in turn causes

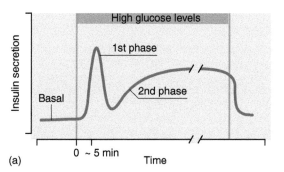

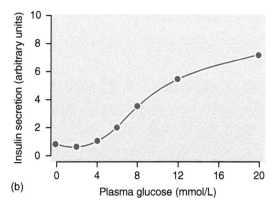

Figure 5.11 (a) The biphasic glucose-stimulated release of insulin from pancreatic islets. (b) The glucose–insulin dose–response curve for islets of Langerhans.

depolarisation of the β cell plasma membrane, leading to an influx of extracellular calcium through cell-surface voltage-gated channels. The increase in cytosolic calcium triggers translocation of insulin granules and exocytosis.

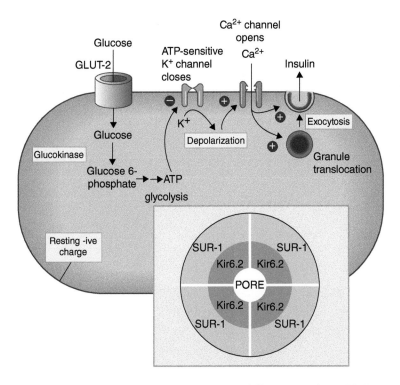

Figure 5.12 The mechanism of glucose-stimulated insulin secretion from the β cell. The structure of the KATP channel is shown in the inset.

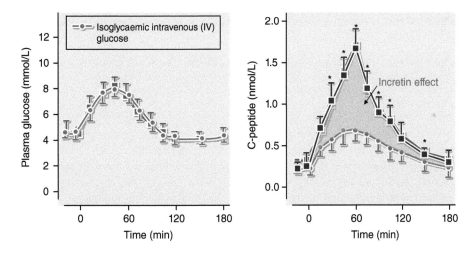

Figure 5.13 The classic experiment illustrating the incretin effect in normal subjects who were studied on two separate occasions. On one occasion, they were given an oral glucose load and on the second occasion an IV glucose bolus was administered in order to achieve identical venous plasma glucose concentration-time profiles on the two study days (left panel). The insulin secretory response (shown by C-peptide) was significantly greater after oral compared with IV glucose (right panel). Adapted from Nauck et al. J Clin Endocrinol Metab 1986; 63: 492–498.

Sulfonylureas stimulate insulin secretion by binding to a component of the K_{ATP} channel (the sulfonylurea receptor, SUR-1) and closing it. The K_{ATP} channel is an octamer that consists of four K⁺-channel subunits (called Kir6.2) and four SUR-1 subunits.

The incretin effect

There is a significant difference between the insulin secretory response to oral glucose compared with the response to intravenous glucose – a phenomenon known as the 'incretin effect' (Figure 5.13). The incretin effect is mediated by

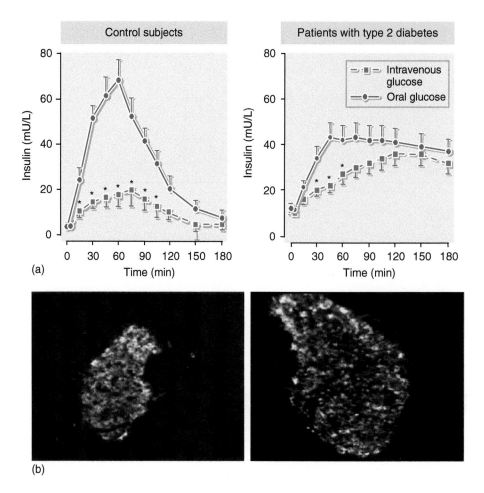

(a)

(b)

Figure 5.14 (a) The incretin effect is greatly diminished in patients with type 2 diabetes compared with normal subjects. This contributes to the impaired insulin secretory response observed in type 2 diabetes. (b) GLP-1 has a trophic effect on pancreatic islets. Shown here is an islet from a db/db mouse before (*left*) and after (*right*) 2 weeks treatment with synthetic GLP-1. Adapted from Stoffers et al. Diabetes 2000; 49: 741–748.

gut-derived hormones, released in response to the ingestion of food, which augment glucose-stimulated insulin release. In particular, there are two incretin hormones: glucagon-like peptide-1 (GLP-1) and gastric inhibitory polypeptide (GIP). Both augment insulin secretion in a dose-dependent fashion. GLP-1 is secreted by L cells and GIP is secreted by K cells in the wall of the upper jejunum.

In patients with type 2 diabetes, GLP-1 secretion is diminished (Figure 5.14). However, in contrast to GIP, GLP-1 retains most of its insulinotropic activity. GIP secretion is maintained in type 2 diabetes, but its effect on the β cell is greatly reduced.

GLP-1 also suppresses glucagon secretion from pancreatic α cells and exerts additional effects on satiety and gastric emptying. There is also considerable interest in the trophic effects of GLP-1 on β cells.

Insulin receptor signalling

Insulin exerts its main biological effects by binding to a cell surface insulin receptor, a glycoprotein that consists of two extracellular α subunits and two transmembrane β subunits. The receptor has tyrosine kinase enzyme activity (residing in the β subunits), which is stimulated when insulin binds to the receptor. The tyrosine kinase domain phosphorylates tyrosine amino acid residues on various intracellular proteins, such as insulin receptor substrate (IRS)-1 and IRS-2, and the β subunit itself (Figure 5.15) (autophosphorylation). The tyrosine kinase activity of the insulin receptor is essential for insulin action.

Post-receptor downstream signalling events are complex but insulin binding to its receptor leads to phosphorylation of a number of intracellular proteins including IRS-1 and IRS-2 (Figure 5.16). Phosphorylated tyrosine residues on these proteins act as docking sites for the non-covalent binding of proteins with specific 'SH2' domains, such as phosphatidylinositol 3-kinase (PI 3-kinase), Grb2 and phosphotyrosine phosphatase (SHP2). Binding of Grb2 to IRS-1 initiates a cascade that eventually activates nuclear transcription factors via activation of the proteins Ras and mitogen-activated protein (MAP) kinase. IRS–PI 3-kinase binding generates phospholipids that modulate other specific kinases and regulate insulin-stimulated effects such as glucose transport, and protein and glycogen synthesis.

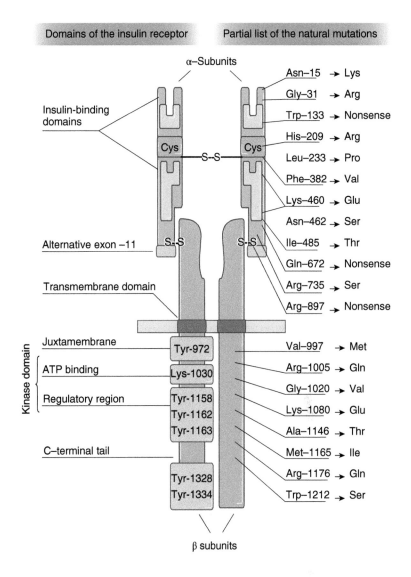

Figure 5.15 The insulin receptor and its structural domains. Many mutations have been discovered in the insulin receptor, some of which interfere with insulin's action and can cause insulin resistance; examples are shown in the right column.

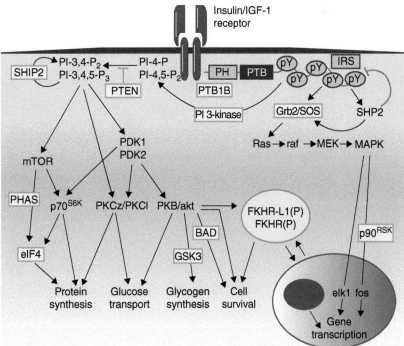

Figure 5.16 The insulin signalling cascade. Insulin binding and autophosphorylation of the insulin (and IGF-1) receptor results in binding of the IRS-1 protein to the β subunit of the insulin receptor via the IRS phosphotyrosine-binding domain (PTB). There is then phosphorylation of a number of tyrosine residues (pY) at the C-terminus of the IRS proteins. This leads to recruitment and binding of downstream signalling proteins, such as PI-3 kinase, Grb2 and SHP2.

The family of GLUT transporters

Glucose is transported into cells by a family of specialised transporter proteins called glucose transporters (GLUTs) (Figure 5.17). The process of glucose uptake is energy independent.

The best characterised GLUTs are:

- GLUT-1: ubiquitously expressed and probably mediates basal, non-insulin mediated glucose uptake.
- GLUT-2: present in the islet β cell, and also in the liver, intestine, and kidney. Together with glucokinase, it forms the β cell's glucose sensor and, because it has a high Km, allows glucose to enter the β cell at a rate proportional to the extracellular glucose level.
- GLUT-3: together with GLUT-1, involved in non-insulin mediated uptake of glucose into the brain.
- GLUT-4: responsible for insulin-stimulated glucose uptake in muscle and adipose tissue, and thus the classic hypoglycaemic action of insulin.
- GLUT-8: important in blastocyst development.
- GLUT-9 and 10: unclear functional significance.

Most of the other GLUTs are present at the cell surface, but in the basal state GLUT-4 is sequestered within vesicles in the cytoplasm. Insulin causes these vesicles to be translocated to the cell surface, where they fuse with the plasma membrane. The inserted GLUT-4 unit then functions as a membrane pore that allows glucose entry into the cell. The process is reversible: when insulin levels fall, the plasma membrane GLUT-4 is removed by endocytosis and recycled back into intracellular vesicles for storage (Figure 5.18).

In normal subjects, blood glucose concentrations are maintained within relatively narrow limits at around 5 mmol/L (90 mg/dL) (Figure 5.19). This is achieved by a balance between glucose entry into the circulation from the liver and from intestinal absorption, and glucose uptake into the peripheral tissues such as muscle and adipose tissue. Insulin is secreted at a low, basal level in the non-fed state, with increased, stimulated levels at mealtimes (Figure 5.20).

At rest in the fasting state, the brain consumes about 80% of the glucose utilised by the whole body, but

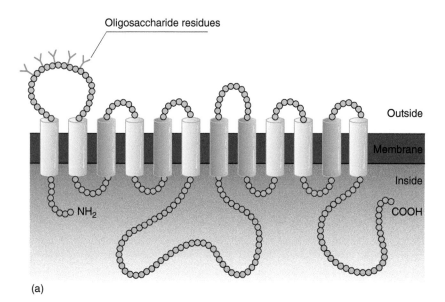

Oligosaccharide residues

Outside

Membrane

Inside

NH₂

COOH

(a)

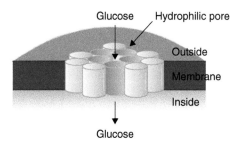

Glucose   Hydrophilic pore

Outside

Membrane

Inside

Glucose

(b)

Figure 5.17 (a) The structure of a typical glucose transporter (GLUT). (b) The intramembrane domains pack together to form a central hydrophilic channel through which glucose passes.

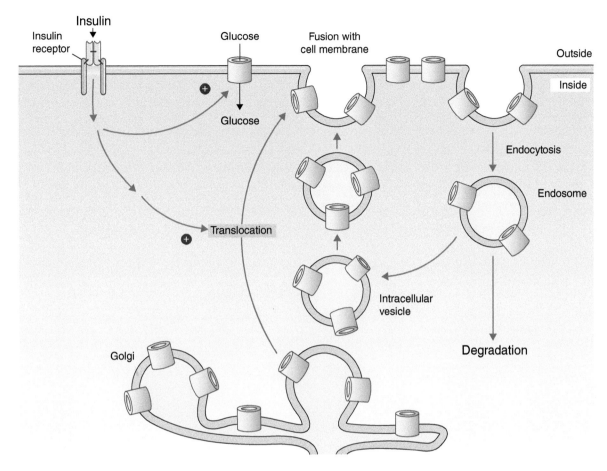

Figure 5.18 Insulin regulation of glucose transport into cells.

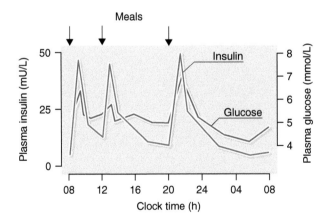

Figure 5.19 Profiles of plasma glucose and insulin concentrations in individuals without diabetes.

brain glucose uptake is not regulated by insulin. Glucose is the main fuel for the brain, such that brain function critically depends on the maintenance of normal blood glucose levels.

Insulin lowers glucose levels partly by suppressing glucose output from the liver, both by inhibiting glycogen breakdown (glycogenolysis) and by inhibiting gluconeogenesis (i.e. the formation of 'new' glucose from sources such as glycerol, lactate and amino acids, like alanine). Relatively low concentrations of insulin are needed to suppress hepatic glucose output in this way, such as occur with basal insulin secretion between meals and at night. With much higher insulin levels after meals, GLUT-4 mediated glucose uptake into the periphery is stimulated.

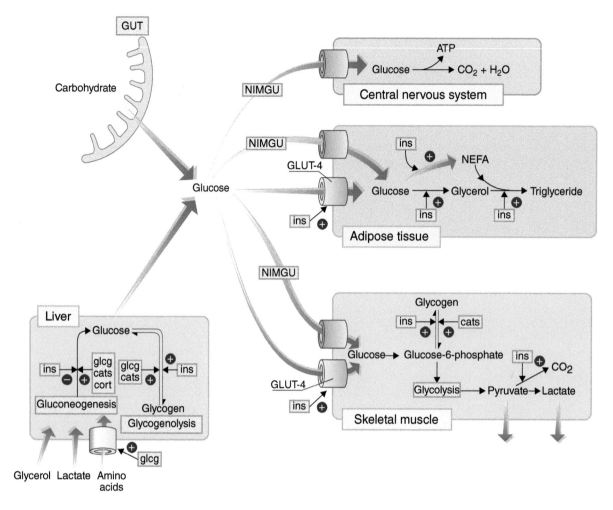

Figure 5.20 Overview of carbohydrate metabolism. cats, catecholamines; cort, cortisol; glcg, glucagon; ins, insulin; NIMGU, non-insulin mediated glucose uptake.

FURTHER READING

Drucker DJ, Habener JF, Holst JJ. Discovery, characterization and clinical development of the glucagon-like peptides. *J Clin Invest* 2017;127:4217–4227.

Fu Z, Gilbert ER, Liu D. Regulation of insulin synthesis and secretion and pancreatic Beta-cell dysfunction in diabetes. *Curr. Diabetes Rev.* 2013;9:25–53.

Henquin JC. Regulation of Insulin Secretion: A matter of phase control and amplitude modulation. *Diabetologia* 2009;52: 739–751.

Henquin JC, Dufrane D, Gmyr V, et al. Pharmacological approach to understanding the control of insulin secretion in human islets. *Diab. Obes. Metab.* 2017;19:1061–1070.

Kojima I, Medina J, Nakagawa Y. Role of the glucose-sensing receptor in insulin secretion. *Diab. Obes. Metab.* 2017;19(Suppl. 1):54–62.

Rorsman P, Braun M. Regulation of insulin secretion in human pancreatic islets. *Annu. Rev. Physiol.* 2013;75:155–179.

Tengholm A, Gylfe E. cAMP signalling in insulin and glucagon secretion. *Diab. Obes. Metab.* 2017;19(Suppl. 1):42–53.

Chapter 6

Epidemiology and aetiology of type 1 diabetes

KEY POINTS

- Type 1 diabetes is one of a number of autoimmune endocrine diseases with a genetic and familial basis, although the majority of cases occur sporadically.
- Incidence rates vary from <5 to >60 per 100,000, generally being highest in northern latitudes.
- These rates are increasing more rapidly than can be explained by genetic factors alone.

- The autoimmune and genetic processes underpinning the disease are being unravelled.
- Environmental factors such as viruses and diet are responsible for some of the increase.
- Preventative trials have been disappointing but more targeted approaches are ongoing.

Introduction

The most common cause of type 1 diabetes (over 90% of cases) is T cell-mediated autoimmune destruction of the islet β cells leading to a failure of insulin production. The exact aetiology is complex and still imperfectly understood. However, it is probable that environmental factors trigger the onset of diabetes in individuals with an inherited predisposition. Unless insulin replacement is given, absolute insulin deficiency will result in hyperglycaemia and ketoacidosis, which is the biochemical hallmark of type 1 diabetes. This is now sometimes termed type 1A. Type 1B or non-autoimmune diabetes is also the result of an absolute insulin deficiency but from a range of possible causes such as monogenic diabetes (see Chapter 8) or pancreatic disease.

Epidemiology

There is a striking variation in the incidence of type 1 diabetes between and within populations. Part of the problem has been the lack of full case ascertainment in carefully defined populations. Historically, the highest incidence rates have been in Northern Europe, but rates are rapidly increasing in other regions such as the Middle East (Figure 6.1 and Table 6.1). The variation in incidence by geographical position in Europe is striking (Figure 6.2) and might reflect the impact of environmental factors. Incidence rates themselves have been increasing over the past three decades. In Europe the average rate of increase from 1989–2013 was 3.4% per annum reflecting a doubling in 20 years. However, the average hides considerable variation with rates of increase slowing in Scandinavia, Ireland, Italy, and Spain and some UK centres, and increasing in others (Poland, Romania, Lithuania, and Macedonia). Lower rates of increase in the decade 2002–2012 have been reported in in the USA (1.8% pa), Canada (1.3% pa) and Australia (0.4% pa); but much higher rates in China (with historically a very low incidence) of 12% pa in Zhejiang province from 2007–2013. These rates of increase must be mediated by environmental factors as they are occurring too rapidly to reflect changes in genetic susceptibility. One explanation of the observed increase in incidence in global regions with a historically low rate has correlated the change to an increased life expectancy at birth and a mathematical model of how this would translate into natural selection.

Handbook of Diabetes, Fifth Edition. Rudy Bilous, Richard Donnelly, and Iskandar Idris.
© 2021 John Wiley & Sons Ltd. Published 2021 by John Wiley & Sons Ltd.

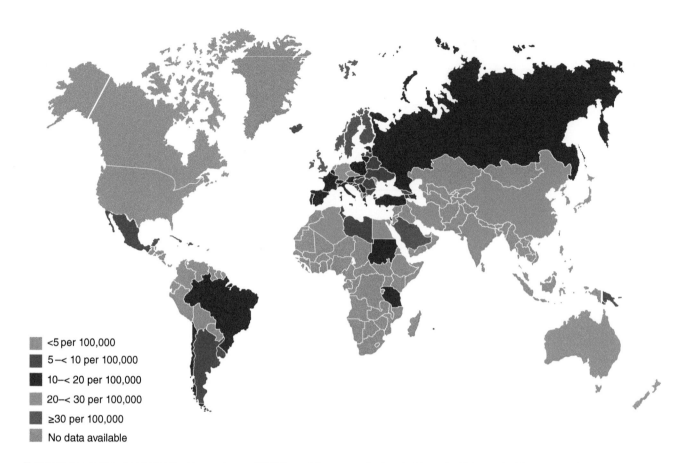

■	<5 per 100,000
■	5 –< 10 per 100,000
■	10 –< 20 per 100,000
■	20 –< 30 per 100,000
■	≥30 per 100,000
■	No data available

Figure 6.1 Age and sex standardised incidence rates per 100,000 population per year for type 1 diabetes in children and adolescents aged 0–14 years. Reproduced from the IDF Diabetes Atlas 9th edition 2019 with permission.

Table 6.1 Highest global rates of incidence per annum of type 1 diabetes in children aged 0–14 years per 100,000 population.

Rank	Country	Incidence Rates /100,000 Population / Year
1	Finland	62.3
2	Sweden	43.2
3	Kuwait	41.7
4	Norway	33.6
5	Saudi Arabia	31.4
6	Canada	29.9
7	United Kingdom	29.4
8	Qatar	28.4
9	Ireland	27.5
10	Denmark	27.0

Data from the IDF Diabetes Atlas 9th edition 2019 with permission.

These scientists suggest that as more individuals live to reproductive age then the likelihood of transmitting diabetes (and other disease) susceptibility genes increases.

There is some evidence of a cyclical variation in incidence from some, but not all, centres in the EURODIAB epidemiological study with a periodicity of 4–6 years, and may reflect exposure to infectious agents such as H1N1 influenza A.

Evidence for environmental influences comes from studies that show a seasonal variation in the onset of type 1 diabetes in some populations, with the highest frequency in the colder autumn and winter months (Figure 6.3). This is often thought to reflect seasonal exposure to viruses, but food or chemicals might also be involved. Moreover, people who have migrated from an area of low to an area of high incidence for type 1 diabetes seem to adopt the same level of risk as the population to which they move. For example, children of Asian families (from the Indian subcontinent and Tanzania) who moved to the UK traditionally have a low frequency of type 1 diabetes, but now have a rising incidence of the disease, which is approaching that of the background population.

Familial clustering of type 1 diabetes provides evidence for complex genetic factors in its aetiology. The lifetime risk for type 1 diabetes in monozygotic twins is >75%; for children with a mother with type 1 diabetes it is 1.3–4.0%; 6.0–9.0% if their father has type 1, and 15% if both have the condition (the background population risk is <0.4%).

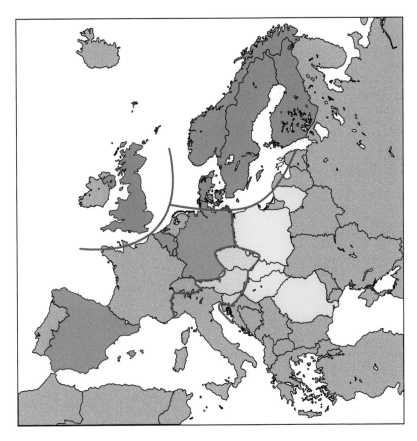

Figure 6.2 Incidence rates (1999–2003) of type 1 diabetes in 0–14-year-olds in 17 European countries grouped into regions with roughly homogeneous rates. Purple 22.9–52.6/100,000; pink 22.4–29.8/100,000; orange 13–18.3/100,000; green 11.1–17.2/100,000; and blue 11.3–13.6/100,000. Reproduced from Patterson et al. Lancet 2009; 373: 2027–2033).

The reasons for the gender differences in inheritability and incidence are unknown. In (European) siblings of children with type 1 diabetes the lifetime risk is 6.0–7.0%, and this is much greater if they share the same human leucocyte antigen (HLA) DR3–DQ2 and DR4–DQ8 haplotype. However, only 10–15% of type 1 diabetes occurs in families with the disease ('multiplex') and most cases are said to be 'sporadic'. The incidence has an equal gender distribution below age 10, thereafter there is a male preponderance although the reasons for these sex differences remain unknown.

Aetiology
Autoimmunity
Evidence for autoimmunity in the pathogenesis of type 1 diabetes originally came from postmortem studies in patients who have died shortly after presentation, and pancreatic biopsies from living patients. They have revealed a chronic inflammatory mononuclear cell infiltrate ('insulitis') (Figure 6.4) associated with the residual β cells in the islets of recently diagnosed type 1 diabetic patients. The infiltrate consists of T cell lymphocytes and macrophages. Later in the disease, there is complete loss of β cells, while the other islet cell types (α, δ and PP cells) all survive. The discovery of islet cell antibodies confirmed the autoimmune basis of the inflammation (Figure 6.5).

Since these original observations, four circulating autoantibodies have been found in people with newly diagnosed type 1 diabetes. They are antibodies to the insulin molecule (IAAs), tyrosine phosphatase (insulinoma antigen-2 protein IA–2), zinc transporter 8 (ZnT8) and glutamic acid decarboxylase 65 (GAD 65). However, less than 10% of individuals with a single autoantibody go on to develop type 1 diabetes, although the proportion increases dramatically in those with two or more autoantibodies (Figure 6.6). The sequence of appearance of autoantibodies differs, the first to appear is IAA (sometimes GAD65) at a median age of 15 (range 6–24) months in prospective studies in high risk children. The second antibody is usually detected within the next 2–4 years, following which the likelihood of developing multiple autoantibodies appears to decline. In first degree relatives of probands with type 1 diabetes, 75% of seroconversions occur before 13 years of age.

The lifetime risk of type 1 diabetes approaches 100% in genetically at-risk children with two or more autoantibodies.

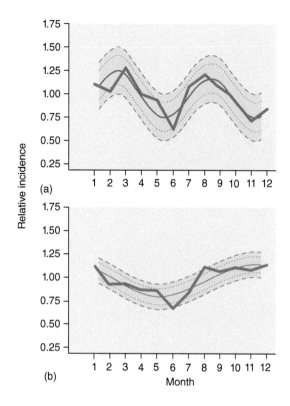

(a)

(b)

Relative incidence

Month

Figure 6.3 Seasonal variation of type 1 diabetes among Finnish children (a) 0–9 years of age, (b) 10–14 years of age during 1983–92. (The observed monthly variation in incidence is the solid line with dots.) The inner interval is the 95% confidence interval (CI) for the observed seasonal variation and the outer interval is the 95% CI for the estimated seasonal variation. Data from Padaiga et al. Diabetic Med 1999; 16: 1–8.

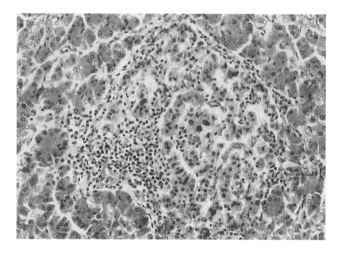

Figure 6.4 Insulitis. There is a chronic inflammatory cell infiltrate centred on this islet. Haematoxylin–eosin stain, original magnification ×300.

The rate of progression to symptomatic disease in these children depends upon the number of autoantibodies (more = faster), the age of seroconversion (earlier = faster), and the type of antibody (IAA and IA–2 = earlier onset; IA–2

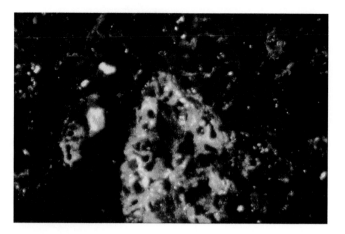

Figure 6.5 ICA demonstrated by indirect immunofluorescence in a frozen section of human pancreas.

and ZnT8 = faster). In first degree relatives, 78% of those developing symptomatic type 1 diabetes have IA–2 and ZnT8 autoantibodies.

The detection of ICAs and GAD antibodies in older persons with type 2 diabetes in Finland and the UKPDS, who were shown subsequently to be more likely to require insulin therapy, has led to the concept of latent autoimmune diabetes of adults (LADA). Although GAD positivity had a specificity of 94.6% for early insulin use in the UKPDS, its sensitivity was only 37.9%. Moreover, the positive predictive value for GAD-positive antibodies was only 50.8% (i.e. only half of those positive went on to need insulin). Nonetheless, it is now accepted that LADA represents a distinct entity on the spectrum of autoimmune diabetes. It is now thought that LADA may represent 4–14% of people diagnosed as type 2 diabetes, which would make it more prevalent than childhood type 1 diabetes in Europe, and it is the most common cause of autoimmune diabetes in China. GAD65 autoantibodies are positive in 7–14%, IA–2 and ZnT8 are less common. It shares genetic features of both type 1 and 2 diabetes but is phenotypically closer to type 2. However, LADA is characterised by a lower age of onset, lower BMI, greater need for insulin within 6 months of diagnosis, and a tendency for worse glycaemic control. Thyroid peroxidase antibodies were positive in 27% of patients in one Italian study. There may be value in screening people who are thought to have LADA for autoantibodies as early insulin therapy is indicated, although there are no trials of specific therapeutic strategies to guide treatment.

The autoimmune basis for type 1 diabetes is underlined by its association with other diseases such as hypothyroidism, Graves' disease, pernicious anaemia, coeliac disease and Addison's disease which are all associated with organ-specific autoantibodies (Box 6.1). Up to 30% of people with type 1 diabetes have autoimmune thyroid disease. NICE

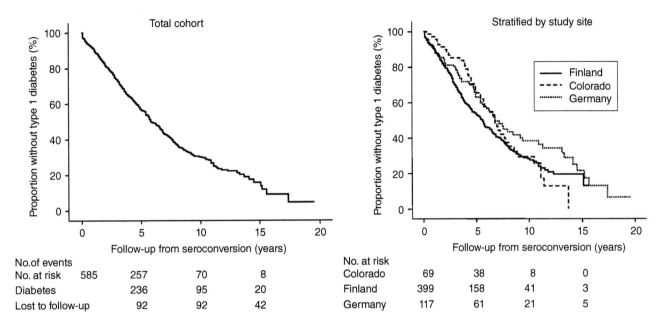

Figure 6.6 Progression to symptomatic Type 1 Diabetes in 585 children with two or more antibodies enrolled into three prospective studies in Finland (DIPP), USA (DAISY) and Germany (BABYDIAB & BABYDIET). Symptomatic diabetes developed in 43.5% at 5 years, 69.7% at 10 years and 84.2% at 15 years follow-up. Reproduced from Insel RA et al. Diabetes Care 2015; 38: 1964–74.

> **Box 6.1** Autoimmune disorders associated with type 1 diabetes.
>
> - Addison's disease
> - Graves' disease
> - Hypothyroidism
> - Hypogonadism
> - Pernicious anaemia
> - Vitiligo
> - Autoimmune polyglandular syndromes, types 1 and 2
> - Coeliac disease

guidance recommends screening all newly diagnosed children with type 1 diabetes for coeliac disease.

The mechanisms leading to autoimmunity have not been elucidated, and are almost certainly multiple with different factors operating in different individuals. What is clear is that exposure to environmental factors impacts upon genetically susceptible individuals to trigger an inflammatory response that ultimately leads to β cell loss and symptomatic diabetes.

Genetics

Genetic susceptibility to type 1 diabetes is most closely associated with HLA genes that lie within the major histocompatibility complex (MHC) region on the short arm of chromosome 6. HLAs are cell surface glycoproteins that show extreme variability through polymorphisms in the genes that code for them. Both high- and low-risk HLA haplotypes have been identified. HLA DR4–DQ8 and DR3–DQ2 confer high risk: the odds ratios for developing type 1 diabetes are 8–11 and 3.6 respectively for each, and 16 for both. 90% of Europid people with type 1 diabetes carry one or the other, and 30% carry both, compared to just 2% in the general population. Siblings sharing the exact DR3–DQ2 and DR4–DQ8 haplotypes with the proband have a >85% risk of developing diabetes before the age of 15 years. HLA DR3 and DR4 susceptibility haplotypes account for around 50% of the heritability of type 1 diabetes. Protective alleles include DQB1*0602, DQA1*0102 and DRB1*1501. DQB1*0602 is present in around 20% of the non-Hispanic white population but only 2% of people with type 1 diabetes. HLA susceptibility and protective haplotypes differ across ethnic groups. In African–Americans, the DR3 haplotype versions are very similar to those seen in non-Hispanic white populations, yet are protective, whereas the DR7 haplotype which is protective in non-Hispanic whites confers susceptibility.

Class II HLAs (HLA–D) play a key role in presenting foreign and self-antigens to T-helper lymphocytes and therefore in initiating the autoimmune process. Polymorphisms in the DR and DQ genes will encode for different amino acids in the peptide binding pockets of the HLA molecules. This affects the binding affinity and range of peptides that are presented to T cells, including potential autoantigens derived from the β cell. This is a likely critical step in 'arming' T lymphocytes, which initiate the immune attack against the β cells. Class I HLA alleles (A, B and C) also modify risk for type 1 diabetes but much less so than class II and usually in interaction. Class I/peptide antigen complexes play a role in CD8 T cell mediated cytotoxicity.

The current understanding of the events leading to β cell damage is as follows: Insulitis represents activation of CD4 and CD8 lymphocytes, CD 68 macrophages, and CD 20 B cells. CD 4 cell activation is related to HLA Class II protein expression, whilst CD 8 cells are related to HLA Class I; both are involved in initiation of insulitis and β cell loss, whereas CD 20 B cells appear to determine progression, and high or low expression results in fast or slow development of symptomatic type 1 diabetes.

Over 50 other regions of the human genome have been identified as being associated with type 1 diabetes using the candidate gene and genome-wide scanning (GWAS) approaches, and together these explain around 80% of heritability. Some of the major genetic polymorphisms and their likely role in Type 1 diabetes are shown in Table 6.2. Combination of the HLA susceptibility genes and PTPN22 and UBASH3A polymorphisms improved the predictability

Table 6.2 Main non- HLA polymorphisms that have been used in predictive modelling, and their possible role in type 1 diabetes. PTNP22 polymorphisms are shared with other autoimmune diseases such as rheumatoid arthritis and inflammatory bowel disease.

Genetic polymorphism	Possible impact
Insulin gene (INS)	Affects amount of insulin mRNA in thymus and influences immune tolerance
Protein tyrosine phosphatase non-receptor type 22 (PTPN22)	Promotes survival of auroreactive T cells in thymus and functional effects on circulating effector and regulator T cells and B cells
Cytotoxic T lymphocyte associated protein (CTLA-4)	Negative regulator of cytotoxic T cells Target for Abatacept therapy
Interleukin-2 receptor subunit α (IL2RA)	Affects sensititvity to IL2
Protein tyrosine phosphatase non-receptor type 2 (PTPN2)	β cell apoptosis after interaction with interferon
Interferon induced helicase (IFIH1)	Binds to virus RNA and moderates interferon mediated viral response
Basic leucine zipper transcription factor 2 (BACH2)	Regulates apoptotic pathways in β cells in conjunction with PTNP2
Ubiquitin associated and SH3 domain-containing protein A (UBASH3A)	Downregulates Nfκβ signaling pathway in response to T cell stimulation decreasing IL-2 gene expression
erb-b2 receptor tyrosine kinase 3 (ERBB3)	Uncertain role in diabetes. Encodes a member of the epidermal growth factor receptor family receptor tyrosine kinase

of developing type 1 diabetes by age 15 years to 45%, compared to only 3% in children who had the other combined genotypes. Prospective studies have shown that different genetic polymorphisms affect different stages of the disease process; DR3–DQ2 and DR4–DQ8 together with PTPN22 and UBASH3A seem to influence the development of autoantibodies, whereas INS, UBASH3A and IFIH1 impact upon the progression to symptomatic diabetes.

Intriguingly, there seems to be cross-talk with the type 2 diabetes susceptibility gene transcription factor 7 like-2 (TCF7L2). People with type 1 diabetes and only a single autoantibody, or who do not have HLA susceptibility haplotypes, are more likely to have the genetic variant TCF7L2 associated with type 2 diabetes, even though its overall frequency in people with type 1 diabetes is not increased.

The genetics of type 1 diabetes are obviously complex and polygenic. The interaction with environmental factors (see below) which results in an orchestrated T cell mediated and B cell facilitated autoimmune destruction of β cells is likely mediated by a range of different mechanisms, some of which will be more prominent in different individuals, and some of which will operate in sequence or together at different stages in the evolution of type 1 diabetes. It is also worth noting that the majority of those who carry genetic polymorphisms that predispose them to developing type 1 diabetes never do so.

Environmental and maternal factors

Although genetic factors are undoubtedly important, the rapidly increasing incidence rates for type 1 diabetes at a younger age strongly suggest that external or environmental factors are playing a part. Much of the evidence that links environmental factors with the aetiology of type 1 diabetes is circumstantial and associative, based upon epidemiology and animal research. The factors most often implicated are viruses, and diet and toxins, but a number of other influences, such as early feeding with cow's milk have been investigated (Table 6.3). These associations remain unexplained but may add support to the hygiene and accelerator hypotheses (see below).

Viruses

The viruses that have been implicated in the development of human diabetes have been deduced from temporal and geographical associations with a known infection. For example, mumps can cause pancreatitis and occasionally precedes the development of type 1 diabetes in children. Intrauterine rubella infection induces diabetes in up to 20% of affected children. However, the strongest associations have been with enteroviruses. A meta-analysis of 26 studies found an OR of 3.7 (95% CI 2.1, 6.8) for enterovirus serological positivity in patients with islet cell autoantibodies and symptomatic

Table 6.3 Associated foetal, maternal, dietary and environmental factors with the strength of the relationship (where known) on the development of type 1 diabetes (T1DM).

Associated factor	Strength of relationship
Shorter gestation	RR 1.18 (95%CI 1.09, 1.28) for gestational age 33–36 weeks and 1.12 (95% CI 1.07, 1.17) for 37 & 38 weeks
Birth weight	SGA RR 0.83 (95% CI 0.75, 0.93) LGA RR 1.14 (95% CI 1.04, 1.24) Severe SGA reduced risk for T1DM
Greater linear growth	Children diagnosed aged 5–10 years taller than peers but growth may be slowed with T1DM onset around puberty
Maternal age	5–10% increase odds per 5 year increase in maternal age
ABO blood group incompatability	Frequency of HLA DR3 similar in children with ABO incompatability and those with T1DM. OR 2.7 compared to controls
Birth order	Weak evidence that 2nd or later child are less likely to develop T1DM < 5 yrs of age
Delivery by caesarean section	Adjusted OR 1.19 (95% CI 1.04, 1.36)
Breast feeding (bf)	OR 0.75 (95% CI 0.64, 0.88) for 2 weeks bf; weaker for 3 months. No benefit of non-exclusive bf beyond 2 weeks
Dietary cereals	Later exposure (>7 months) to gluten HR for T1DM 3.33(95% CI 1.54, 7.18). Early exposure (<3 months) increases risk of coeliac disease.
Vitamin D supplements	OR 0.71 (95% CI 0.60, 0.84) but marked heterogeneity in studies
Omega 3 fatty acids	Lower intake associated with higher rates in Norway. Clinical trials underway
Atopy	OR 0.82 (95% CI 0.68, 0.99) for asthma in children with T1DM, but not eczema or rhinitis (see hygiene hypothesis)
Child day care	Inconclusive data but some association between attending day care and lower T1DM risk

OR = odds ratio; RR = relative risk; HR = hazard ratio; CI = confidence interval; SGA = small for gestational age; LGA = large for gestational age.

type 1 diabetes, and the virus most commonly identified is coxsackie B. There was, however, a significant heterogeneity in these studies. In prospective cohort studies, patients with positive enterovirus antibodies had accelerated progression to symptomatic diabetes, but they did not seem to initiate islet autoimmunity.

In a few cases, coxsackie viral antigens have been isolated in islets postmortem, and viruses isolated from the pancreas have been shown to induce diabetes in susceptible mouse strains. Electron microscopy of the pancreas in some subjects who died shortly after the onset of type 1 diabetes identified retrovirus-like particles within the β cells, associated with insulitis. There have also been case reports of multiple family members developing type 1 diabetes after contracting enteroviral infection.

Viruses may target the β cells and destroy them directly through a cytolytic effect or by triggering an autoimmune attack (Figure 6.7). Autoimmune mechanisms may include 'molecular mimicry'; that is, immune responses against a viral antigen that cross-react with a β cell antigen (e.g. a coxsackie B4 protein (P2–C) has sequence homology with GAD, an established autoantigen in the β cell). Also, anti-insulin antibodies from patients with type 1 diabetes cross-react with the retroviral p73 antigen in about 75% of cases. Alternatively, viral damage may release sequestered islet antigens and thus restimulate resting autoreactive T cells, previously sensitised against β cell antigens ('bystander activation'). Persistent viral infection could also stimulate interferon-α synthesis and hyperexpression of HLA class I antigens, and the secretion of chemokines that recruit activated macrophages and cytotoxic T cells.

Apoptosis

One model of β cell destruction is via the process of apoptosis or programmed cell death (Figure 6.8). This is effected by the activation of cellular caspases triggered by extrinsic means, including the interaction of cell surface Fas (the death-signalling molecule) with its ligand FasL, on the surface of infiltrating CD4 and CD8 cells. There is an intrinsic pathway mediated by a balance between anti- and pro-apoptotic mitochondrial pathways and both converge via the caspase activation pathway to cause β cell death. Other factors that induce apoptosis include macrophage derived nitric oxide (NO) and toxic free radicals, and disruption of the cell membrane by perforin and granzyme B produced by cytotoxic T cells. T cell cytokines (e.g. interleukin–1, tumour necrosis factor–α, interferon–γ) have been shown to up-regulate Fas and FasL and induce NO and toxic free radicals.

Dietary factors

Wheat gluten is a potent diabetogen in animal models of type 1 diabetes (BB rats and NOD mice; see below), and 5–10% of patients with type 1 diabetes have gluten-sensitive enteropathy (coeliac disease). Recent studies have demonstrated that patients with type 1 diabetes and coeliac disease share disease-specific alleles. Wheat may induce subclinical gut inflammation and enhanced gut permeability to lumen antigens in some patients with type 1 diabetes, which may lead to a breakdown in tolerance for dietary proteins. Other possible diabetogenic factors in diet include N–nitroso compounds, speculatively implicated in Icelandic smoked meat, which was a common dietary constituent in winter months.

Toxins

The notion that there may be environmental β cell toxins is supported by the existence of chemicals that cause an insulin-dependent type of diabetes in animals. Examples are

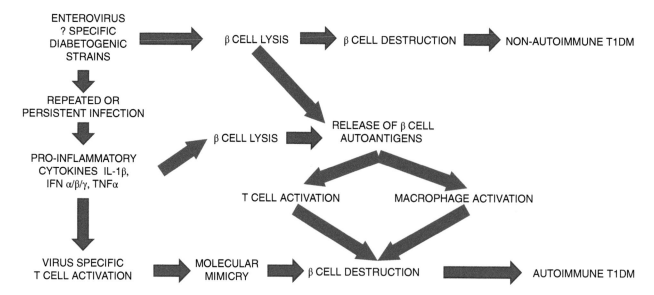

Figure 6.7 Potential mechanisms of viral aetiology of autoimmune and non-autoimmune type 1 diabetes. IL = Interleukin; IFN = Interferon; TNF = Tumour Necrosis Factor. Adapted from Craig ME et al Pediatr Diabetes 2013;14:149–58.

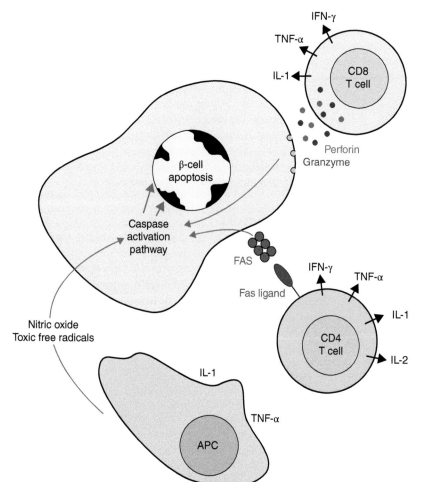

Figure 6.8 Proposed mechanisms of β cell death. β cells die through a process known as apoptosis, characterised by condensation and fragmentation of nuclear chromatin, loss of cytoplasm and expression of surface receptors that signal macrophages to ingest the apoptotic cell. Apoptosis is effected by activation of the caspase pathway.

alloxan and streptozocin, both of which damage the β cell at several sites, including membrane disruption, enzyme interaction (e.g. with glucokinase) and DNA fragmentation. The rat poison vacor causes type 1 diabetes in humans, possibly because it has a similar action to streptozocin.

Animal models

Spontaneous diabetes that resembles type 1 diabetes in humans occurs in some animals, notably the BioBreeding (BB) rat and the non-obese diabetic (NOD) mouse. These 'animal models' have many of the same characteristics as human autoimmune diabetes, including a genetic predisposition, MHC association, insulitis, circulating islet cell surface and GAD autoantibodies, a long prediabetic period that precedes overt hyperglycaemia and environmental factors that trigger or accelerate the appearance of diabetes, such as wheat and cow's milk proteins. Many hypotheses of the causes of type 1 diabetes have been developed and tested in these animals.

Hygiene hypothesis

The increasing incidence of atopy as well as early-onset type 1 diabetes in Western societies may be a consequence of a lack of exposure to common pathogens such as helminth worms (so called 'old friends'), or lactobacilli (microflora). Chronic exposure might include a more tolerant T cell response to antigens, while a cleaner, more sterile early environment would result in an exaggerated response in subsequent months or years. Some of the associated factors listed in Table 6.3 would support this hypothesis.

Pregnancy is thought to have a Th2 lymphocyte orientation whilst early environmental antigen exposure stimulates Th1 responses. The first line immune response in children comprises immature dendritic cells which are primed to respond to specific antigens, and they also carry innate pattern recognition receptors that bind to viral or bacterial cell surfaces. T-cell receptors are highly cross reactive so an immune response to common allergens or self antigens might be activated by infection. It was originally thought that an imbalance in Th1 and 2 cells would lead to a different balance in cytokine release predisposing to either autoimmunity (Th1 predominance) or allergy (Th2 predominance). However, this construct has not been supported by the observation that helminth (pinworm) exposure actually leads to a more pronounced Th2 response but lower rates of atopy. Thus, the hygiene hypothesis, despite supportive associative data, remains unproven.

Accelerator hypothesis

The observed increase in non-autoimmune type 1 diabetes and its links to type 2 diabetes susceptibility genes, as well as the increasing rates of obesity in children, has led to the concept of increasing insulin resistance as a cause of β cell loss. It is generally believed that β cell loss is a feature of ageing, and

obesity related insulin resistance could accelerate this loss through apoptosis and be partly responsible for the increasing incidence of both type 1 and type 2 diabetes. Much of the supportive evidence remains cross sectional rather than prospective, however.

Stages of Diabetes

The increasing understanding of the processes leading to symptomatic type 1 diabetes has resulted in a consensus model in individuals who have a genetic susceptibility and comprises 3 stages (Figure 6.9). Stage 1 individuals have positive autoantibodies but normal glucose tolerance. As mentioned above, increasing numbers of islet autoantibodies and increasing titres represent disease progression. Stage 2 is reached as β cell loss results in glycaemic responses to a glucose challenge becoming abnormal, but there is no universal agreement as to what the glucose stimulus should be or what threshold of blood glucose (or HbA1c) would define 'dysglycaemia'. Both the presence of impaired fasting glucose or glucose intolerance (see Chap 3) following a 75g OGTT and a 20% increase in baseline HbA1c have a positive predictive value (PPV) of 98% for symptomatic type 1 diabetes within 5 years in prospective studies in high risk individuals, and it is known that the first phase insulin response to intravenous glucose declines rapidly 18–6 months before diabetes symptoms. Stage 3 is the development of symptomatic diabetes.

Prevention Trials

This staging has helped in the design of clinical prevention trials. Early studies focused on antigen specific (by early exposure to intravenous or oral insulin), or immunosuppressive approaches. Neither proved to be successful, partly because of the difficulty in recruiting patients at a potentially reversible stage of their disease. The most successful study used an anti-CD3 antibody which decreased the actions of CD8 T lymphocytes on target β cells. Teplizumab was given for 14 days in a randomised controlled trial to 76 high risk (Stage 2) individuals. The intervention delayed the diagnosis of type 1 diabetes by a median of 24 months and was well tolerated, although there was a significant reactivation of EB virus disease in those with evidence of previous infection. This proof of concept trial will likely lead to further studies of this and other agents, and several are ongoing.

Screening for Type 1 Diabetes

The improvement in assays for islet autoantibodies and the development of genetic prediction models has raised the possibility of population screening for individuals at high type 1 diabetes susceptibility. The problem is that the numbers needed to be screened to identify a single case are prohibitive (Figure 6.10) and the absence of an effective treatment means that conventional criteria for screening are not fully satisfied. The TrialNet and other research programmes aims

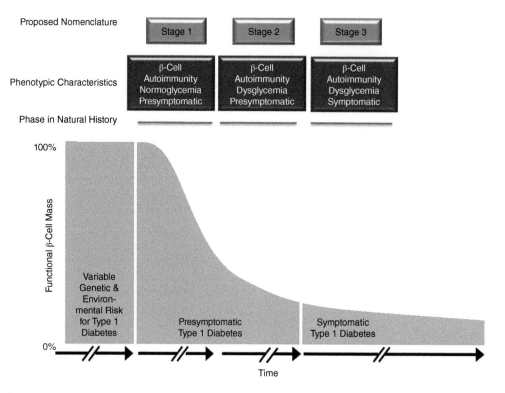

Figure 6.9 Stages of Type 1 Diabetes as proposed by the Juvenile Diabetes Research Foundation, Endocrine Society and American Diabetes Association and adopted by TrialNet for preventative studies. Autoantibodies are present many years prior to development of symptomatic diabetes (Stage 3). Prior to this those in Stage 1 have normal glucose tolerance and those in Stage 2 varying levels of hyperglycaemia below the diagnostic thresholds of diabetes. Intervention and prevention studies have largely focused on Stage 2 and 3 patients. Reproduced from Insel RA et al. Diabetes Care 2015; 38: 1964–74 with permission.

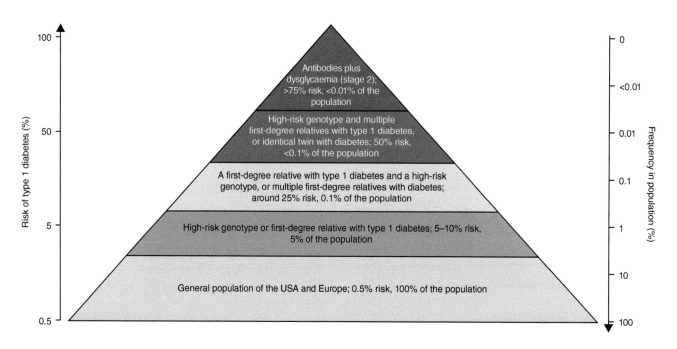

Figure 6.10 Lifetime risk of developing Type 1 diabetes (left axis) compared to prevalence of risk in the overall population (right axis). Individuals in the apex have the highest risk of developing diabetes (>75% within 5y) but represent 0.01% (1 in 10,000) of the overall population. From Dayan CM et al Lancet 2019 with permission.

to recruit first degree relatives of probands with type 1 diabetes and as our understanding of heritability develops, the argument for more widespread but focused screening may become stronger.

CASE HISTORY

A 4-year-old boy whose mother has had type 1 diabetes since age 13 years developed thirst, polyuria, hyperphagia, and weight loss shortly after recovering from a head cold. His mother tested his capillary blood glucose with her own meter and found it to be 25.3 mmol/L. His birth weight was 4.1 kg and he was bottle fed with cow's milk from birth.

Comment: This case illustrates several cardinal features of type 1 diabetes. A positive family history, age of onset <5 years, symptoms beginning after a minor infection, and early exposure to cow's milk. Birth weight >4 kg is linked to type 2 diabetes in some populations.

LANDMARK STUDY

The Barts–Windsor study was the first prospective family study in type 1 diabetes and was created by the fortuitous collaboration between Andrew Cudworth (then at St Bartholomew's Hospital) and John Lister who was the diabetologist in Windsor and who kept a file index of all new cases of type 1 diabetes that he had seen in the district. Around 200 families with a proband with type 1 diabetes and an unaffected sibling were identified and serum collected from as many family members as possible. The findings contributed to what Edwin Gale termed a paradigm shift in the thinking around the aetiology of type diabetes (see 2001 reference below for masterful description). The original objective was to detect the viral culprit for type 1 diabetes. Instead, they confirmed the autoimmune basis of the disease; the clinically silent but immunologically active stage in individuals who had islet cell and GAD autoantibodies years before developing diabetes; and the causative links with some HLA antigens and the protective nature of others. Sadly, Andrew died just as the study was producing its most impressive results, but it remains a fine example of how happenchance and clinical diligence can combine to change our thinking about disease in fundamental ways.

KEY WEBSITES

- Diabetes Atlas: www.diabetesatlas.org
- www.Trialnet.com International network of scientists and clinicians exploring cause and treatment of type 1 diabetes

FURTHER READING

Craig ME, Nair S, Stein H et al. Viruses and diabetes: a new look at an old story. *Pediatr Diabetes* 2013; 14: 149–58.

Dayan CM, Korah M, Tatovic D et al. Changing the landscape for type 1 diabetes: the first step to prevention. Lancet 2019; dx.doi.org/10.1016/S0140–6736919032127–0

Gale EAM. The discovery of type 1 diabetes. *Diabetes* 2001; 50:217–226.

Gomez–Taurino I, Arif S, Eichmann M, Peakman M. T cells in type 1 diabetes: instructors, regulators and effectors: a comprehensive review. *J Autoimmunity* 2016; 66: 7–16.

Insel RA, Dunne JL, Atkinson MA et al. Staging presymptomatic type 1 diabetes: a scientific statement of JDRF, the Endocrine Society, and the American Diabetes Association. *Diabetes Care* 2015; 38: 1964–74 doi:10.2337/dc15-1419

International Diabetes Federation. *Diabetes Atlas*, 9th edn. Brussels: International Diabetes Federation, 2019.

Laugsen E, Ostergaard JA, Leslie RDG. Latent autoimmune diabetes of the adult: current knowledge and uncertainty. *Diabetic Medicine* 2015; 32: 843–52 doi:10.1111/dme.12700

Patterson CC, Dahlquist GG, Gyurus E, Green A, Soltesz G and the EURODIAB Study Group. Incidence trends for childhood type 1 diabetes in Europe during 1989–2003 and predicted new cases 2005–20: a multicentre prospective registration study. *Lancet* 2009; 373: 2027–2033.

Patterson CC, Harjutsalo V, Rosenbauer J et al. Trends and cyclical variation in the incidence of childhood type 1 diabetes in 26 European centres in the 25 year period 1989–2013: a multicentre prospective registration study. *Diabetologia* 2019; 62: 408–17 doi.org/10.1007/s00125-018-4763-3

Redondo MJ, Steck AK, Pugliese A. Genetics of type 1 diabetes. *Pediatr Diabetes* 2018; 19: 346–53.

Stiemsa LT, Reynolds LA, Turvey SE, Finlay BB. The hygiene hypothesis: current perspectives and future therapies. *Immunotargets Ther* 2015; 4: 143–57.

Epidemiology and aetiology of type 2 diabetes

Prevalence rates and global burden

Globally, an estimated 422 million adults were living with diabetes in 2014 (85–95% is type 2). According to the WHO Global Report on diabetes, the global prevalence of diabetes (aged-standardised) has nearly doubled since 1980, rising from 4.7% to 8.5% in the adult population. This reflects the increasing prevalence of type 2 diabetes risk factors, particularly obesity (Figures 7.1–7.3). In people with type 2 diabetes, 90% are overweight or obese.

Diabetes prevalence has risen faster in low- and middle-income countries than in high-income countries. The highest prevalence rates are currently in the Eastern Mediterranean and Middle East with North and South America close behind (Figure 7.4 and 7.5). Conversion rates from impaired glucose tolerance (IGT) to type 2 diabetes are 5–11% per annum. In terms of absolute numbers, the Western Pacific region (particularly China) will see almost a 50% increase to 100 million people with diabetes by 2025.

The largest number of people with type 2 diabetes is currently in the 40–59-year age group, where numbers will almost reach parity with 60–79-year olds by 2025.

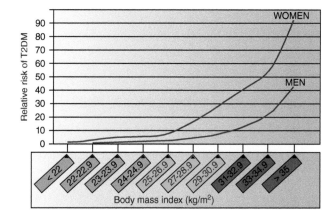

Figure 7.1 The relationship between body mass index (BMI) and risk of type 2 diabetes in men and women.

There is however considerable variation between IDF regions and within each region. For example, in the Western Pacific, the tiny island of Nauru has a comparative prevalence in 2007 of 30.7%, whilst nearby Tonga has less than half that rate at 12.9%, the Philippines 7.6% and China 4.1% (Figure 7.6).

Handbook of Diabetes, Fifth Edition. Rudy Bilous, Richard Donnelly, and Iskandar Idris.
© 2021 John Wiley & Sons Ltd. Published 2021 by John Wiley & Sons Ltd.

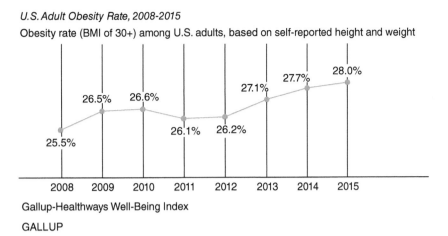

Figure 7.2 Rising obesity rates in the USA (2008-2015) based on self-reported height and weight and using BMI>30 as a cut-off. U.S. Obesity Rate Climbs to Record High in 2015, Gallup. © 2016 Gallup, Inc.

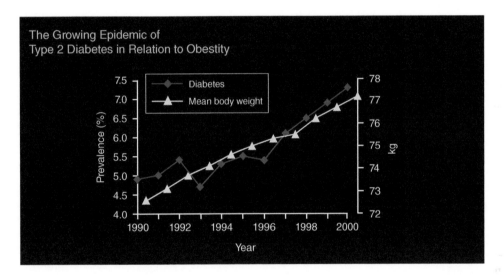

Figure 7.3 The rising Prevalence of type 2 diabetes parallels the rising incidence of overweight and obesity. This trend has continued in more recent years. Mokdad AH et al. JAMA, 1999, 282: 1519–1522; Mokdad AH et.al Diabetes Care, 2000, 23:1278–1283.

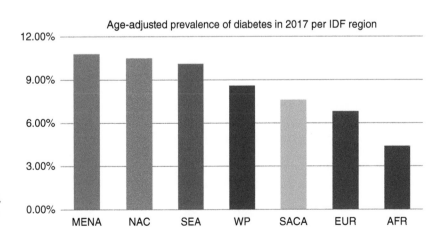

Figure 7.4 Age-adjusted prevalence rates of type 2 diabetes in different geographical regions of the world, as monitored by the International Diabetes Federation (IDF). IDF 2017. © International Diabetes Federation.

Prevalence* of diabetes and IGT (20-79 years) by IDF region, 2017 and 2045

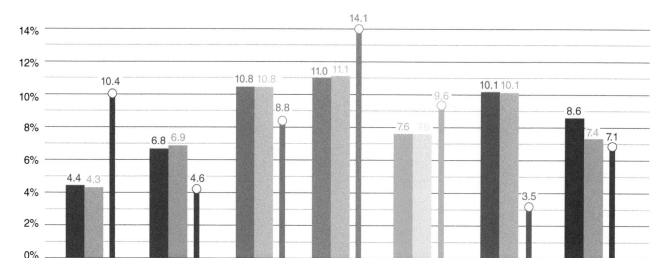

Figure 7.5 The IDF atlas also monitors the rising prevalence of prediabetes (impaired glucose tolerance) in different geographical regions. IDF Diabetes Atlas. © 2017 International Diabetes Federation.

In Europe, comparative prevalence rates vary from 1.6% in Iceland to 7.9% in Germany, Austria and Switzerland. The UK prevalence rate is 2.9% (age adjusted) and 4.0% (absolute), increasing to 3.5% and 4.6% respectively by 2025.

Diabetes caused 1.5 million deaths in 2012. Higher-than-optimal blood glucose caused an additional 2.2 million deaths (Figure 7.7 and 7.8). Of these deaths, 43% occur before the age of 70, and the proportion of deaths attributable to high glucose is highest in low- and middle-income countries.

Urban versus rural

There is a clear trend for rates of diabetes to increase in populations as they move from a rural to an urban existence. The reasons are unclear but probably relate to both decreasing physical activity as well as dietary changes. For example, rural Chinese have a prevalence of type 2 diabetes of 5%, which is less than half the rate of Singaporean Chinese (10.5%). Much larger differences are seen in South Asian, Hispanic, African, and Polynesian peoples (Figure 7.9).

Impaired glucose tolerance

Comparative prevalence for IGT vary by region with rates almost double those for type 2 diabetes in Africa, but slightly lower elsewhere (Figure 7.5). These differences are almost certainly a reflection of socio-economic factors as well as a paucity of studies in many African countries where extrapolation is necessary between very different populations. In Europe, the comparative prevalence will increase slightly from 9.1% in 2007 to 9.6% in 2025, representing an absolute change from 65.3 to 71.2 million (UK figures 4.7% to 4.9%, 2.17 to 2.4 million respectively).

Incidence

The reported incidence rates for type 2 diabetes vary according to the population under study and the year of observation. For white Europid populations, rates of 0.1–1% per annum have been reported. For Hispanic populations in the USA, rates of 2.8% were recorded in the San Antonio Study, which are similar to those of the Pima Indians in Arizona (approximately 2.5%) and the Australian aborigines (2.03%). Over the last 20 years, incidence rates among the Pima Indians has not changed, although the age of onset of type 2 diabetes has been declining.

The occurrence of type 2 diabetes in adolescence is a great cause for concern worldwide. In US Asian and Pacific Islanders, for example, rates of 12.1/100,000 patient–years have been reported in 10–19-year-olds, which is similar to rates reported for type 1 diabetes. In the UK, the overall incidence for <16-year-olds is much lower, at 0.53 per/100,000 patient–years, but 10 times more common in South Asian or black African compared to white children.

The rural–n ratio remains for diabetes incidence rates even in the presence of other risk factors such as central obesity. In Japan, there is an approximately threefold increase in the incidence among obese urban compared to rural populations (15.8 versus 5.8% over 10 years). Similarly, there

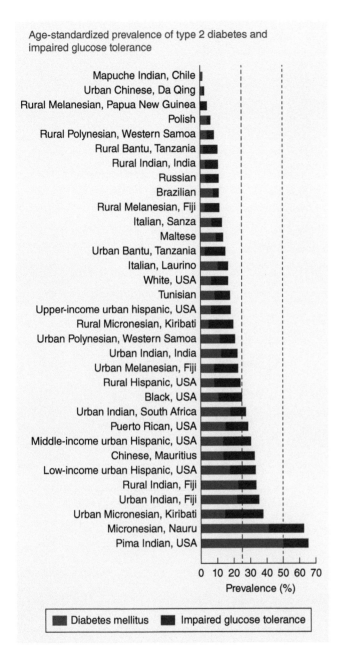

Age-standardized prevalence of type 2 diabetes and impaired glucose tolerance

- Mapuche Indian, Chile
- Urban Chinese, Da Qing
- Rural Melanesian, Papua New Guinea
- Polish
- Rural Polynesian, Western Samoa
- Rural Bantu, Tanzania
- Rural Indian, India
- Russian
- Brazilian
- Rural Melanesian, Fiji
- Italian, Sanza
- Maltese
- Urban Bantu, Tanzania
- Italian, Laurino
- White, USA
- Tunisian
- Upper-income urban hispanic, USA
- Rural Micronesian, Kiribati
- Urban Polynesian, Western Samoa
- Urban Indian, India
- Urban Melanesian, Fiji
- Rural Hispanic, USA
- Black, USA
- Urban Indian, South Africa
- Puerto Rican, USA
- Middle-income urban Hispanic, USA
- Chinese, Mauritius
- Low-income urban Hispanic, USA
- Rural Indian, Fiji
- Urban Indian, Fiji
- Urban Micronesian, Kiribati
- Micronesian, Nauru
- Pima Indian, USA

0 10 20 30 40 50 60 70
Prevalence (%)

■ Diabetes mellitus ■ Impaired glucose tolerance

Figure 7.6 A league table of countries showing widely different prevalence rates of type 2 diabetes and impaired glucose tolerance. A mixture of genes and environment account for these differences. Forouhi NG and Wareham NJ. Medicine, 2006; 34(2): 57–60.

is a twofold increase in incidence for USA versus Mexican Hispanic people corrected for age and economic circumstance, probably a reflection of changes in diet and lifestyle.

Risk factors for type 2 diabetes
Obesity
About 80% of people with type 2 diabetes are obese, and the risk of developing diabetes increases progressively as the

BMI (weight (kg)/height (m)²) increases (Figure 7.1). A BMI >35 kg/m² increases the risk of type 2 diabetes developing over a 10-year period by 80-fold, as compared to those with a BMI <22 kg/m². Small increments in body weight translate into large increases in type 2 diabetes risk (Figure 7.10).

The latest data from the US NHANES survey confirms a 6–10-fold higher lifetime risk of type 2 diabetes for 18-year-olds with a BMI >35 kg/m² compared to those with BMI <18.5 kg/m², with an associated 6–7 year reduction in overall life expectancy.

Obesity is still widely defined as a BMI >30 kg/m² although BMI is not an accurate reflection of fat mass or its distribution, particularly in Asian people. A simple waist circumference may be better. The pattern of obesity is also important in that central fat deposition is associated with greater insulin resistance and confers a much higher risk for developing diabetes compared to gluteofemoral deposition (Figure 7.11). In clinical practice, 'central' obesity can be assessed by measuring the ratio of waist:hip circumference, but it is unclear whether this has any advantage over a simple measurement of waist circumference alone.

Fat deposition at other sites, particularly in skeletal muscle, liver and in the pancreatic islets, may contribute to metabolic defects and insulin resistance. This 'ectopic' fat deposition leads to lipotoxicity, which in turn causes insulin resistance and (in islets) impairs insulin secretion.

Physical exercise and diet
Low levels of physical exercise also predict the development of type 2 diabetes, possibly because exercise increases insulin sensitivity and helps prevent obesity (Figure 7.12). People who exercise the most have a 25–60% lower risk of developing type 2 diabetes regardless of their other risk factors such as obesity and family history.

The Diabetes Prevention Programme and the Diabetes Prevention Study have shown that lifestyle modifications with moderate exercise and modest weight loss can dramatically reduce the number progressing from IGT to type 2 diabetes and reinforce the importance of lifestyle factors in the cause of diabetes.

Insulin resistance
Whole-body 'insulin resistance' can be estimated from the amount of glucose that needs to be infused intravenously in order to maintain a constant blood glucose level during a simultaneous intravenous infusion of insulin. This (euglycaemic hyperinsulinaemic 'clamp') method is cumbersome, so for studying populations the HOMA (homeostasis model assessment) methods are more practical for estimating steady-state beta-cell function (HOMA B) and insulin sensitivity (HOMA S) as percentages of normal. These estimates can be derived from a single fasting measurement of plasma C-peptide, insulin and glucose concentrations.

Deaths attributable to diabetes by age (20–79 years)

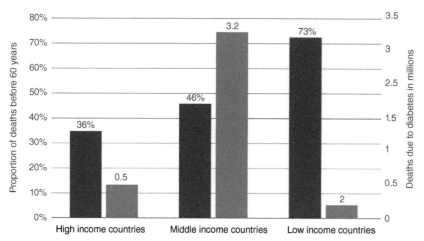

"Half of the 4 million people who die from diabetes are under the age of 60"

Figure 7.7 Deaths attributable to diabetes are highest in low- and middle-income countries. IDF Diabetes Atlas. © 2017 International Diabetes Federation.

The Relationship Between Glycaemic Control (Updated HbA1c) and the Incidence of Cardiovascular Disease

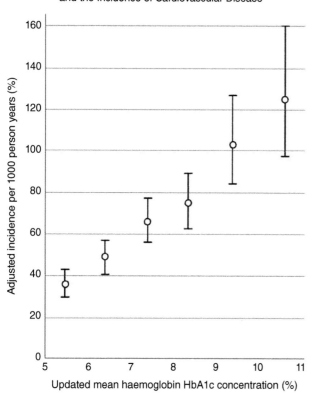

Figure 7.8 The relationship between HbA1c and the incidence of cardiovascular disease. This is a linear relationship which extends down into the prediabetic range (i.e HbA1c<6.5%). Bain et al. Diabetes, Obesity and Metabolism, 2016; 18(12): 1157–1166.

Insulin resistance (or, more correctly, diminished insulin sensitivity) precedes the onset of diabetes and can worsen with increasing duration (Figure 7.13). Insulin resistance is a major factor in the aetiology of type 2 diabetes, and affects the muscle, liver, and adipose tissues (Figure 7.14).

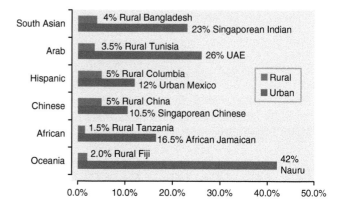

Figure 7.9 Varying prevalence rates of type 2 diabetes by ethnicity/region and location (red, rural; blue, urban) for 2007. UAE, United Arab Emirates. Data from *Diabetes Atlas*.

Hormones and cytokines

Visceral fat liberates large amounts of non-esterified fatty acids (NEFAs) through lipolysis, which increases gluoconeogenesis in the liver and impairs glucose uptake and utilisation in muscle. NEFAs may also inhibit insulin secretion, possibly by enhancing the accumulation of triglycerides within the β cells. In addition, adipose tissue produces cytokines, such as TNF-α, resistin and IL-6, all of which have been shown experimentally to interfere with insulin action. TNF-α has been shown to inhibit tyrosine kinase activity at the insulin receptor and decrease expression of the glucose transporter GLUT-4.

Adiponectin is a hormone with anti-inflammatory and insulin-sensitising properties that is secreted solely by fat cells. It suppresses hepatic gluconeogenesis and stimulates fatty acid oxidation in the liver and skeletal muscles, as well as increasing muscle glucose uptake and insulin release from the β cells. Circulating adiponectin is reduced in obesity and a recent meta-analysis showed that the relative risk for

Relationships Between Body Weight and Diabetes

Relationship Between Increasing
Body Weight and Diabetes
Prevalence: 1990–2000

Relationship Between
Weight Gain in Adulthood
and the Risk of Type 2
Diabetes in Men and Women

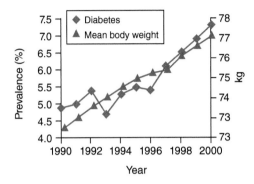

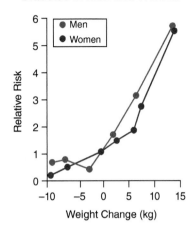

Figure 7.10 Weight gain is a particularly strong driver of type 2 diabetes risk (right panel). Small increments in body weight translate into large increases in relative risk. Haffner SM. Obesity, 2006; 14(6s): 121S–127S.

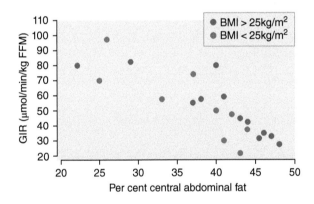

Figure 7.11 Insulin resistance (as assessed by glucose infusion rate (GIR) to maintain constant blood glucose during simultaneous insulin infusion) is proportional to visceral fat mass, independent of BMI. FFM, fat-free mass. Data from Pan et al. Diabetes 1997; 46: 983–988.

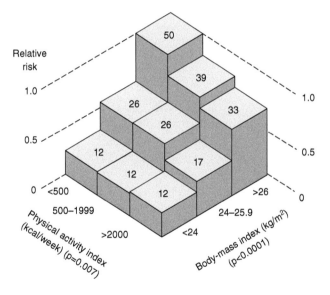

Figure 7.12 Age-adjusted risk of type 2 diabetes among 5990 men. The figure shows data for the physical activity index in relation to BMI. Each block represents the relative risk of type 2 diabetes per 10,000 man-years of follow-up, with the risk for the tallest block set at 1.0. The numbers on the blocks are incidence rates of type 2 diabetes per 10,000 man-years. From Helmrich et al. N Engl J Med 1991; 325: 147–152.

diabetes was 0.72 for every 1-log μg/mL increment in adiponectin level.

Resistin is an adipocyte-secreted hormone that increases insulin resistance and was first described in rodents, being found in increased levels in experimental obesity and diabetes. In humans, it appears to be derived largely from macrophages, however, and its precise role in human diabetes is uncertain, although higher circulating levels have been found in some people with type 2 diabetes.

Leptin is an adipokine that was found to be absent in the ob/ob mouse model of obesity and diabetes. Its normal function is to suppress appetite, thus providing a candidate mechanism linking weight gain and appetite control.

Although abnormal leptin function has been described in humans, these defects are very rare and paradoxically high levels have been found in type 2 diabetes.

Ghrelin is a recently described peptide secreted from the stomach and may act as a hunger signal. Circulating levels are negatively correlated with BMI and are suppressed by

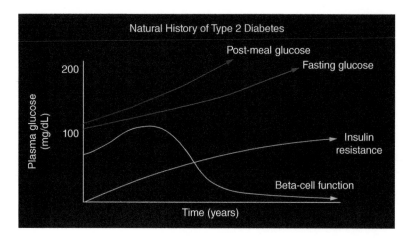

Figure 7.13 The natural history of type 2 diabetes development often begins with rising insulin resistance due to obesity, diet and low levels of exercise. This insulin resistance results in a compensatory rise in circulating insulin concentrations which, initially, maintains normal or near-normal glycaemia. But over time the pancreas becomes exhausted and the compensatory increase in insulin secretion falls. When beta cell secretion of insulin decreases blood glucose levels rise to meet the diagnostic cut-off for type 2 diabetes. DeFronzo R.Diabetes Care, 1992, 15: 318–368; Haffner S, et al. Diabetes Care, 1999, 22: 562–568.

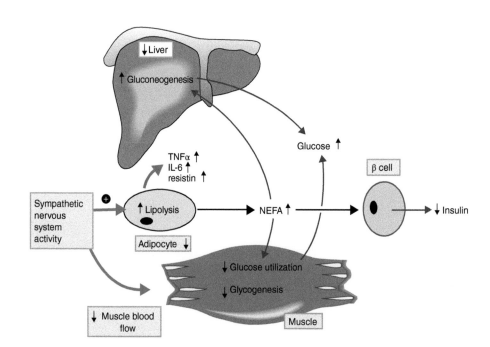

Figure 7.14 Mechanisms of insulin resistance in type 2 diabetes.

food intake. It has no known role in human diabetes, but antagonism may provide a therapeutic target.

Finally, there is often increased sympathetic nervous system activity in obesity, which might also increase lipolysis, reduce muscle blood flow and thus glucose delivery and uptake, and therefore directly affect insulin action.

Inflammation

Many of these cytokines are involved in the acute-phase response and it is therefore not surprising that circulating markers such as C-reactive protein and sialic acid are increased in type 2 diabetes patients, as well as in those who later go on to develop the condition. Because these markers have also been found to be elevated in patients with atherosclerosis, a unifying hypothesis has evolved proposing that inflammation may be a common precursor and link between diabetes and coronary artery disease.

Genetics

Evidence for a genetic basis for type 2 diabetes comes from a clear familial aggregation, but it does not segregate in a classic Mendelian fashion. About 10% of patients with type

2 diabetes have a similarly affected sibling. The concordance rate for identical twins is variously estimated to be 33–90% (17–37% in non-identical twins), but the interpretation of this is difficult because siblings may have similar lifestyles and diets. Thus, the explanation for the high concordance may be environmental rather than genetic.

Unlike type 1, type 2 diabetes is not associated with genes in the HLA region. So far, 19 gene variants have been described and validated as being associated with type 2 diabetes. Of these, the strongest is TCF7L2; 15% of European adults carry two copies of the abnormal gene and they have double the lifetime risk of developing type 2 diabetes compared to the 40% who carry no copies. Carriers of the T risk allele have impaired insulin secretion and enhanced hepatic glucose output. Nearly all of the other described genes affect either β cell mass or function; few appear to have potential effects on insulin resistance.

Thrifty phenotype hypothesis

A link between low birthweight and later development of type 2 diabetes in a UK population has led to a hypothesis linking foetal malnutrition to impaired β cell development and insulin resistance in adulthood. Abundant adult nutrition and consequent obesity would then expose these problems, leading to IGT and eventually type 2 diabetes. This has been called the thrifty phenotype hypothesis (Figure 7.15).

A meta-analysis of 31 populations involving 152,084 individuals from varying ethnic groups and 6090 cases of diabetes was published in 2008. This confirmed a negative association between birthweight and diabetes in 23, but found a positive association in eight studies. The combined odds ratio for type 2 diabetes was 0.8 (95% CI 0.72–0.89) for each 1 kg increase in birthweight. This relationship was strengthened if macrosomic (birthweight >4 kg) and offspring of mothers with known type 2 diabetes were excluded (odds ratio (OR) 0.67, 95% CI 0.61–0.73). Notably there was a tendency for a positive relationship in North American populations largely due to higher rates of maternal obesity and gestational diabetes. Adjustment for socio-economic status had no effect, but adjustment for achieved adult BMI attenuated the relationship.

With increasing maternal obesity and gestational diabetes mellitus (GDM), it is conceivable that the relationship will change to the pattern currently seen in Native Americans which is more U-shaped. However, it is still unclear whether low birthweight is a causative factor or a sign of other potential mechanisms which may predispose to later diabetes.

Metabolic syndrome

The aggregation of obesity, hyperglycaemia, hypertension, and dyslipidaemia (high TG's and low HDL-cholesterol) in people with both type 2 diabetes and cardiovascular disease is termed the metabolic syndrome (Table 7.1).

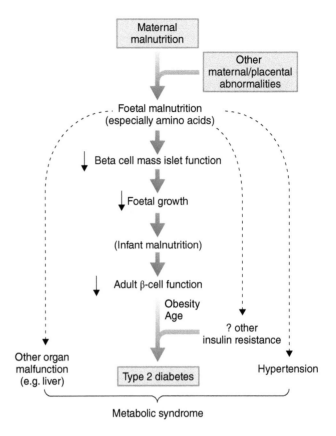

Figure 7.15 The 'thrifty phenotype' hypothesis.

Since several definitions appeared, there has been considerable debate as to their relative strengths and weaknesses. Indeed, there is some debate as to whether this constitutes a true syndrome at all and whether they add anything to predictive models for type 2 diabetes and coronary artery disease. A major problem is the correlation of many of the features. In prospective studies, fasting plasma glucose (FPG) is overwhelmingly linked to subsequent development of diabetes, but much less so with coronary artery disease. Thus, the predictive utility of the metabolic syndrome as a concept adds little to its constituent risk factors when they are used individually. The long-term usefulness of the definition of the metabolic syndrome for identification and intervention in order to prevent diabetes and cardiovascular disease has yet to be demonstrated.

β cell dysfunction

Type 2 diabetes develops because of a progressive deterioration of β cell function, coupled with increasing insulin resistance for which the β cell cannot compensate. At the time of diagnosis β cell function is already reduced by about 50% and continues to decline regardless of therapy (Figure 7.16).

The main defects in β cell function in type 2 diabetes are a markedly reduced first- and second-phase insulin response

Table 7.1 Definition of metabolic syndrome.

Risk factor	Defining level	
	NCEP ATP III	IDF
Abdominal obesity (waist circumference)		
Men	>102 cm	≥94 cm (Europid) ≥90 cm (others)
Women	>88 cm	≥80 cm for all
Plasma triglycerides	≥1.7 mmol/L	≥1.7 mmol/L
Plasma HDL cholesterol		
Men	<0.9 mmol/L	<1.03 mmol/L
Women	<1.1 mmol/L	<1.29 mmol/L
Blood pressure	≥130/≥85 mmHg	≥130/≥85 mmHg or on treatment
Plasma fasting glucose	≥6.1 mmol/L	≥5.6 mmol/L or pre-existing type 2 diabetes
Diagnostic criteria	3 or more of the above	Obesity plus 2 others

Source: NCEP ATP III, National Cholesterol Education Programme – 3rd Adult Treatment Panel; IDF, International Diabetes Federation.

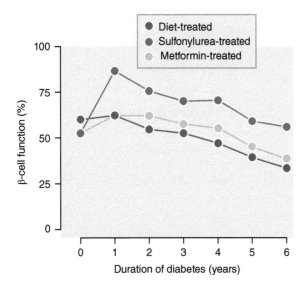

Figure 7.16 β-cell function as measured by the homeostasis model assessment (HOMA) method (calculated from the fasting blood glucose and insulin concentrations) in patients with type 2 diabetes from the UKPDS. β cell function is already reduced to 50% at diagnosis and declines thereafter, despite therapy. Data from Hales and Barker. Diabetologia 1992; 35: 595–601.

to intravenous glucose, and a delayed or blunted response to mixed meals (Figure 7.17). There are also alterations in pulsatile and daytime oscillations of insulin release. Some researchers have also found increases in the proportions of plasma proinsulin and split proinsulin peptides relative to insulin alone. Many of these abnormalities can be found in people with IGT and even in normoglycaemic first-degree relatives of people with type 2 diabetes, indicating that impaired β cell function is an early and possibly genetic defect in the natural history of type 2 diabetes (Figure 7.18).

The most common histological abnormality found in the islets of patients with type 2 diabetes is the presence of insoluble amyloid fibrils lying outside the cells. These are derived from islet amyloid polypeptide (IAPP, also sometimes known as amylin). This is co-secreted with insulin in a molar ratio of 1:10–50. Although IAPP is reported to

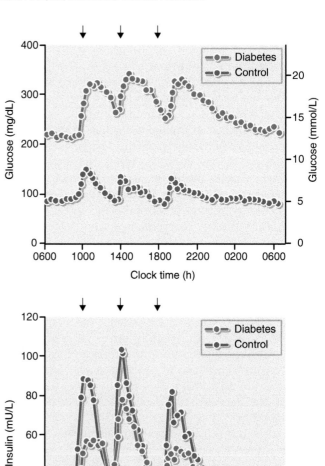

Figure 7.17 Plasma concentrations of glucose and insulin in subjects with type 2 diabetes and control subjects without diabetes in response to mixed meals. Data from UK Prospective Diabetes Study Group. Diabetes 1995; 44:1249–1258.

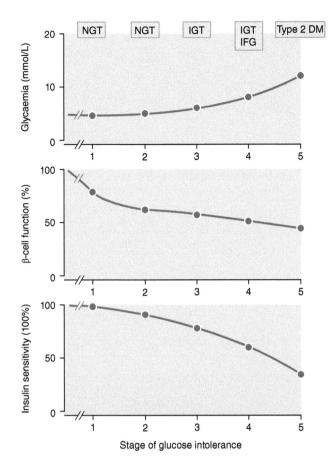

Figure 7.18 The stages of glucose tolerance and associated β cell function and insulin sensitivity, from normal glucose tolerance (NGT) through impaired glucose tolerance (IGT), with or without impaired fasting glucose (IFG), and finally type 2 diabetes mellitus (DM). Courtesy of Dr H Lewis Jones, Liverpool University, UK.

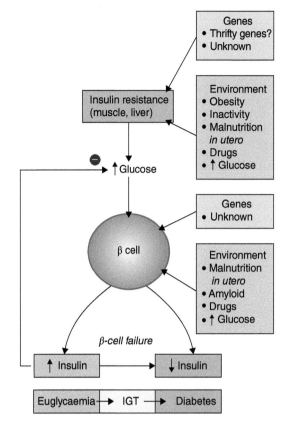

Figure 7.19 Pathogenesis of type 2 diabetes. Both genetic and environmental factors contribute to both insulin resistance and β cell failure.

impair insulin secretion and to be toxic to the β cell, its precise role in the pathogenesis of type 2 diabetes is uncertain because deposits can be found in up to 20% of elderly people who had completely normal glucose tolerance in life (See Figure 7.19).

β Cell mass is thought to be decreased by only 20–40% in type 2 diabetes and this clearly cannot explain the >80% reduction in insulin release that is observed. There must therefore be additional functional defects in the β cell, perhaps mediated by glucose or lipid toxicity. It is likely that IAPP contributes to this process.

Conclusion

Both insulin resistance and β cell dysfunction are early features of glucose intolerance and type 2 diabetes. There has been much debate as to whether one is the primary defect that precedes the other. In practice, the contribution of insulin resistance and β cell dysfunction varies considerably

between patients, as well as during the course of the disease. Usually, there is a decline in both insulin sensitivity and insulin secretion in patients who progress from IGT to type 2 diabetes and undoubtedly environmental and genetic factors contribute to this process (Figure 7.11).

LANDMARK CLINICAL TRIALS

Diabetes Prevention Program Research Group. Reduction in incidence of type 2 diabetes with lifestyle intervention or metformin. N Engl J Med 2002; 346: 393–403.

Lindstrom J, Ilanne-Parikka P, Peltonen M, et al. Sustained reduction in the incidence of type 2 diabetes by lifestyle intervention: follow-up of the Finnish Diabetes Prevention Study. Lancet 2006; 368: 1673–1679.

KEY WEBSITES

• Diabetes atlas for prevalence/incidence: www.eatlas.idf.org
• HOMA calculator: www.dtu.ox.ac.uk

FURTHER READING

Alberti KG, Zimmet P, Shaw J. Metabolic syndrome – a new worldwide definition. A consensus statement from the International Diabetes Federation. Diabetic Med 2006; 23: 469–480.

Expert Panel On Detection, Evaluation And Treatment Of High Blood Cholesterol In Adults (Adult Treatment Panel III). Executive summary of the 3rd report of the National Cholesterol Education Programme (NCEP). JAMA 2001; 285: 2486–2497.

International Diabetes Federation. *Diabetes Atlas*, 5th edn. Brussels: International Diabetes Federation, 2017.

Kahn R, Buse J, Ferrannini E, Stern M. The metabolic syndrome: time for a critical appraisal. Joint statement from the American Diabetes Association and the European Association for the Study of Diabetes. Diabetes Care 2005; 28: 2289–2304.

Li S, Shin HJ, Ding EL, van Dam RM. Adiponectin levels and risk of type 2 diabetes. A systematic review and meta-analysis. JAMA 2009; 302: 179–188.

Maleciki MT. Genetics of type 2 diabetes mellitus. Diabet Res Clin Pract 2005; 68(Suppl 1): S10–S21.

Nomi SL, Kansagara D, Bougatsos C, Fu R, US Preventive Services Task Force. Screening adults for type 2 diabetes: a review of the evidence for the US Preventive Services Task Force. Ann Intern Med 2008; 148: 855–868.

Sparso T, Grarup N, Andreasen C, et al. Combined analysis of 19 common validated type 2 diabetes susceptibility gene variants shows moderate discriminative value and no evidence of gene-gene interaction. Diabetologia 2009; 52: 1308–1314.

Waugh N, Scotland G, McName P, et al. Screening for type 2 diabetes: literature review and economic modelling. Health Technol Assess 2007; 11: 1–125.

Whincup PH, Kaye SJ, Owen CG, et al. Birth weight and risk of type 2 diabetes mellitus. JAMA 2008; 300: 2886–2897.

Other types of diabetes

KEY POINTS

- Other types of diabetes can be of genetic origin, secondary to pancreatic or other endocrine disease, or drug related.
- Of the monogenic causes, maturity-onset diabetes of the young is probably the best characterised, but abnormalities in mitochondrial DNA and other genes are also important.
- Secondary pancreatic dysfunction due to pancreatitis, calculous disease, cystic fibrosis and haemochromatosis can also occur.

- Excess of counter-regulatory hormones such as glucocorticoids, growth hormone, catecholamines, and glucagon are also associated with hyperglycaemia.
- Long term drug therapy with cardiovascular disease medications, steroids, antipsychotic therapies, immunosuppressive agents, and protease inhibitors is associated with diabetes development.

Introduction

Type 1 and type 2 account for over 95% of all cases of diabetes. The remaining 5% can be divided into four broad categories: (1) monogenic causes, (2) causes secondary to pancreatic disease, (3) associations with other endocrinopathies, and (4) associations with long-term drug therapies. This chapter will cover the main conditions and syndromes in each of these categories but as our understanding of the genetic basis of what is now termed type 2 diabetes grows, then more specific sub-types are likely to be characterised.

Monogenic Diabetes and association with other Inherited Conditions
Maturity-onset diabetes of the young

Maturity-onset diabetes of the young (MODY) owes its name to a time when diabetes was defined by age of onset. The nomenclature has stuck, however, and MODY defines usually non-insulin dependent diabetes occurring before the age of 25 years and with a striking autosomal dominant inheritance. β cell dysfunction is usually present but in contrast to type 2 diabetes, obesity and insulin resistance are unusual. Abnormalities in >10 different genes have been described,

but only four account for >95% of cases (Table 8.1). The previous numerical nomenclature (MODY 1,2,3 etc) has now been superseded by the specific gene abnormality in most reviews. MODY accounts for about 1–4% of paediatric patients with diabetes in most white Europid populations. The diagnostic criteria which should suggest a diagnosis of MODY are listed in Box 8.1.

A recent survey of newly presenting non-type 1 diabetes in children <16 years of age in the UK revealed 17 cases of MODY, giving an incidence of 0.13/100,000 patient-years. This is almost certainly an underestimate as changes in glucokinase (GCK)(MODY 2) are often undetected for many years because it is largely asymptomatic. An online calculator to estimate likelihood of MODY and help guide decision making for genetic testing is available at www.diabetesgenes.org.

The most common causes (accounting for >60% of cases) are mutations in nuclear transcription factors that control insulin production and secretion. They are listed in Table 8.1 together with associated clinical features. Defects in the glucose-sensing GCK enzyme account for around 32% of cases and cause insulin release at higher than usual circulating blood glucose levels, usually leading to a raised fasting blood glucose (5.5–9.0 mmol/L) with an HbA1c of 38–58 mmol/mol

---

Handbook of Diabetes, Fifth Edition. Rudy Bilous, Richard Donnelly, and Iskandar Idris.
© 2021 John Wiley & Sons Ltd. Published 2021 by John Wiley & Sons Ltd.

Table 8.1 Different genetic aetiologies of main types of MODY.

Genetic basis	Clinical and biochemical features	Frequency
HNF1A	Raised HDL cholesterol. Responds well to sulfonylureas	30–50%
Glucokinase	β cell response to high blood glucose impaired. Mild fasting hyperglycaemia, can present as gestational diabetes. Usually does not require treatment	30–50%
HNF4A	Low fasting triglycerides. Increased birthweight. Reduced apolipoproteins apo A11 and apo C111. Responds to sulfonylureas	5–10%
HNF1-B	Renal abnormalities (cysts, dysplasia). Uterine and genital abnormalities. Short stature and low birthweight. Pancreatic atrophy	2–5%
IPF-1	Pancreatic agenesis with homozygous mutations. Average age of onset 35y Renal abnormalities (cysts, dysplasia). Uterine and genital abnormalities. Short stature and low birthweight. Pancreatic atrophy	<1%
NEURO D1	None described but probably reduced β cell formation. Very rare	<1%
CEL	Pancreatic atrophy with exocrine deficiency. Very rare	<1%

HNF, hepatocyte nuclear factor; IPF, insulin promotor factor; NEURO D1, neurogenic differentiating factor 1; CEL, carboxyl-ester-lipase.

Box 8.1 Diagnostic criteria for MODY. (Adapted from ISPAD Guidelines Pediatric Diabetes 2014; 15: Suppl 20: 47-64)

- Early diagnosis of diabetes – usually before age 25 years in at least one family member and evidence of an autosomal inheritance pattern through 2 and preferably 3 generations with similar phenotype in affected individuals
- Absent autoimmune markers for type 1 diabetes
- Preserved β cell function for > 5 years post diagnosis (prolonged "honeymoon period" of insulin independence)
- Absent features for type 2 diabetes (obesity, acanthosis nigricans)

(5.5–7.5%). These patients are commonly detected either in pregnancy during screening for gestational diabetes, or as part of a health screening programme. GCK deficiency needs no treatment, is largely benign and not associated with diabetes complications.

HNF1A and 4A gene mutations lead to progressive loss of β cell function and, as a result, patients have more severe hyperglycaemia and are prone to develop microvascular complications. Initial treatment with sulfonylureas can be effective but >25% do not respond and most eventually require insulin therapy. Mutations in HNF1B cause generalised cystic abnormalities and often present initially with renal tract problems.

Neonatal diabetes

Autoimmune mediated type 1 diabetes is almost never diagnosed <6 months of age so any neonate presenting with hyperglycaemia without islet cell antibodies should undergo genetic testing. Monogenic neonatal diabetes is rare affecting 1 in 100,000 births. Around 50% have permanent hyperglycaemia (PNDM) caused by a mutation in the gene coding the

Kir 6.2 and SUR1 sub-units of the KATP channel on the β cell. This defect results in an inability to release insulin and consequent ketoacidosis, usually occurring before 6 months of age. Sulfonylurea therapy closes this channel by an ATP-independent route and is effective in over 90% of cases of PNDM.

Transient neonatal diabetes (TNDM) is characterised by severe intra-uterine growth restriction, and a mutation in chromosome 6q24 accounts for most cases. Hyperglycaemia resolves after a median of 12 weeks of age, but recurs in puberty in about 60%. Not all of those who relapse respond to sulfonylurea treatment.

Mitochrondrial diabetes

Mitochrondrial DNA is inherited maternally. A heteroplasmic mutation at position 3243 results in type 2 diabetes and sensorineural deafness. Around 20% of cases present acutely and some develop ketoacidosis. Presentation usually occurs before middle age. Other features include myopathy, pigmented retinopathy, cardiomyopathy and neurological abnormalities. Its most severe form comprises the MELAS syndrome (Myopathy, Encephalopathy, Lactic Acidosis and Stroke-like episodes). Prevalence studies suggest that Mt 3243 accounts for 1–2% of Japanese and 0.2–0.5% of European type 2 diabetes. Many patients can be treated with oral agents initially, but metformin is not recommended because of its links to lactic acidosis.

Monogenic insulin resistance syndromes

There are 3 main categories: primary insulin signalling defects; insulin resistance secondary to adipose tissue problems (lipodystrophies); and insulin resistance as part of a complex syndrome.

Insulin signalling defects

Genetic abnormalities in the insulin receptor can give rise to rare but well-described syndromes characterised by severe insulin resistance. Autosomal recessively inherited mutations

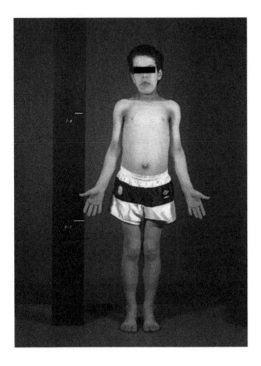

Figure 8.1 Rabson–Mendenhall syndrome in a 12-year-old boy, showing growth retardation, prominent acanthosis nigricans affecting the axillae, neck and antecubital fossae, and typical facies.

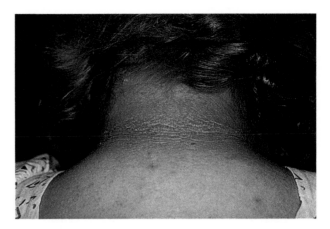

Figure 8.2 Acanthosis nigricans on the nape of the neck of a 26-year-old woman with the type A insulin resistance syndrome.

of the gene encoding the α subunit of the insulin receptor can lead to Donohue syndrome (leprechaunism) or the slightly less severe Rabson–Mendenhall syndrome (Figure 8.1). Affected children present with failure to thrive and other syndromic features and have a very poor prognosis.

Autosomal dominant insulin resistance presents during puberty with oligomenorrhoea, hyperandrogenism, and acanthosis nigricans, features shared with polycystic ovary syndrome (Figure 8.2). This has been termed type A insulin resistance and is more common in females, although is almost certainly underdiagnosed in males. In 25% of cases there is a mutation of the tyrosine kinase domain of the β subunit of the insulin receptor.

Rare mutations of the human preproinsulin gene can lead to abnormal levels of insulin precursors. Such patients are heterozygous (homozygosity would be incompatible with life), and develop diabetes in later life in response to other factors such as obesity.

Insulin resistance secondary to adipose tissue problems
Lipodystrophies
These are rare inherited conditions characterised by a partial or total absence of adipose tissue and have an associated insulin resistance. In many cases, the genetic basis has been discovered, leading to new insights into the causes of insulin resistance. 50% of patients with partial lipodystrophy

(sometimes called the Kobberling–Dunnigan syndrome) have an autosomally dominant inherited abnormality in the LMNA (encoding lamin A/C which is a constituent of nuclear lamina) or PPAR γ gene. These changes result in defective adipocyte differentiation and/or cell death. Apart from type 2 diabetes, some of these patients also have problems with severe hypertriglyceridaemia, hepatic steatosis and pancreatitis.

Generalised lipoatrophy usually presents in early childhood and several different genetic causes have been described. Severe insulin resistance, diabetes and hyperlipidaemia are the norm.

Insulin resistance as part of complex syndromes
These are rare inherited conditions of which the Alstrom and Bardet-Biedl syndromes are best characterised with defects in the centrosomal protein leading to centripetal obesity.

Management of monogenic insulin resistance syndromes
For those with insulin receptor abnormalities, high dose insulin is the only therapy and is often ineffective at achieving satisfactory glycemic control. U500 insulin (sometimes given by continuous subcutaneous infusion) is often necessary.

For those with adipose tissue abnormalities then calorie restriction and weight loss to decrease insulin resistance is important but often difficult to achieve. Insulin sensitising agents such as metformin and thiazolidinediones can be effective but most will also require high doses of U500 insulin. Subcutaneous leptin is effective for those with generalised lipodystrophies and for some with partial fat cell depletion.

Other monogenic causes
Wolfram syndrome
This rare autosomal recessive disorder was first described in 1938 and has a mean age of onset of 6 years. The most common features are Diabetes Insipidus, type 1 Diabetes Mellitus,

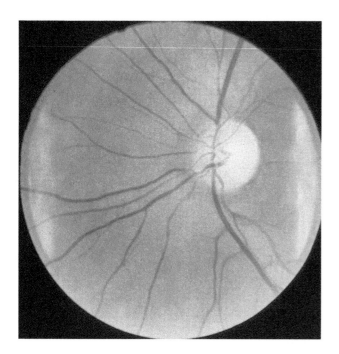

Figure 8.3 Optic atrophy (note white optic disc) in a patient with Wolfram's syndrome.

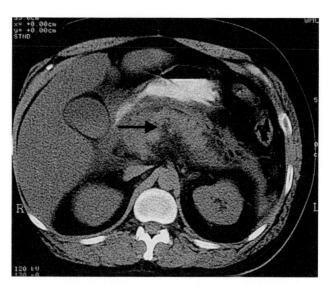

Figure 8.4 Acute pancreatitis. CT scan of the abdomen, showing marked oedema and swelling of the gland (arrow). Subsequently, a pancreatic pseudocyst developed.

Optic Atrophy (Figure 8.3) and Deafness (DIDMOAD). There are many other features, notably psychiatric illness. A gene defect on chromosome 4 coding for a transmembrane protein (wolframmin) has been described, causing mitochondrial dysfunction leading to abnormal function of the endoplasmic reticulum. Diabetes usually occurs in the second decade and prevalence has been estimated as between 1 in 100,000 – 800,000 of the population.

Myotonic dystrophy

This autosomal dominant disorder is the most common adult form of muscular dystrophy (prevalence 1 in 8000 population) and is characterised by abnormal insulin secretion, insulin resistance and type 2 diabetes. The abnormal mutation is in the protein kinase gene on chromosome 19 and this may affect insulin receptor RNA and protein expression or perhaps calcium-dependent insulin release from the β cells.

Friedreich's ataxia

This autosomal recessively inherited condition presents before age 25 and is associated with overt diabetes in 10% and impaired glucose tolerance in 20% of cases.

Klinefelter's syndrome

Occurs in 1–2/100 male births and affected individuals have an additional X chromosome. Glucose intolerance is reported in up to 40%.

Genetic associations with autoimmune endocrinopathies

Both Turner's (partial or whole deletion of an X chromosome) and Down syndrome (trisomy21) are associated with an increased incidence of autoimmune endocrinopathies including type 1 diabetes.

Type B autoimmune insulin resistance is very rare and the result of circulating antibodies to the insulin receptor. There is a link with other autoimmune diseases, and shares with these a female preponderance. Patients may have fluctuating hyper- and hypoglycaemia and are very difficult to treat.

Pancreatic disease

Many pancreatic diseases can cause diabetes, but in total they account for <1% of all cases. Acute pancreatitis (commonly associated with alcoholism or gallstones) (Figure 8.4) usually results in transient hyperglycaemia, but permanent diabetes occurs in up to 15% of patients.

Chronic pancreatitis, which is commonly caused by alcoholism in Western countries, leads to IGT or diabetes in 40–50% of cases. Intraductal protein plugs subsequently calcify as characteristic calcite stones, with cyst formation, inflammation, and fibrosis (Figure 8.5a). One-third require insulin, but ketoacidosis is rare. Many patients are extremely insulin sensitive, requiring small doses to prevent ketosis and weight loss; higher doses are often associated with hypoglycaemia.

Tropical calcific pancreatitis (Figure 8.5b) is confined to India and developing nations, and results in diabetes in 90% of cases. Even in these countries, it accounts for only 1% of diabetes. It usually presents in the 3rd and 4th decade of life

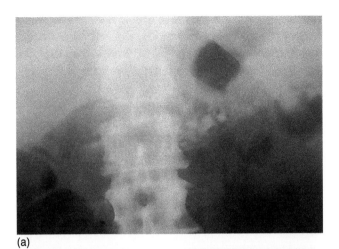

(a)

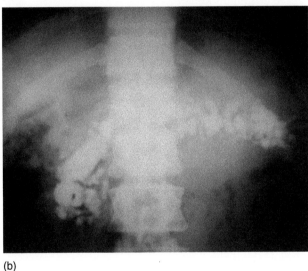

(b)

Figure 8.5 Pancreatic calculi, showing characteristic patterns in alcoholic chronic pancreatitis (a), and fibrocalculous pancreatic diabetes (b).

and rarely leads to ketoacidosis. It is often associated with malnutrition, but its aetiology is not understood, and most patients require insulin.

Cystic fibrosis (CF)

This is a common autosomal recessive condition which results in abnormal chloride and water transport across epithelial membranes. Over 1500 mutations in the cystic fibrosis transmembrane conductance regulator gene have been described and they result in differing severities of the condition. Pancreatic and pulmonary disease predominate, and better treatment has resulted in much improved survival. Diabetes results from β cell failure secondary to exocrine pancreatic damage. A UK survey of 8029 patients on the cystic fibrosis register studied from 1996 to 2005 revealed an annual incidence of diabetes of 3.5%, but this was 1–2%

in the first decade of life, and 6–7% in the fourth. At least 20% of adolescents, and 40–50 % of adults with CF have glucose intolerance of some degree, and it is estimated that 70–90% of those surviving to age 40 will have overt diabetes. Female sex, more severe lung dysfunction, liver disease, exocrine pancreatic insufficiency, steroid use, and severity of gene expression were all positively related to diabetes development. Annual screening using an oral glucose tolerance test is recommended from age 12 in the UK and age 10 in the USA, HbA1c does not appear to be uniformly sensitive as a screening tool in CF patients. Cardiovascular disease rates do not seem to be increased, but microvascular complications can occur and need screening and surveillance as for people with type 1 diabetes. The majority of patients require insulin treatment, and many are very sensitive and require small doses. Increasing numbers of women with CF are having babies and their care during pregnancy is the same as for women with type 1 diabetes.

Haemochromatosis

This is an autosomal recessive inborn error of metabolism, usually caused by a mutation in the haemochromatosis gene (HFE) on chromosome 6. Around 1 in 2-300 of white northern European descent are homozygous for the HFE mutation. The HFE protein is expressed on duodenal enterocytes and modulates iron uptake. Haemochromatosis is associated with increased iron absorption and tissue deposition, notably in the liver, pancreatic islets, skin, and pituitary gland and hypothalamus. The classic clinical triad is one of hepatic cirrhosis, glucose intolerance (with insulin-requiring diabetes in 25%), and skin hyperpigmentation, which has led to the term 'bronzed diabetes'. Presentation is usually in the 4th - 6th decades. Serum iron and ferritin concentrations are raised. Secondary haemochromatosis may occur in patients who undergo frequent blood transfusions, for example those with β-thalassaemia or other haemoglobinopathies.

Pancreatic cancer

Rarely, diabetes can be a presenting feature of pancreatic cancer. Usually, however, there are other features such as profound weight loss and back pain. The prognosis is very poor; insulin treatment is usual.

Diabetes complicating other endocrine diseases

Several endocrine conditions are associated with diabetes mellitus. Cushing's syndrome is the result of glucocorticoid excess from any cause, including steroid drug induced, pituitary adenomas, adrenal tumours, and ectopic ACTH production. Glucocorticoid excess results in central obesity which causes insulin resistance. This in turn stimulates hepatic gluconeogenesis, peripheral adipose tissue lipolysis, and fatty acid release. All of these inhibit peripheral glucose uptake and the net result is hyperglycaemia. Most patients have some degree of glucose intolerance, with overt diabetes in 10–20% of cases.

Acromegaly is a condition of growth hormone excess arising from an anterior pituitary tumour. This causes glucose intolerance by inducing insulin resistance. Overt diabetes and impaired glucose tolerance each affect around one-third of patients with acromegaly. Glucose tolerance returns to normal with reduction of circulating growth hormone levels.

Phaeochromocytomas are tumours that arise from the chromaffin cells of the sympathetic nervous system, usually in the adrenal medulla but they can occur anywhere along the sympathetic nervous chain. They secrete excess catecholamines, and typically the clinical presentation is that of high blood pressure, headache, tachycardia, and sweating, sometimes occurring in paroxysms. Up to 75% have evidence of glucose intolerance which occasionally needs treatment with insulin. Resolution is usual with removal of the tumour.

Glucagonomas are rare tumours of the islet α cells (Figure 8.6). They are slowly growing but often malignant. The most striking clinical features are weight loss and a characteristic rash, termed 'necrolytic migratory erythema' affecting skin flexures and the perineum. There is also a tendency to thromboembolism and neuropsychiatric disorders.

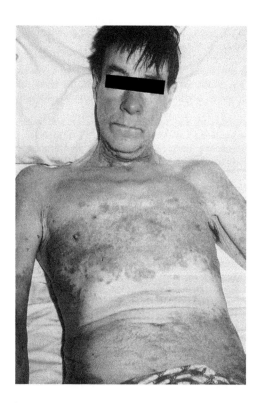

Figure 8.6 A patient with glucagonoma, showing characteristic necrolytic migratory erythema. Non-ketotic diabetes was controlled with low doses of insulin.

Diabetes is common and the result of enhanced gluconeogenesis and glycogenolysis induced by high circulating glucagon levels. It usually resolves with removal of the tumour.

Medication associated diabetes

Many therapeutic agents can adversely affect glucose tolerance. Sometimes it is uncertain whether the medication itself caused the hyperglycaemia or exposed a pre-existing problem when it was prescribed. Moreover, people with cardiovascular disease have an increased incidence of diabetes which may have developed with or without the medication. Post transplant diabetes (PTDM – previously termed new onset diabetes after transplantation – NODAT) is increasingly recognised as an entity in its own right and is probably part caused by immunosuppressive therapy.

Cardiovascular medications

Thiazide diuretics inhibit insulin release from the β cell, and the effect is dose dependent. Non-selective β blockers have a similar effect on the β cell, but by a different mechanism. The magnitude of the diabetogenic effect has led, in part, to their no longer being recommended in guidelines as first line therapy for hypertension. Statins are associated with an excess risk of < 10% for diabetes resulting in around 2 cases/100 person years of use. However, this problem is significantly outweighed by the 25% risk reduction in cardiovascular event rate associated with their use.

Steroids

Long term steroid use, particularly in supra physiological doses (>7.5 mg/d prednisolone equivalent) is associated with a high risk of diabetes and screening for glucose intolerance should be part of long-term surveillance. The lowest possible dose should be used for maintenance.

Antipsychotic medications

Diabetes is much more common in people with schizophrenia, particularly in those from black or ethnic minorities. There is a 10-fold increased relative risk for diabetes in 18–34 year olds with a severe mental illness (Chapter 28). It is thought that this is due, in part, to long term antipsychotic therapy, and the newer agents such as olanzapine, clozapine, and risperidone may be more of a problem in this regard. The precise mechanism is unclear but may be related to the associated weight gain with these agents, or due to changes in neurotransmitters and their action on the hypothalamus.

Immunosuppressive agents and post-transplant diabetes (PTDM)

Steroids have already been mentioned and their long-term use post-transplant is being discouraged. The calcineurin inhibitors, tacrolimus and cyclosporin A, affect β cell growth and function and have high rates of associated diabetes. Sirolimus (an mTOR inhibitor) is also associated with PTDM, especially when used in combination with tacrolimus. Sirolimus increases insulin resistance and impairs β cell response to hyperglycaemia. Reported rates of PTDM are 10–74% in kidney, 11–38% in heart, and 7–30% in liver transplant recipients. There is no universal agreement on a screening strategy for PTDM, although the diagnostic criteria are the same as for non-transplant-associated diabetes. The validity of an HbA1c is uncertain because of altered red blood cell production and turnover in transplant recipients. PTDM is associated with a two- or threefold increase in fatal and non-fatal cardiovascular events in kidney transplant recipients, and also seems to be linked to poorer overall transplant survival. Current management is based upon type 2 guidelines, but some recommend a more rigorous approach with early insulin therapy. Most patients with PTDM will become insulin requiring.

Protease inhibitors

Patients taking highly active antiretroviral therapy (HAART) are more likely to develop diabetes, probably because of a direct effect of the agents on the β cell as well as increasing insulin resistance. There is a >threefold increased incidence of diabetes in men receiving HAART and many will require insulin treatment.

CASE HISTORY

A 22-year-old woman was referred to the medical obstetrics clinic for booking at 6 weeks gestation of her first pregnancy. She had had diabetes for 10 years, initially on sulfonylureas for 6 months but now on insulin. She had never been ketotic. Her control was fair (HbA1c 64 mmol/mol (8.2%)). She had a strong family history of diabetes; her mother had type 2 diabetes and was now on insulin and currently an inpatient, having required a below-knee amputation for neuroischaemia and gangrene. Her brother was in the army and had recently been diagnosed with type 2 diabetes at the age of 19 years. Another brother aged 24 years had had diet-controlled diabetes for 6 years.

DNA testing revealed a mutation in the HNF1A gene, confirming a diagnosis of MODY. During pregnancy her glycaemic control improved dramatically but unfortunately she developed rapidly progressive retinopathy requiring laser photocoagulation. Postpartum she was tried again on sulfonylureas but her glycaemia worsened and she was recommenced on insulin. Three years later she had established nephropathy and has required vitreoretinal surgery.

Comment: This case shows many of the typical features of MODY as outlined in Box 8.1. Not all can be managed on oral agents and many are prone to severe complications. This woman and her family have received counselling from the UK Regional MODY Service.

KEY WEBSITES

- Diagnostic criteria and details of how to request genetic tests for MODY in the UK: http://projects.exeter.ac.uk/diabetesgenes/mody/
- Information on monogeneic form of diabetes: http://diabetes.niddk.nih.gov/dm/pubs/mody/
- Diagnostic probability calculator for MODY www.diabetesgenes.org
- Cystic Fibrosis Trust www.cysticfibrosis.org.uk

FURTHER READING

Adler AI, Shine BSF, Chamnan P, Haworth CS, Bilton D. Genetic determinance and epidemiology of cystic fibrosis-related diabetes: results from a British cohort of children and adults. Diabetes Care 2008; 31: 1789–1794.

American Diabetes Association. Classification and diagnosis of diabetes. Diabetes Care 2020; 43(Suppl 1): S14 – 31. doi.org/10.2337/dc20-S002

Gardner DSL & Tai ES. Clinical treatment and features of maturity onset diabetes of the young (MODY). Diabetes, Metabolic Syndrome and Obesity: Targets and Therapy 2012; 5: 101–8. http://dx.doi.org/10.2147/DMSO.S23353

Garg A. Acquired and inherited lipodystrophies. N Engl J Med 2004; 350: 1220–1234.

McCarthy MI, Hattersley AT. Learning from molecular genetics. Diabetes 2008; 57: 2889–2898.

Moran A, Brunzell C, Cohen RC et al. Clinical care guidelines for cystic fibrosis-related diabetes, Diabetes Care 2010; 33: 2697–2709. doi 10.2337/dc10-1768

Rubio-Cazezas O, Hattersley AT, Njolstad PR, Mlynarski W, Ellard S, White W, Chi DV, Craig ME. The diagnosis and management of monogenic diabetes in children and adolescents. Pediatr Diabetes 2014; 15 Suppl 20: 47 – 64 doi 10.1111/pedi.12192

Semple RK, Savage DB, Cochran EK, Gorden P, O'Rahilly S. Genetic syndromes of severe insulin resistance. Endocrine Reviews 2011; 32: 498–514. doi.org/10.1210/er.2010-0020

Shivaswamy V, Boerner B, Larsen J. Post-transplant diabetes mellitus: causes treatment and impact on outcomes. Endocrine Reviews 2016; 37: 37–61 doi 10.1210/er2015-1084

The UK Cystic Fibrosis Trust Diabetes Working Group. The management of cystic fibrosis related diabetes mellitus. 2004; https://www.cysticfibrosis.org.uk

Part

2

Metabolic control and complications

Chapter
9

Diabetes control and its measurement

KEY POINTS

- Assessment of diabetic control is based upon estimates of glycaemia. Capillary blood glucose monitoring is relatively convenient and easy to perform and is a critical adjunct to modern insulin treatment regimens. Its role in diet or tablet-controlled type 2 diabetes is less certain.
- Glycated haemoglobin concentrations estimate average blood glucose over the preceding 8–12 weeks. Its measurement is now subject to international standardisation and the units have changed in the UK from percent to mmol/mol. Many national bodies are recommending the use of an HbA1c-derived estimated average blood glucose.
- Continuous glucose monitoring systems are now widely available and their role in management is growing. The development of an international consensus for target ranges and interpretation and utilisation of the results is welcome. There is increasing use of these technologies in combination with insulin delivery systems.

Introduction

'Diabetic control' defines the extent to which the metabolism of the person with diabetes differs from that in the person without diabetes. Measurement usually focuses on blood glucose: 'good' control implies maintenance of near-normal blood glucose concentrations throughout the day. However, many other metabolites are disordered in diabetes and some, such as ketone bodies, are now more easily measurable and clinically useful, particularly during acute illness or periods of poor blood glucose control.

In addition to blood and urine glucose concentrations, there are indicators of longer-term glycaemic control over the preceding weeks using glycated haemoglobin (HbA1c or fructosamine concentrations (Table 9.1). Over the last decade, the development of continuous monitoring of subcutaneous interstitial glucose concentrations has enabled much finer tuning of treatment. The monitoring of glucose concentrations in 'real time' and linkage to insulin delivery devices has led to the development of 'closed loop' systems that vary insulin delivery according to the glucose reading (Chapter 10). A clear understanding of the relationship between interstitial and circulating blood glucose concentrations is crucial, however.

Capillary blood glucose monitoring

Single blood glucose measurements are of little use as an assessment of overall control in type 1 diabetes because of unpredictable variations throughout the day and from day to day, although they are important in order to detect and confirm hypoglycaemia. In order to assess control more meaningfully, serial, timed blood glucose samples are usually needed. In diet- or stable tablet-controlled type 2 diabetes, although blood glucose levels are elevated, they tend not to vary widely throughout the day. In these patients a fasting or random blood glucose relates reasonably well to mean blood glucose concentration and to glycated haemoglobin and is probably adequate (Table 9.1).

Self-monitoring of capillary blood glucose by patients at home using special enzyme-impregnated reagent strips and a meter is now an integral part of modern diabetes management, especially for those who are on insulin therapy. Strips usually contain a combination of glucose oxidase and peroxidase. Colorimetric tests have been superseded by newer electrochemically based strips which generate a current rather than a colour change. Meters vary in their need for standardisation, their accuracy, their memory, and their ability to generate blood glucose profiles when connected to

Handbook of Diabetes, Fifth Edition. Rudy Bilous, Richard Donnelly, and Iskandar Idris.
© 2021 John Wiley & Sons Ltd. Published 2021 by John Wiley & Sons Ltd.

Table 9.1 Available measures of glycaemic control and their main clinical uses.

Measure of control	Clinical use
Urine glucose	In people with stable control and who are unable/unwilling to perform blood tests
Capillary blood glucose – fasting	Correlates with HbA1c particularly in T2DM
	Estimate of insulin deficiency in T2DM
Capillary blood glucose – post meal	Correlates with CV risk
	Correlates with foetal growth in pregnant women
	Estimate of insulin resistance in T2DM
Continuous glucose monitoring	Provides real time estimates of blood glucose
	Enables closer matching of therapy to control by establishing pattern of glycaemia throughout the day enabling more precise adjustments of insulin
	Early warning of hypoglycaemia especially at night
Estimated average glucose (from HbA1c)	More accessible information for patients/carers than HbA1c alone
Glycated haemoglobin (HbA1c)	Estimate of glycaemic control over preceding 3 months
Glycated serum proteins (albumin, fructosamine)	Estimate of glycaemic control over preceding 2 weeks
Urine/blood ketones	Early warning/diagnosis of developing DKA
	Measure of response of DKA to treatment

DKA = Diabetic Ketoacidosis; T2DM = Type 2 Diabetes.

a computer or wirelessly with a smart phone or the cloud. Some contain algorithms that can give advice on insulin dosage prior to a meal, depending on its carbohydrate content. Some meters require more blood than others, but most now use a fraction of a microlitre and give results within seconds. Meters are often made freely available by the manufacturers in the UK, and most of the testing strips are available on prescription.

It is worth remembering that all meters tend to be less accurate at lower blood glucose values and usually have an upper limit of detection following which they read 'high'. They also vary in accuracy, and readings may differ from plasma glucose by as much as 15–20%.

There are many devices which contain a spring-loaded lancet in order to obtain a capillary blood sample. This is usually obtained from the fingers; the sides of the fingertip are less sensitive than the pulp, and the ring and little fingers are less sensitive than the index and middle fingers. A major reason for poor compliance and low frequency of testing is finger discomfort. In recent years strips require less blood and many lancet devices have a depth adjustment. Some offer the option of testing at alternative sites to the fingers such as the forearm, abdomen, calf, and thigh. However, there can be discrepancies in values measured at the finger and these sites, particularly during times of rapid change in blood glucose such as after meals or exercise.

Frequency of testing

Initial trials of home blood glucose monitoring were nothing short of revelatory for patients previously used to urine tests. Latterly, as part of clinical trials (e.g. Diabetes Control and Complications Trial (DCCT) in type 1 and UK Prospective Diabetes Study (UKPDS) in type 2) and structured educational programmes (e.g. Diet Adjustment For Normal Eating (DAFNE) for type 1 diabetes and Diabetes Education Self-Management for Ongoing and Newly Diagnosed (DESMOND) type 2 diabetes in the UK), they have been shown to help patients achieve sustained long-term improvements in glycaemic control. However, systematic reviews have failed to confirm that home blood glucose monitoring alone results in significant glycaemic improvement. NICE guidance uses it as an essential component of care management in type 1 diabetes, with a frequency dependent upon the clinical circumstances (at least 4 times a day, 5 for Children and Adolescents, 7 in pregnancy), whereas for type 2 diabetes home blood glucose monitoring should be available for the indications listed in Box 9.1 Both NICE type 1 and type 2 guidelines suggest that knowledge and skills of interpretation, and action taken based upon home blood glucose monitoring results should be assessed at least annually. The American Diabetes Association guidelines suggest 6–10 tests per day in people with type 1 diabetes on multiple daily injections or pump therapy, and for pregnant women. Otherwise their advice is concordant with that from NICE.

Urine glucose monitoring

Glycosuria occurs when blood glucose levels exceed the renal threshold for glucose (usually 10 mmol/L–180 mg/dL). However, urine glucose testing is unreliable in the assessment of blood glucose control because the renal threshold varies between and within patients (Box 9.2). Fluid intake can affect urine glucose concentrations and importantly, the result does not reflect blood glucose at the time of the test but over the duration that the urine has accumulated in the

---

Box 9.1

Indications for capillary blood glucose monitoring in type 2 diabetes
- Insulin therapy.
- On oral therapy with a risk of hypoglycaemia (e.g. sulfonylureas, glinides).
- Assessment of response of glycaemia to changes in management or lifestyle.
- Monitoring of glycaemia during intercurrent illness.
- Avoidance of hypoglycaemia during driving, employment or physical activity.
- Planning or established pregnancy.

bladder. A negative urine test cannot distinguish between hypoglycaemia, normoglycaemia, and modest hyperglycaemia. For these reasons, urine testing is rarely performed as part of routine diabetes care, except in those who are unable or unwilling to perform blood glucose monitoring, and in these cases it should be supplemented with periodic HbA1c testing. It is no longer mentioned in current guidelines.

Glycated haemoglobin

Haemoglobin A comprises over 90% of most adult haemoglobin and is variably glycated by the non-enzymatic attachment of circulating sugars, mostly glucose. HbA1c comprises the major glycated component and historically has been shown in numerous studies to correlate with average blood glucose (Figure 9.1).

As the average life span of the red cell is 90–120 days, the percentage glycated haemoglobin is a reflection of glycaemic control over the 8–12 weeks preceding the test. However, the level of glycation is not linear with time – 50% of the value reflects the 30 days prior to the test, and only 10% the initial 30 days of red cell life.

This is important to remember because if the life span of a patient's red cell is less than 90 days (e.g. in haemolytic anaemias or pregnancy) then theoretically the HbA1c could be only 50% of the expected value. Although high-pressure liquid chromatography (HPLC) methodology and the new International Federation for Clinical Chemistry and Laboratory Medicine (IFCC) standard have largely eliminated the confounding problems of aberrant haemoglobins, these can still cause falsely high values in some populations where they exist in high prevalence.

The more common causes of misleading HbA1c values are shown in Box 9.3. Many of these have been eliminated by refinements of modern assays but it is important to check with the local providing laboratory. Carbamylation due to uraemia increases HbA1c by 0.7 mmol/mol (0.063%) for every 1 mmol/L increase in plasma urea concentration so is of relatively minor consequence.

Of more importance is the observation that there is considerable inter-individual variation in the correlation between average blood glucose and HbA1c. Analysis of the DCCT

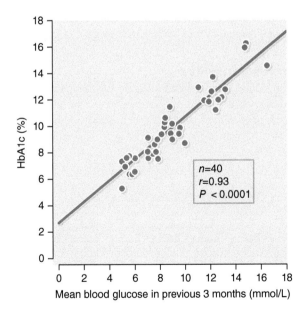

Figure 9.1 Correlation in patients with type 1 diabetes between blood glucose concentration over the preceding 3 months and glycated haemoglobin (HbA1c) level. Source: Adapted from Paisey et al. Diabetologia 1980; 19: 31–34.

In figure: HbA1c (%) on y-axis (0–18); Mean blood glucose in previous 3 months (mmol/L) on x-axis (0–18). $n=40$, $r=0.93$, $P<0.0001$

cohort showed that for a mean blood glucose of 10 mmol/L based upon 7-point home blood glucose monitoring profiles over 24 hours, the HbA1c can range from 42–86 mmol/mol (6% to 10%). A concept of rapid and slow glycators has been proposed to explain this phenomenon, but it is more likely to reflect variable red blood cell membrane transport of glucose. Research has shown a range of approximately 0.7–1.0 for this property between individuals and could explain HbA1c differences of 16–25 mmol/mol (1.5–2.3%) for any given mean blood glucose value. These observations question whether a universal target HbA1c should be set in guidelines, and perhaps explains some of the often observed discrepancy between recorded home blood glucose tests and glycated haemoglobin concentrations.

The recommended frequency of testing of HbA1c is twice per year in stable patients and 4–6 times for those with type 1 diabetes or those undergoing treatment changes.

IFCC standard

Most HbA1c assays have been standardised to that used in the DCCT as part of work carried out by the National Glycohaemoglobin Standardisation Programme (NGSP) in the USA. However, Sweden and Japan have each had their own standard. The IFCC has developed a new reference method that specifically measures only one molecular species of HbA1c and relates this to total haemoglobin. This method is expensive and laborious and can only be used to standardise local assays. It reports in units of mmol/mol and the absolute values are quite different from the current familiar percentage (Table 9.2). However, it has been decided internationally that there should be a gradual switch to the IFCC standard with its new units. An international consensus agreed the following, although the USA and many other countries continue to report in percent units.

- HbA1c results would be standardised worldwide to the new IFCC standard.
- The IFCC method is currently the only valid anchor that permits such standardisation.

- HbA1c would be reported in both new and old units initially (no longer in the UK) sometimes together with estimated average glucose (eAG see below).
- Glycaemic goals should be expressed in IFCC units, NGSP percent and eAG mmol/L or mg/dL.

Estimated average glucose (eAG)

Many patients have difficulty relating HbA1c to their results of home blood glucose monitoring, sometimes confusing the numerical value with blood glucose concentration (although this is less of a problem at least in the UK with the new IFCC standard using mmol/mol–Table 9.2). Because of this, glycated haemoglobin levels are often reported together with an estimated average blood glucose (eAG) derived from it. The initial equations were based upon the DCCT cohort, but the more recently used conversion has come from the A1c-Derived Average Glucose (ADAG) Trial (Table 9.3) utilising frequent capillary blood glucose measurements and continuous subcutaneous glucose monitoring. However, the strongly positive correlation ($r = 0.92$) has not been reproduced in children and there may also be differences in African Americans. Moreover, eAG is a population-based estimate, the wide confidence intervals demonstrate the wide inter-individual variability (Table 9.3). There are differing views on the utility of eAG and there are as yet no data to suggest it has clinical benefit over and above HbA1c. It is also important to remember that eAG relates to plasma, not whole blood, so there will inevitably be some discrepancy with meter-based home blood glucose measurements. However, eAG provides a more accessible estimate of control for patients and may create the basis for more meaningful discussions about management, although it has to some extent been superseded by continuous glucose monitoring (see below).

Glucose variability

Attempts have been made to obtain an estimate of blood glucose variability based upon the ranges or standard deviations of the mean of profiles, or continuous subcutaneous

Table 9.2 Guide to values of HbA1c (IFCC) and DCCT (NGSP) standardised assay.

DCCT (%)	IFCC method (mmol/mol)
4.0	20
5.0	31
6.0	42
6.5	48
7.0	53
7.5	58
8.0	64
9.0	75
10.0	86

Conversion equation IFCC HbA1c (mmol/mol) = [DCCT HbA1c (%) – 2.15] × 10.929.

Table 9.3 Estimated average blood glucose concentration derived from HbA1c reported by the ADAG Trial. Overall correlation was 0.92 but note wide 95% CI particularly at higher blood glucose values.

HbA1c mmol/mol (%)	Mean blood glucose mmol/L (95% CI)	Mean blood glucose mg/dl (95% CI)
42 (6.0)	7.0 (5.6,8.4)	126 (100,152)
53 (7.0)	8.6 (6.3,10.3)	154 (123,185)
64 (8.0)	10.2 (8.2,12.1)	183 (127,217)
75 (9.0)	11.8 (9.4,13.8)	212 (170,219)
86 (10.0)	13.4 (10.7,15.7)	240 (193,282)
97 (11.0)	14.9 (12.0,17.5)	269 (217,314)
108 (12.0)	16.5 (13.3,19.3)	298 (240,347)

monitoring. So far, these analyses using the DCCT and other data sets have not been shown to provide advantages over HbA1c alone, and have largely been superseded by continuous glucose monitoring technologies.

Fructosamine

Serum fructosamine is a measure of glycated serum protein, mostly albumin, and is an indicator of glycaemic control over the preceding 2–3 weeks (the lifetime of albumin). Colorimetric assays for fructosamine, which are now adapted for automated analysers, give a normal reference range of 205–285 μmol/L. Fructosamine generally correlates well with HbA1c, except when control has changed recently.

It has potential advantages over HbA1c, particularly in situations such as haemoglobinopathies or pregnancy when the glycated haemoglobin is hard to interpret. However, standardisation is difficult: uraemia, lipaemia, hyperbilirubinaemia and vitamin C use can affect the assay, and there may be an effect of high or low circulating blood proteins.

Urine and blood ketone measurements

Ketones can be measured in urine using a colorimetric test or in capillary blood using an electrochemical sensor similar to those now used for glucose (Figure 9.2).

Acetoacetate and acetone are detected by the urine test (Figure 9.3), β hydroxybutyrate by the blood strips. As the ratio of β hydroxybutyrate to acetoacetate is around 6:1 in human ketoacidosis, the blood test offers a more appropriate way to

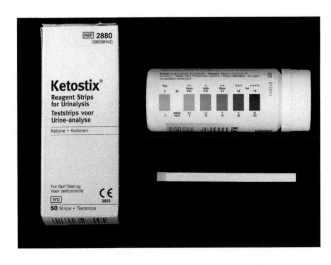

Figure 9.3 Urine ketone testing strips. NOTE these detect urinary acetoacetate whereas the blood ketone meter detects b hydroxy butyrate.

monitor diabetes control during intercurrent illness; or in situations that may predispose to ketoacidosis, such as pregnancy; or where it can occur relatively quickly, such as in patients using continuous subcutaneous insulin infusion pump therapy. As yet there is little evidence on which to form a consensus but blood ketone testing should be available in acute medical and obstetric assessment units, as well as for inpatients with diabetes with intercurrent illnesses and as a means of monitoring response to treatment for diabetic ketoacidosis. NICE guidance recommends universal provision of blood ketone testing for children and adolescents. Many units also provide their insulin pump users with blood ketone monitoring.

Continuous glucose monitoring (CGM) systems

A major objective of diabetes research has been to provide continuous real-time monitoring of blood glucose so that insulin therapy can be matched to glycaemia. Unfortunately, there are significant problems of infection and thrombosis with long term intravascular sensors. Glucose sensors placed subcutaneously avoid these complications and have been refined over the last 20 years so that they can be placed for up to 14 days, and can communicate wirelessly with insulin delivery devices (or smart phones or the cloud), thus making possible a closed-loop artificial pancreas (Figures 9.4 and 9.5 and see Chapter 10).

The measurement technology is similar to capillary blood glucose monitoring and utilises the glucose oxidase reaction and electron transfer detection. Measurements are made every 1–5 minutes and transmitted every 5–15 minutes. There are also devices that are blinded to the user which can be used to detect patterns of glycaemia without the confounding of patient response to the results. Although the current devices are more accurate and sophisticated, they

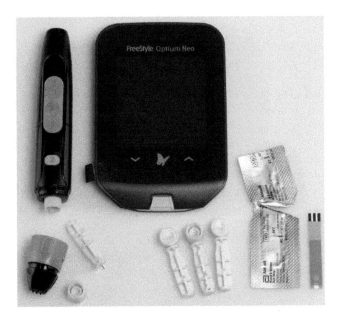

Figure 9.2 Example of combined blood glucose and blood ketone meter together with sampling device and lancets. Testing strips are foil wrapped and must be used before expiry date.

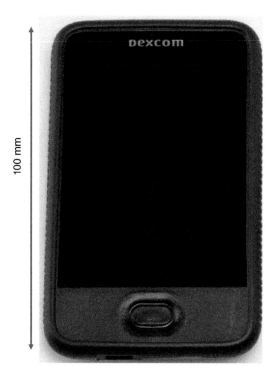

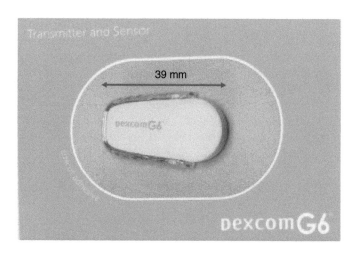

Figure 9.4 Continuous Glucose Sensor and Transmitter and associated Meter. The sensor has a fine cannula around 4 mm long and 0.3 mm wide (not seen as it is on the opposite side) and is inserted using an applicator usually on the anterior abdominal wall. Estimates of interstitial fluid glucose concentrations are transmitted to the meter and a read out appears on the screen. Most modern systems no longer require calibration from capillary blood glucose tests.

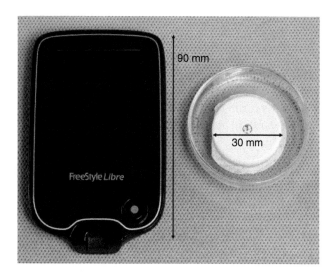

Figure 9.5 Flash (intermittent) glucose monitoring system. Sensor and transmitter (right) are inserted via an applicator usually onto the posterior surface of the upper arm. The cannula (not seen, on the other side of sensor) is 0.4 mm wide and 5 mm long. The sensor communicates wirelessly with the meter and does not need calibration. Glucose readings are obtained by either holding the meter within 4 cm of the sensor or via mobile phone app. Data are downloadable to a computer.

still have some drawbacks. Firstly, they are based upon measures of interstitial fluid, not blood glucose. This inevitably means that there is a delay or lag between detecting changes in blood glucose (mean delay 4 minutes, historical range 2–45 minutes). This lag can be affected by level of blood glucose, exercise, food intake and blood flow to the interstitial sampling site. Accuracy of the current devices tends to be less good at lower blood glucose levels. Secondly, such systems are by definition invasive as they require subcutaneous sensor insertion, usually on the abdominal wall, especially when linked to an insulin pump, or on the upper arm. Thirdly, linkage to subcutaneous insulin infusion pumps introduces a further time lag in responsiveness (that of insulin absorption from the subcutaneous site). The technology is also expensive and requires replacement every 10–14 days. Some of these problems have been overcome by using alarms if glucose is rising or falling quickly, or if the readings cross preset thresholds. Most now show a trend arrow with the reading, further alerting the patient of impending hyper or hypoglycaemia. A fully implantable device (Senseomics) that lasts 90–180 days has now been licensed for use in both Europe and the USA but clinical experience is limited.

The accuracy of blood glucose monitoring devices including CGM has been the subject of a great deal of research. The Clarke error grid was devised in 1987 for this purpose and plots the correlation between the device under investigation and a reference method (usually a laboratory blood glucose analyser). The resulting graph is then divided into a series of zones with preset parameters of recommended blood glucose control targets. There are 5 zone categories: Zone A <20% deviation from true blood glucose or both readings are <4 mmol/L; Zone B deviation from true blood glucose is >20% but no action is needed; Zone C potential over correction of acceptable blood glucose values; Zone D potential dangerous failure to detect and treat abnormal true blood glucose; and Zone E potentially inappropriate treatment contradictory to requirements. An example of such an analysis is shown in Figure 9.6 where a continuous monitoring device (in this case the no longer used Navigator) is compared with venous blood glucose. Although this method of comparison has its critics because of its a priori assumptions of ideal control and appropriate patient responses, the Clarke Error Grid is almost universally applied to all methods of glucose monitoring as an assessment of accuracy.

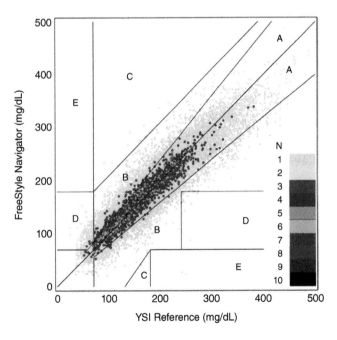

Figure 9.6 Clarke error grid showing the density of paired FreeStyle Navigator (a continuous glucose monitoring system) and YSI (Yellow Springs Instrument) benchtop venous blood glucose analyser as reference. Colour coded measurements are shown in 1 mg/dl squares from 1 (grey) to 10 (black) times per square.

The 5 zones of the error grid are labelled A – E. For explanation and significance please see text. 81.7% of points were within the A zone and 16.7% in B. Reproduced from Richard L. Weinstein et al. Diabetes Care 2007;30:1125–1130 with permission

Clinical trials of CGM have shown benefit for patients in terms of time spent in target range, avoidance of hypoglycaemia, and lower HbA1c. Most guidelines support their use for two broad indications in type 1 diabetes. Firstly, short-term (2–4 weeks) diagnosis of problems in glycaemic control by revealing patterns of blood glucose in response to meals or exercise for example (Figure 9.7). This may also be of benefit in people with type 2 diabetes and poor control, but is only helpful during stable periods (not on vacation or during intercurrent illness for example); and secondly, in patients with problematic hypoglycaemia and unawareness (Figure 9.8). It is clear from clinical trials that patients obtain maximum benefit the more they use the data and adjust their insulin dose, and a minimum of 70% usage is currently recommended.

There are some downsides to CGM use, however. The need for checking and responding can induce anxiety, some patients feel the need to switch off or escape. A more difficult problem is that of data overload which can also overwhelm the patient, and, until recently, there were no universally agreed target glucose ranges. In order to get around these problems a consensus on how to report, interpret, and use continuous monitoring data was recently published. Glucose data are to be divided into three categories, time in range (TIR), time above range (TAR) and time below range (TBR). The ranges can be set individually depending on the patient (less strict for those with co-morbidities, more strict in pregnancy for example) (Figure 9.9). Objectives can then be set using the 'SMART' principles (Box 9.4) helping patients feel in control. It is suggested that by addressing TBR first there is the potential for immediate relief from the unpleasant symptoms and consequences of hypoglycaemia, thus providing the patient with a real sense of achievement and reinforcing engagement. Much more needs to be done to develop decision support advice and the Endocrine Society has provided recommendations for real time adjustment. CGM has been endorsed as a means of monitoring glycaemic control by the ADA, American Association of Clinical Endocrinologists (AACE), and the International Society for Paediatric and Adolescent Diabetes (ISPAD). Both of the regulatory authorities in the USA (FDA) and Europe have now approved CGM systems as a replacement for intermittent capillary blood glucose monitoring. NICE guidance is summarised in Box 9.5.

It is clear that the development of CGM has provided both patient and health care professional with a wealth of information to underpin recommendations for treatment, but in order to achieve maximum benefit both parties need to invest a great deal of time and effort. It is important not to set unrealistic expectations and inadvertently induce a sense of failure in both patient and professional.

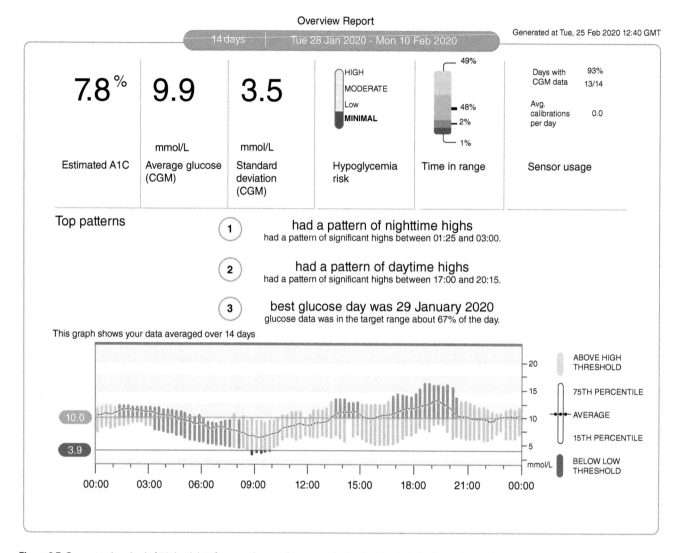

Figure 9.7 Computer download of 14 days' data from continuous glucose monitoring (real-time) device in a patient with type 1 diabetes showing average daily profile and percentile ranges. The pattern shows a problem with post prandial hyperglycaemia in the evenings. 49% of readings were outside target requiring an evening insulin dose increase.

Box 9.4

SMART Objectives

Specific–sets out what needs to be achieved
Measurable–uses tangible evidence
Achievable–but needs to provide a challenge
Relevant–addresses patient priorities and needs
Timely–should be attainable within realistic time frame

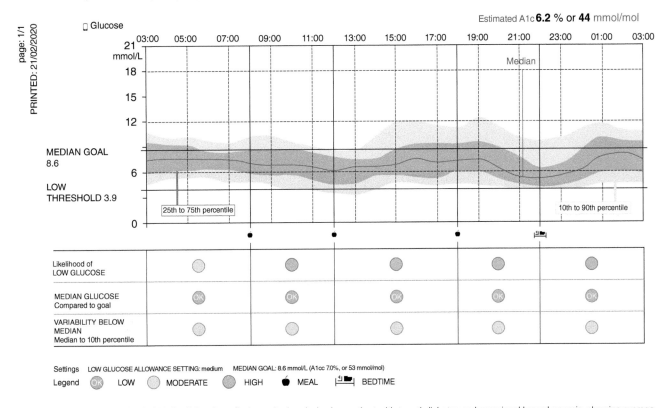

Figure 9.8 Computer download of 14 days' data from flash monitoring device in a patient with type 1 diabetes and occasional hypoglycaemia, showing average daily profile and percentile ranges. Overall control is excellent but with increased possibility of hypoglycaemia particularly at bedtime. Increasing long acting carbohydrate at his evening meal was recommended.

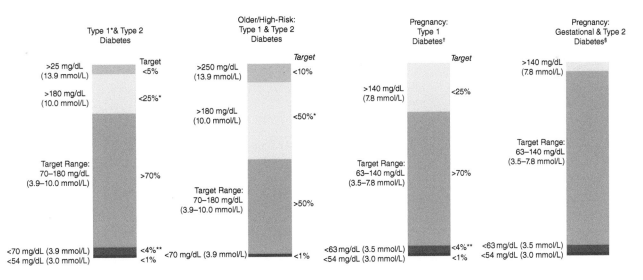

⇔ For age <25 yr., if the A1C goal is 7.5%, then set TIR target to approximately 60%, (See *Clinical Applications of Time in Ranges* section in the text for additional information regarding target goal setting in pediatric management.)

↑ Percentages of time in ranges are based on limited evidence. More research is needed.

§ Percentages of time in ranges have not been included because there is very limited evidence in this area. More research is needed. Please see *Pregnancy* section in text for more considerations on targets for these groups.

* Includes percentage of values >250 mg/dL(13.9 mmol/L).

** Includes percentage of values <54 mg/dL(3.0 mmol/L).

Figure 9.9 CGM Target Ranges for different groups of patients as agreed by international consensus. Green = Time In Range (TIR); Yellow/Orange = Time Above Range (TAR); Red = Time Below range (TBR). Reproduced from Tadej Battelino et al. Diabetes Care 2019;42:1593–1603 with permission.

Box 9.5 NICE Guidance on the use of continuous glucose monitoring.

What NICE says about CGM for adults (From NG17):
- It is not recommended for all adults with Type 1 diabetes.
  - They say it should be considered for people who have:
  - had >1 severe hypoglycaemic episode a year with no obvious cause
  - complete hypoglycaemic unawareness
  - >2 hypoglycaemic episodes a week, with no symptoms and which affect day to day life
  - extreme fear of hypoglycaemia
  - an HbA1c ≥75 mmols/mol (≥9.0%) despite testing at least 10 times a day.
- A person must be prepared to use it at least 70 % of the time.
- Real-time CGM should be provided by a centre who are expert in using it, as part of strategies to improve a person's HbA1c levels and reduce hypoglycaemia.

What NICE says about CGM for children (from NG18):
- It should be offered to children who:
  - have frequent, severe hypoglycaemia
  - have hypoglycaemia unawareness with serious consequences (e.g. fits, anxiety)
  - cannot recognise, or tell somebody about hypo symptoms (e.g. because of developmental or neurological issues).
- It should be considered for children who:
  - are under school age
  - are elite athletes (e.g. compete at regional or national or international level)
  - have other issues that make diabetes management more difficult (e.g. anorexia or steroid treatment)
  - have high blood glucose levels despite full support and insulin adjustment.

What NICE says about CGM in pregnancy (from NG3):
- It should be offered to all women:
  - with type 1 diabetes
  - who are on insulin and experiencing problematic severe hypoglycaemia and/or unstable blood glucose levels.

CASE HISTORY

A 24-year-old white Europid man developed classic symptoms of type 1 diabetes and was commenced upon insulin as a basal–bolus regimen. His initial HbA1c was 82 mmol/mol (9.7%). Six months later at regular review his home blood glucose monitoring showed excellent control with readings between 3.8 and 8.9 mmol/L (68–160 mg/dL) and he only reported occasional, mild, effort-related hypoglycaemia. However, his HbA1c value came back the next day at 67 mmol/mol (8.3%). He was con-

tacted at home and an increase in his insulin of 2 units per dose was recommended and a repeat HbA1c ordered for 6 weeks' time. This was reported as 65 mmol/mol (8.1%) and a further insulin increase was instituted. Five days later he was admitted to hospital following a profound nocturnal hypoglycaemic episode during which he was found fitting.

Haemoglobin electrophoresis revealed the presence of HbS. The laboratory used an HbA1c assay that was sensitive to HbS, particularly at lower HbA1c concentrations. On direct questioning, it transpired that his parents were from the Mediterranean area.

Comment: Several learning points emerge. HbS can occur in non-African populations, so a family history in all people with diabetes is important. Secondly, it is important to know the limitations of the assays used by local laboratories. Lastly, in the presence of discrepancies between home monitoring and laboratory, do not always assume the patient's tests are incorrect. In this case continuous glucose monitoring may have helped but was not available at the time.

LANDMARK CLINICAL TRIAL

Koenig RJ, Peterson CM, Jones RL, Saudek C, Lehrman M, Cerami A. Correlation of glucose regulation and hemoglobin A1c in diabetes mellitus. N Engl J Med 1976; 295: 417–420.

Although abnormal haemoglobin electrophoresis had been described in diabetes since the 1950s, this was the first correlation between a change in glycaemia and a change in HbA1c. Five patients with a fasting blood glucose ranging from 280 to 450 mg/dL (15.6–25.0 mmol/L) were hospitalised and their values corrected to 70–100 mg/dL (3.9–5.6 mmol/L). HbA1c was 50–109 mmol/mol (6.8–12.1%) initially, falling to 22–60 mmol/mol (4.2–7.6%) after glycaemic improvement. Later, much larger studies confirmed the linear relationship (Figure 9.2) but the author's conclusion was spot on: 'Periodic monitoring of hemoglobin A1c levels provides a useful way of documenting the degree of control of glucose metabolism in diabetic patients . . .'.

KEY WEBSITES

- National Glycohemoglobin Support Program. Excellent information on HbA1c, eAG and the new IFCC standards: www.ngsp.org
- National Institute for Health and Care Excellence (NICE). All UK guidelines available on this site (FreeStyle Libre for blood glucose monitoring MIB110; Type 1 Diabetes in adults: diagnosis and management NG17; Diabetes (type 1 and type 2) in children and adolescents: diagnosis and management NG18; Type 2 diabetes in adults: management NG 28): www.nice.org.uk
- Diabetes UK. Guidance on monitoring: www.diabetes.org.uk
- American Diabetes Association. Standards of care published in *Diabetes Care* as a supplement each January: http://professional.diabetes.org/
- SIGN Guidelines: www.SIGN.ac.uk

FURTHER READING

American Diabetes Association. Standards of medical care in diabetes – 2020. Diabetes Care 2020; 43(Suppl 1): S66–S76.

American Diabetes Association, European Association for the Study of Diabetes, International Federation of Clinical Chemistry and Laboratory Medicine, and International Diabetes Federation. Consensus statement on the world-wide standardisation of the HbA1c measurement. Diabetologia 2007; 50: 2042–2043.

Battelino T, Danne T, Bergenstal RM et al. Clinical targets for continuous glucose monitoring data interpretation: recommendations from the international consensus on time in range. Diabetes Care 2019; 42: 1593–1603

Beck RW, Bergenstal RM, Laffel LM, Pickup JC. Advances in technology for management of type 1 diabetes. Lancet 2019; dx.doi. org/10.1016/S0140-6736(19)31142-0

DAFNE Study Group. Training in flexible, intensive insulin management to enable dietary freedom in people with type 1 diabetes: dose adjustment for normal eating (DAFNE) randomized controlled trial. BMJ 2002; 325:746–751.

DESMOND Type 2 diabetes education www.desmond-project.org.uk

Khera PJ, Joiner CH, Carruthers A, et al. Evidence for individual heterogeneity in the glucose gradient across the human red blood cell membrane and its relationship to hemoglobin glycation. Diabetes 2008; 57: 2445–2452.

Nathan DM, Kunen J, Borg R, Zheng H, Schoenfeld D, Heine RJ, for the A1C Derived Average Glucose (ADAG) Study Group. Translating the A1c assay into estimated average glucose. Diabetes Care 2008; 31: 1473–1478.

Management of type 1 diabetes

KEY POINTS

- The objective of insulin treatment is to try and reproduce the physiological pattern of insulin production using subcutaneous injections. This usually entails multiple daily injections of short-, and intermediate- or long-acting insulins, together with regular capillary blood glucose testing.
- There is no clear evidence-based superiority of the newer short- or long-acting insulin analogues in terms of glycaemic control, although hypoglycaemia rates tend to be lower.

- Continuous subcutaneous insulin infusion can improve glycaemia and reduce hypoglycaemia in patients struggling on conventional therapy, and the latest devices linked to continuous glucose monitoring systems and insulin delivery suspend or enhance algorithms offer further benefits.

Modern management of type 1 diabetes comprises a package of measures including multiple daily injections or continuous insulin infusion (pump therapy) for a more physiological insulin replacement; assessment of glycaemic control using blood glucose self-monitoring as well as clinic tests such as glycated haemoglobin (HbA1c); insulin dosage adjustment according to diet and exercise; a healthy diet with carbohydrate counting; and intensive diabetes education. The landmark Diabetes Control and Complications Trial (DCCT) randomised 1441 patients to either intensive treatment (including all the elements listed above plus regular contact with a named healthcare professional) or to conventional therapy with one or two injections of insulin a day. Significant improvements in HbA1c and a reduction in microvascular complications were seen in the intensively managed group. In practice, it is difficult to sustain the level of intensive healthcare professional support in the DCCT, but providing patients with self-management tools such as the Diet Adjustment For Normal Eating (DAFNE) Programme in the UK has been shown to significantly reduce HbA1c at 6 and 12 months. Educational aspects of management such as these will be dealt with later (Chapter 33), and monitoring was the subject of Chapter 9. This chapter will focus on the different available insulins and how to use them and continuous insulin delivery systems. Islet and whole organ pancreas transplantation is covered in Chapter 34.

Insulin replacement

The objective of insulin replacement is to mimic the insulin secretion pattern in the person without diabetes by utilising multiple subcutaneous injections or boluses. In the person without diabetes, there is normally a rapid increase in plasma insulin after meals, triggered by glucose absorption into the bloodstream. This surge in insulin limits postprandial glycaemia by stimulating hepatic and peripheral glucose uptake. During fasting and between meals, insulin measurements drop to much lower levels (often called basal or steady state) which are sufficient to maintain blood glucose in the range 3.5–5.5 mmol/L. Even after a prolonged fast, it is possible to detect circulating insulin.

Basal insulin levels tend to be highest in the early morning, probably in response to the well-described surge in growth

Handbook of Diabetes, Fifth Edition. Rudy Bilous, Richard Donnelly, and Iskandar Idris.
© 2021 John Wiley & Sons Ltd. Published 2021 by John Wiley & Sons Ltd.

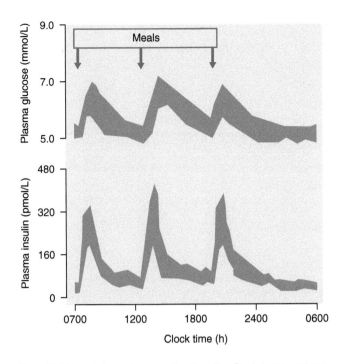

Figure 10.1 Normal plasma glucose and insulin profiles. Shaded areas represent mean ± 2 SD. Modified from Owens et al. Lancet 2001; 358: 739–746.

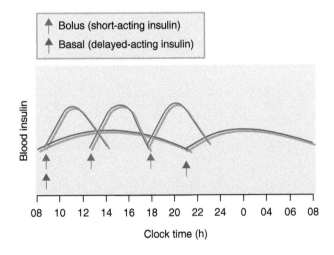

Figure 10.2 Basal-bolus insulin regimen.

hormone and cortisol at that time of day (Figure 10.1). These counter-regulatory hormones tend to increase blood glucose and this has been termed the 'dawn phenomenon'.

For practical reasons, insulin is usually injected subcutaneously and regimens comprise short-acting insulin (soluble (regular) human or analogue) to simulate the normal mealtime surge, together with a longer acting insulin which is used to provide the background or basal concentration. This combination is commonly called a 'basal-bolus' regimen or sometimes multiple daily injection (MDI) therapy (Figure 10.2).

Other routes of insulin administration such as intravenous infusion or intramuscular injection have not proven practical in the long term and despite intensive research, oral insulin preparations are not yet available. Inhaled preparations of short-acting insulin are available in the USA and they have been shown to be effective, although there have been concerns in the past about their possible long-term effects on the respiratory tract.

Until the 1980s, insulin was extracted and purified from animal sources. Porcine insulins are still available but have been largely replaced by human-sequence insulin produced from genetically engineered bacteria. Recently modified human insulin molecules (so-called analogues) have now been developed (Figure 10.3).

Essentially, insulins can be divided into short-acting and intermediate to long-acting preparations, and those currently available in the UK are listed in Table 10.1. The usual total daily dose ranges from 0.4–1.0 u/kg body weight and is usually given as 50% short (further divided according to meals) and 50% intermediate/long acting (usually given once at night or in the morning but not infrequently twice daily).

Short-acting insulins

Achieving normoglycaemia with insulin injections is frustrated by several pharmacological problems. Firstly, subcutaneously injected insulin is absorbed into the peripheral rather than the portal bloodstream; thus, effective insulinisation of the liver can be achieved only at the expense of systemic hyperinsulinaemia. Moreover, human short-acting insulins are absorbed too slowly to mimic precisely the normal prandial peaks, and must therefore be injected up to 20–30 minutes before the meal so that the peak of blood insulin corresponds with postprandial glycaemia.

Some of the delay in absorption of subcutaneous insulin is a result of the formation of hexamers following injection (Figure 10.4). The hexamers need to dissociate into dimers or monomers so that insulin can be absorbed into the bloodstream. In order to get around this problem, the insulin molecule has been modified using genetic and protein engineering techniques. These changes in amino acid sequence reduce the tendency to self-associate into hexamers and therefore speed absorption. The first short-acting analogue to be marketed was lispro, closely followed by aspart and glulisine (see Figure 10.3). Their peak action occurs 1–2 hours after injection (compared to 2–3 hours for unmodified human) and they can therefore be injected at the start or even during a meal. Although this is highly convenient for patients, a systematic review by the Cochrane Collaboration of short-acting analogues versus unmodified human insulin demonstrated a modest advantage in terms of glycaemic control (HbA1c −1.7 mmol/mol (95% CI −2.2,−1.1)(−0.15%, 95% CI −0.2,−0.1), with no effect on hypoglycaemia rates. A pattern of lower postprandial and

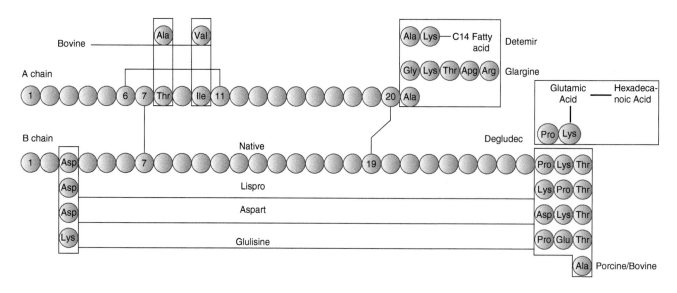

Figure 10.3 Schematic amino acid sequence of native human insulin; porcine and bovine insulin; the short-acting insulin analogues lispro, aspart and glulisine; and the long-acting analogues glargine,degludec and detemir. ALA, alanine; ARG, arginine; PRO, proline; LYS, lysine; ASP, aspartate; THR, threonine; GLU, glutamate; GLY, glycine; ILE, isoleucine; VAL, valine.

Table 10.1 Insulin preparations and their costs in the UK based upon the British National Formulary Drug Tariffs in BNF 78 Sept 2019 – Mar 2020.

Duration	Origin	Type	10 mL vial	5 × 3 mL cartridge	Disposable pen × 5
Short					
4–8 hours	Animal – bovine				
	Animal – porcine	Neutral	£27.72	£41.58	
		Neutral	£31.80	£46.95	
	Human – genetic	Actrapid	£15.68		
		Humulin S	£15.68	£19.08	
		Insuman Rapid		£19.08	£27.90
3–4.5 hours	Analogue	Aspart	£14.08	£28.31	£30.60
		Lispro	£16.61	£28.31	£29.46
		Glulisine	£16.00	£28.30	£28.30
Intermediate					
16 – 22 hours	Animal – porcine	NPH	£31.30	£46.95	
	Human Insulatard	NPH	£15.68	£19.08	£21.70
	Humulin I	NPH	£15.68	£19.08	£21.70
	Insuman Basal	NPH	5 mL £5.61	£19.08	£21.70
Long					
16 – 24 hours	Animal – bovine	Lente	£27.72		
	Animal – bovine	Protamine zinc	£27.72		
21 - 27 hours	Analogues	Detemir		£42.00	£42.00
16 – 23 hours		Glargine	£27.92	£37.77	£37.77
>42 hours		Degludec		£46.60	£46.60
Biphasic	Animal – porcine	30/70	£31.30	£46.95	
		(30% neutral, 70% NPH)			
	Human	Humulin M3	£15.68	£19.08	£21.70
		(30% Humulin S, 70% Humulin I)			
		Insuman Comb 15		£17.50	
		(15% Insuman rapid, 85% Insuman basal)			
		Insuman Comb 25	5 mL £5.61	£17.50	£19.80
		(25% Insuman rapid, 75% Insuman basal)			
		Insuman Comb 50		£17.50	
		(50% Insuman Rapid, 50% Insuman Basal)			
	Analogue	Novomix 30		£28.79	£29.89
		(30% Aspart, 70% Aspart NPH)			
		Humalog Mix 25	£16.61	£29.46	£30.98
		(25% Lispro, 75% Lispro NPH)			
		Humalog Mix 50		£29.46	£30.98
		(50% Lispro, 50% Lispro NPH)			

NPH = Neutral Protamine Hagedorn.

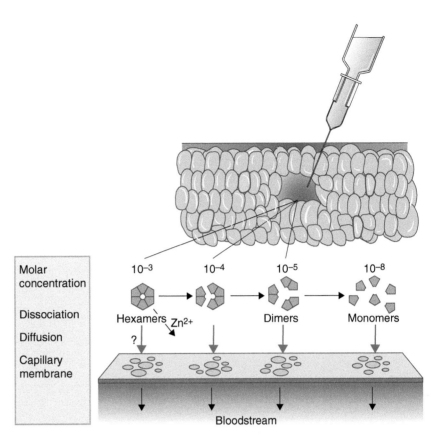

Figure 10.4 What happens in the subcutaneous tissue after subcutaneous injection of regular human insulin.

higher preprandial blood glucose levels has been demonstrated by other reviews.

Some patients who were well controlled on animal insulin felt less well when switched to the human preparation. Many complained that their warning signs of hypoglycaemia were lost. However, carefully controlled studies have failed to show significant differences in the glycaemic response to the two insulins, and under blinded conditions patients were unable to distinguish between them.

Intermediate- and long-acting insulins

There are three main types of intermediate- and long-acting insulins. Isophane (or NPH, neutral protamine Hagedorn, named after its inventor) is an insoluble suspension of human insulin made by combining it with the highly basic protein protamine together with zinc, at a neutral pH. NPH insulin can be derived from animal, unmodified human or analogue insulins. Lente insulins are made by adding excess zinc to soluble insulin, and there is also a combination of protamine and zinc suspended insulin available, although neither are prescribed very often in the UK. Pharmacokinetic studies have shown NPH insulin has a peak action from 4–7 hours, and an overall duration of action 16–22 hours after injection.

Because of the peak action profile of NPH insulin, there was a tendency for patients to develop nocturnal hypoglycaemia.

As a result of this, three longer-acting insulin analogues have been developed which have a flatter absorption profile. The first of these (insulin glargine) was made by adding two arginine molecules to the C-terminal of the B chain and substituting a glycine for alanine at A21 (Figure 10.3). This modification altered the isoelectric point (which is when proteins are least soluble) from pH 5.4 to 7.4. This means that at a slightly acidic pH in the vial, glargine is soluble and clear (in contrast with NPH which is a cloudy solution), but after subcutaneous injection it precipitates as microcrystals and is gradually absorbed. Detemir is human insulin where the C-terminal amino acid on the B chain is substituted with a C14 fatty acid (Figure 10.3). This binds to albumin which slows absorption and also prolongs circulation. Insulin Degludec has a molecule of hexadecanoic acid attached to the lysine residue B29 via a glutamic acid bridge. This preparation forms multi hexamers subcutaneously producing a pool of insulin that is slowly, predictably, and gradually absorbed into the circulation. The pharmacological properties of these insulins are shown in Table 10.2. No consistent benefit in terms of a reduction in HbA1c has been found between NPH and longer acting analogues, but fasting glycaemia and rates of nocturnal hypoglycaemia are reduced. Current NICE guidance for adults with type 1 recommends that insulin detemir twice daily should be first choice, but detemir or glargine once daily can also be considered if patients prefer.

Table 10.2 Pharmacological properties of the available intermediate and long-acting insulins. Variability is expressed as the coefficient of variability of the area under the curve of the glucose infusion rate needed to maintain a steady blood glucose concentration after injection of the same dose in the same individuals on separate days.

Pharmacology	NPH	Glargine	Detemir	Degludec
Onset of action	60 – 120 mins	60 – 120 mins	60 – 120 mins	30 – 90 mins
Duration	16 – 22 hrs	21 – 27 hrs	16 – 23 hrs	>42 hrs
Time of peak	4 – 7 hrs	4 – 12 hrs	7 – 9 hrs	None
Day to day variability	48%	48 – 99%	27%	20%

Data from Rossetti et al Diabetes Obesity and Metabolism 2014; 16: 695 – 706.

The ADA and SIGN do not specify a preparation. A significant drawback of the analogues is their cost which makes them beyond the reach of many in developing countries and even in private health care systems such as the USA.

Premixed or biphasic insulins

A number of these are available (see Table 10.1), but those most commonly in use in the UK comprise 30% quick acting and 70% NPH, although the newer analogues come in 25:75, 30:70 or 50:50 mixtures. These fixed rate combinations give less flexibility than MDI but can be more acceptable to patients with predictable lifestyles and who do not wish to inject more frequently. The evening injection of the NPH component may not be adequate to provide overnight glycaemic control, particularly if it is administered around 6 pm, or if the patient has a significant dawn phenomenon.

A combination of insulins degludec and aspart in a 70:30 proportion has been produced and is available in the USA, and also has a license in Europe.

Injection sites

The recommended injection sites are the subcutaneous tissue of the abdomen, upper outer thighs, upper outer arms, and buttocks (Figure 10.5). Disposable plastic syringes with a fine needle can be reused for several injections, although these have been largely superseded in the UK by insulin pens (see below). There is no need to pinch up the skin prior to injection (in fact, this probably causes more discomfort). Care should be taken to avoid inadvertent intramuscular injection which can be a particular risk in the upper arms and legs of slim people or children.

Insulin absorption is fastest in the abdomen and slowest in the thigh and buttocks, although it can be accelerated from these sites by exercise or taking a sauna or warm bath. Short-acting insulin is usually given into the abdomen, which is less affected by exercise, and longer acting insulins into the thigh.

Repeated injection into the same subcutaneous site may, in the long term, give rise to a local accumulation of fat (lipohypertrophy) because of the local trophic action of insulin (Figure 10.6). Lipohypertrophy can be unsightly and can

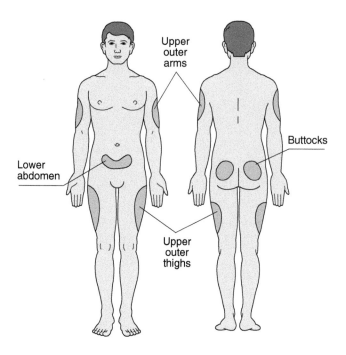

Figure 10.5 Suitable sites for subcutaneous insulin injection.

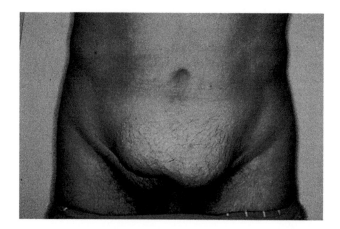

Figure 10.6 Suprapubic lipohypertrophy at habitually used insulin injection sites.

slow insulin absorption and in order to prevent it, patients should be advised to rotate the site of their injections. It is important to remember that lipohypertrophic areas become relatively painless and are thus often favoured by patients who may inadvertently make the problem worse. For this reason, inspection of injection sites is an important part of the annual patient review. Lipodystrophy (localised subcutaneous fat loss) is rarely seen with modern insulins. The MHRA has responded to recent case reports of cutaneous amyloid at insulin injection sites by emphasising the importance of rotation of injection sites.

Insulin pens

Pen needle devices are the most popular option for insulin therapy (Figure 10.7), they are more convenient than using insulin containing vials and separate syringes and needles. There are at least eight currently available in the UK. Whilst they differ slightly, the principles are the same. Insulin is contained in a 3 mL cartridge in the barrel of the pen. There is an adjustable dosage dial which drives a plunger in the cartridge when depressed, and insulin is delivered through a removable fine needle which screws onto the cartridge at the opposite end of the pen (Figure 10.7). Prefilled pens are also available, they are more convenient particularly for those

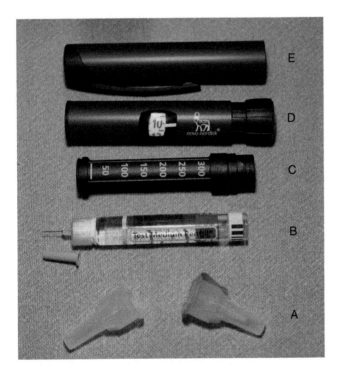

Figure 10.7 Example of disassembled insulin pen. Insulin dose is selected using the dial at the top of the pen (D). The cartridge (B) contains 300 units and is inserted into the barrel (C) which is then connected to the upper unit (D) which contains a plunger. The needles (A) are screwed onto the cartridge after insertion into the barrel. After use, the needle is protected by the pen barrel cap (E).

patients on mixed insulin preparations. Their main drawback is that they cannot be recycled. The advantages of pens are their portability, the needles are often finer than conventional syringes and needles, and they tend to keep their sharpness longer because they are not being continually inserted through the bung of a 10 mL vial. Pen needles also have the advantage of being available in different lengths, which means it is easier to avoid inadvertent intramuscular injection. Some pens now have a wireless transmitter which can record timing and quantity of insulin dosing.

Intensive insulin therapy

Multiple daily injections (MDI) of insulin are only part of intensive or optimised treatment. The other components are patient education, dietary advice and carbohydrate counting, and frequent insulin adjustment based upon the results of glucose monitoring. Moreover, patients need to be in a systematic programme of care and medical surveillance. Education and structured care will be covered later (see Chapter 33).

MDI comprises doses of short-acting, regular or rapid-acting analogue insulins given with meals, at a variable dose depending on the carbohydrate content. Patients are encouraged to monitor carefully and learn by checking the postprandial blood glucose 1½–2 hours after meals to see if their first estimation was correct. Various calculators have been developed to help patients gauge their insulin sensitivity and to estimate the amount of insulin they need per 10g of dietary carbohydrate. One such is the 500 rule which divides 500 by the total daily dose of insulin, and this gives the number of grammes of carbohydrate requiring 1 unit of insulin. For example, a person on 70 units of insulin a day would require 1 unit for 7g carbohydrate. A similar calculation can be made to estimate the amount of insulin needed to correct a high blood glucose. The 100 rule divides 100 by the total daily insulin dose, and in the same example would suggest that 1 unit of insulin would lower blood glucose by 1.4 mmol/L. (for blood glucose units mg/dl use 2000 divided by total daily insulin). These tools are indicative and will need to be refined with experience in individual patients. Many blood glucose monitoring devices now contain algorithms that will estimate the correct mealtime bolus of insulin, only requiring the patient to enter the carbohydrate content.

Isophane or long-acting analogues can be given once at night or morning, or twice daily. As previously mentioned, insulin sensitivity decreases in the few hours before breakfast because of surges of growth hormone and cortisol during sleep. The effect of this, together with the waning of the previous evening's insulin dose, can result in fasting hyperglycaemia (the 'dawn phenomenon'). This problem can often be addressed by using a different, longer lasting preparation, or by injecting later in the evening. The large coefficients of variation for the different medium and long-acting insulins (Table 10.2) demonstrate the need for flexibility, and a degree of trial and error in determining the optimum dose, time and site of injection.

Diet and Carbohydrate counting

Recommended dietary content for people with diabetes is largely based upon the concepts of healthy eating, with a balance between carbohydrate, protein and fat, and the inclusion of foods rich in essential vitamins and minerals. Many use illustrations of typical meals to show the proportions and relative calorie contributions. For people taking insulin, however, the carbohydrate content of a meal is crucial in determining their prandial insulin requirement. Numerous aids have been developed, perhaps the most effective are pictorial representations of common meals relating the carbohydrate content to plate/portion size. Many of these are produced by organisations such as Diabetes UK or the ADA and are often freely available. Some are also available as downloads for smartphones which make them particularly convenient. Their other advantage is that they can take account of different dietary practices of different communities such as those that are based on rice or grains for example. In addition, there are many commercial resources, but some will be based upon their author's opinion and the evidence base should be checked accordingly. The difference between these tools and the older concepts of dietary carbohydrate restriction is that they allow people to choose what they wish to eat and adjust insulin dose accordingly, whereas previously the insulin dose was fixed and the diet had to be limited to match it. The DAFNE strapline sums this up as "Eat what you like, like what you eat".

Glycaemic targets

Glycaemic targets published in the UK and the USA are shown in Table 10.3. These will need to be discussed and agreed with individual patients to take account of their personal and medical circumstances. For example, those with existing microvascular complications may need a lower target HbA1c, whereas patients suffering from regular

hypoglycaemia (particularly if their warnings are blunted and they live alone) may need more relaxed targets. Diabetes UK has come up with the phrase '4 is the floor', suggesting a minimum blood glucose of 4 mmol/L, and the ADA has adopted a definition of hypoglycaemia of ≤3.9 mmol/L (70 mg/dl).

Continuous subcutaneous insulin infusion

Continuous insulin delivery systems can be either 'open loop', in which insulin infusion rates are preselected by the patient, or 'closed loop' in which there is continuous glucose sensing and a computer-regulated feedback control of insulin delivery (the so-called 'artificial pancreas').

Continuous subcutaneous insulin infusion (CSII) was developed over 30 years ago. This was an open-loop delivery system in which a portable pump infused insulin subcutaneously at a fixed rate via a butterfly cannula. The latest devices are much smaller and much more technologically sophisticated (Figures 10.8 and 10.9). They infuse insulin at variable basal rates, usually in pulses, thus reproducing background insulinisation. At mealtimes, patients give a bolus dose taking into account the carbohydrate content of the meal and the prevailing blood glucose concentration (sometimes using the rules of 500 and 100 – see above). A typical strategy for commencing pump therapy is to

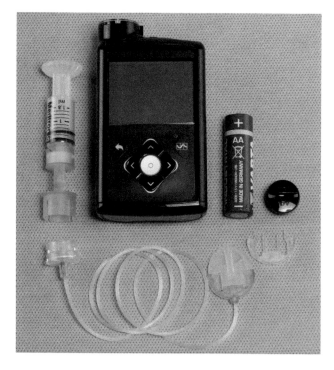

Figure 10.8 Insulin infusion pump, fillable insulin cartridge (left), subcutaneous infusion set (below) and battery (right). Same device as worn by patient in Figure 10.9.

Table 10.3 Glycaemic targets from NICE (National Institute of Health Care Excellence) and the ADA (American Diabetes Association).

Time	NICE	ADA
Fasting adult (child)	5 – 7 mmol/L (4 – 7)	
Pre meal adult (child)	4 – 7 mmol/L (both)	4.4 – 7.2 mmol/L (both) 80–130 mg/dl
Post meal adult (child)	90 – 120 mins 5 – 9 mmol/L (both)	Maximum 90 mins 10 mmol/L (both) 180 mg/dl
HbA1c adult (child)	48 mmol/mol (both) 6.5%	53 mmol/mol (both) 7.0%

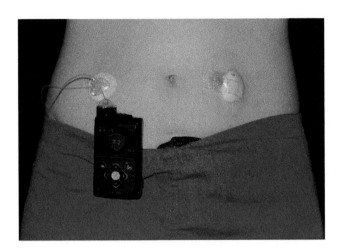

Figure 10.9 Insulin infusion pump and glucose sensor fitted on a patient with type 1 diabetes. The sensor communicates wirelessly with the pump. The current glucose value is shown as 7.2 mmol/L.

reduce the patient's total daily insulin dose on injections by 20–30% and then allocating the remainder, one half to the basal rate and the other split equally between the three main meals. Pumps linked to continuous glucose sensing devices will estimate the correct bolus, only requiring the patient to enter the carbohydrate load into the device and an algorithm estimates the dose. Mealtime boluses can be delivered as a single square wave over a set period of time (taking into account the speed of absorption of the carbohydrate) or as a dual wave. Pumps can all be downloaded onto computers wirelessly or via the cloud. This information can then be discussed in person or virtually with the patient in order to guide management.

Because only short-acting (usually analogue) insulin is used, the problem of variable absorption of intermediate and long-acting preparations is overcome. Moreover, basal rates can be changed hour by hour, and this is particularly useful in individuals who exhibit the dawn phenomenon and during periods of exercise. The latest devices have built-in algorithms that can suspend insulin delivery if the glucose reading drops below a predefined threshold (low glucose suspend), or the trajectory of sensed glucose is downward and likely to cross the hypoglycaemic threshold (Tandem Basal IQ System). The newest pumps also have the capacity to increase insulin delivery if the glucose is rising or crosses a preset upper threshold.

All externally worn pumps have the same essential components (Figure 10.8). They are battery driven using a standard size power source. They have an insulin reservoir of 180–300 units that is topped up from an insulin vial, and this is connected via a flexible cannula (variable lengths are available), which is inserted several millimetres under the skin, either directly by the patient or by using an inserter device. These cannulae need replacing every three days,

after this time there is a risk of infection and local subcutaneous irritation. The abdomen is the most common site.

Another type of delivery system is the patch pump, so called because they are attached directly to the skin. They have an internal reservoir that is filled with insulin and an external handset. After attachment, the handset instructs the pump to insert the cannula. This has the advantage that the wearer does not have to insert the cannula themselves, and this is particularly helpful for those with needle phobia, or for young children. The handset stores 90 days of data and can be downloaded to a computer. The disadvantages are the need to replace the pump every three days or so, and the external handset which is necessary to deliver mealtime boluses.

Totally implantable pumps that deliver insulin into the peritoneal cavity have been used in Europe and the USA for many years. Overall glycaemic control tends to be similar to that during MDI or CSII but with reduced fluctuations and fewer hypoglycaemic episodes. These pumps need to be implanted subcutaneously with a catheter placed in the peritoneal cavity; requiring a general anaesthetic. The insulin pump reservoir is topped up by using a syringe and needle via an injection port. The pump is programmed by a small external device which can be used to deliver variable basal rates and boluses. These devices are only funded in the UK on an individual patient basis and their use is really confined to patients with severe brittle diabetes who have not responded to CSII.

Clinical effectiveness

There have been a number of systematic reviews and meta analyses of pump therapy compared to multiple daily injections. There have also been several clinical trials with inconsistent results but there is broad agreement on the conclusions. Firstly, daily insulin requirements are usually lower on pump therapy (on average 15%). Secondly, the greatest improvement in glycaemic control is experienced by those with poorer control at the time of commencement of pump treatment. Thirdly, hypoglycaemia rates are reduced (Figure 10.10 and Table 10.4) and, finally, most patient surveys favour pump therapy for its flexibility and convenience.

Pump use increased in the UK after it received NICE approval. The latest NHS audit for 2017/18 showed that around 30% of people with type 1 diabetes aged <30 years were using pumps, with a total of 12,900 of all ages in England and Wales in the 63 centres who took part. This represents a likely national proportion of 17% of those with type 1 diabetes, which is much lower than many other countries in Europe and elsewhere. There was, however, a wide range of frequency of use of 5-40%, and a significantly lower use in the most economically deprived areas (16% vs 24% for the least deprived). 34% of pump users had an

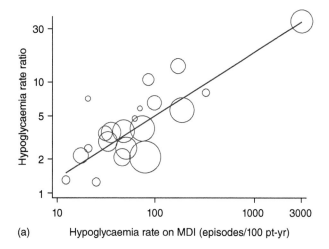

(a)　Hypoglycaemia rate on MDI (episodes/100 pt-yr)

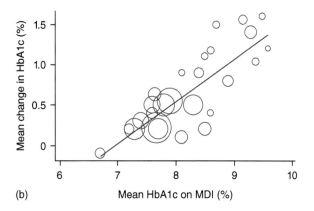

(b)　Mean HbA1c on MDI (%)

Figure 10.10 Meta regression analysis of mean effect size of insulin pump therapy on hypoglycaemia rate ratio (panel a) and HbA1c (panel b) compared to multiple daily injections (MDI) in a meta-analysis of trials comparing the two forms of treatment. Note that the greatest reductions in hypoglycaemia, as assessed by a larger rate ratio, and HbA1c were seen in those with the most episodes or the highest values at baseline. From Pickup JC. Diabetic Medicine 2019; 36: 269 – 78 with permission.

Table 10.4 Incidence of reported ketoacidosis and severe hypoglycaemia over 3 months prior to survey in 22,697 participants (age range 1 – 93 years) in the Type 1 Diabetes Exchange Registry in the USA audited 2016 – 18.

Treatment modality	Ketoacidosis	Severe Hypoglycaemia
Insulin Pump (± CGM)	2 %	5 %
Injections (± CGM)	4 %	9 %
CGM (Pump and Injections)	1 %	7 %
Blood Glucose Monitoring (Pump and Injections)	3 %	5 %

CGM = continuous glucose monitoring. Data from Foster et al Diabetes Technology & Therapeutics 2019; 21: 66 – 72.

Table 10.5 Achieved HbA1c on Multiple Daily Injections (MDI) or Continuous Subcutaneous Insulin Infusion (CSII) with and without Continuous Glucose Monitoring (CGM) in 22,697 people with type 1 diabetes enrolled onto the Type 1 Diabetes registry in the USA in 2016 – 18.

Age Group	MDI Alone	CSII Alone	MDI + CGM	CSII + CGM
< 13 yrs n = 3653	75 mmol/mol (9.0%)	72 mmol/mol (8.7%)	64 mmol/mol (8.0%)	63 mmol/mol (7.9%)
13– 26 yrs n = 10468	81 mmol/mol (9.6%)	75 mmol/mol (9.0%)	73 mmol/mol (8.8%)	67 mmol/mol (8.3%)
>26 yrs n = 6407	66 mmol/mol (8.2%)	62 mmol/mol (7.8%)	56 mmol/mol (7.3%)	57 mmol/mol (7.4%)

Data from Foster et al Diabetes Technology & Therapeutics 2019; 21: 66–72.

intermediate and long acting insulin), there were concerns about a potential increase in rates of ketoacidosis (DKA). These concerns have not been realised by experience, most recent surveys suggest rates of DKA are no more, or possibly less, that those seen with injection therapy (Table 10.4)

To realise the full metabolic potential of pump therapy requires huge effort from patients and professional teams, and, ideally, a 24 hour helpline. Insulin pump manufacturers offer emergency support for mechanical failures, but variable medical advice. Professional bodies have issued guidance on best practice for delivery of an insulin pump service (Box 10.1), and NICE recommends as a minimum, input from doctors, specialist nurses and dieticians.

Not all people with type 1 diabetes either want or are suitable for pump therapy. Many do not like the idea of being connected to a device; some struggle with the technology and the need to download information continually and use it for dose adjustments; and some dislike being reminded of their diabetes all the time. However, psychological or mental health problems alone should not preclude a trial of CSII; one centre reported significant benefit in terms of reduction of hospital admission rates with DKA, together with a reduction in HbA1c, even though the level on CSII was less than ideal at >75 mmol/mol (>9.0%). Estimates of the numbers of patients in the UK who might want or benefit from CSII

HbA1c < 58 mmol/mol (7.5%), compared to 27% on multiple injections. The authors concluded that pump therapy was under-utilised and commissioners needed to expand use, particularly in those areas with the lowest uptake.

In the USA, the Type 1 Diabetes Exchange Registry surveys its patients and care teams every few years and asks for information on control and complications from the preceding three months. In 2016-18, data on 22,697 patients aged between 1 and 93 years were collected. 63% were using pumps, and 30% continuous glucose monitoring (CGM) (either with pumps or injections). Glycaemic control was better on pumps, and pumps and CGM was best in young people (Table 10.5).

Because pump therapy necessarily means that patients have smaller amounts of insulin subcutaneously at any one time than those on injections (who will have variable amounts of

Box 10.1 Essential components of routine consultation with people using insulin pumps with or without continuous glucose monitoring.

Regular follow-up. (Note follow-up frequency can be perceived by patient as reward for best practice – paradoxically patients with best glucose control may prefer to be seen more frequently)

Visualise pump and meter data (preferably using computer) and use as basis of consultation

Discuss: Blood glucose monitoring frequency (or CGM use)
Mealtime bolus frequency and timing
Use of bolus calculators and review carbohydrate counting skills
Use of variable basal rates
Frequency of cannula site change (ideally every 3 days)
Exercise management (including mealtime bolus and basal rate adjustments)

Inspect cannula sites

Consider medical causes of poor control such as coeliac or thyroid disease

Consider group discussion or support

Consider motivational interviewing

Adapted from Pickup JC. Diabetic Medicine 2018; 36: 269–78.

Box 10.2 NICE Technology Guidance 151 on continuous subcutaneous insulin infusion.

Continuous subcutaneous insulin infusion is:
1. Recommended for adults and children over 12 years of age provided that:
   a) attempts to achieve target HbA1c on MDI result in disabling hypoglycaemia *or*
   b) HbA1c levels remain ≥ 69 mmol/mol (≥ 8.5%) on MDI despite high levels of care.
2. Recommended for children <12 years provided that:
   a) MDI is deemed impractical or inappropriate
   b) a trial of MDI should be considered between ages 12–18 years.
3. CSII should be initiated by a trained team comprising a physician with a specialist interest, a diabetes specialist nurse and a dietitian. Teams should provide structured education and advice on diet, lifestyle and exercise.
4. CSII should be continued if there is a sustained improvement in glycaemic control as evidenced by a reduction in HbA1c and/or number of hypoglycaemic episodes.

vary, but it is probable that at least 20% would accept the treatment and thus achieve benefit.

Cost effectiveness

Pump treatment has been estimated to cost 1.4 times that of MDI therapy. There are now several different insulin pumps available; they cost around £3000 in the UK with running costs of approximately £800–1000 per year. For closed loop devices, the sensors and other consumables increase the running costs to around £400 per month (according to NICE). Patch pumps tend to be more costly at index prices than externally worn systems. Part of the problem with comparing costings is that companies negotiate discounts with local providers in the UK and the information is deemed commercially sensitive. Most pumps have a 4 year warranty and life span. Mechanical problems are quite common and a source of patient dissatisfaction. The regulation of therapeutic devices is less stringent than for medications, and there have been initiatives from professional bodies to improve the situation.

For CSII alone compared to MDI therapy, a systematic review of studies of cost effectiveness found an incremental cost effectiveness ratio (ICER) for each quality adjusted life year (QALY) gained to be US$40,143 (95% CI 23,409, 56,876) for patients with poor glycaemic control and/or

hypoglycaemic unawareness with recurrent episodes. NICE assessed CSII in 2008 and found it to be cost effective according to their usual criterion of an ICER of £30,000 per QALY. They found that CSII was effective in terms of cost per QALY of £16,842 to £34,330; this fell to less than £29,000 when improvement associated with the reduction in severe hypoglycaemic rates was taken into account. Their guidance for indications for clinical use is summarised in Box 10.2. CSII should also now be offered to all pregnant women with type 1 diabetes who do not achieve blood glucose control without disabling hypoglycaemia.

Combination therapy of insulin with other hypoglycaemic therapies

Because some patients with type 1 diabetes have insulin resistance (insulin requirements > 1u/kg body weight/day) and obesity there have been studies exploring the use of oral agents as an adjunct to insulin therapy. Metformin has been shown to reduce body weight, but with no significant benefits in terms of insulin dose or glycaemic control. Pramlintide (a synthetic amylin analogue which slows gastric emptying) reduces post prandial hypoglycaemia and HbA1c and is licensed for use in type 1 diabetes in the USA (but not the UK).

Recently, there have been at least 10 studies of the use of Sodium Glucose Co-Transporter 2 (SGLT2) inhibitors in people with type 1 diabetes. Most have been of short duration (maximum 52 weeks) but meta-analysis has shown benefit in terms of reductions in fasting plasma glucose, HbA1c (by around 5mmol/mol (0.45%), body weight (~2.5kg) and total daily insulin dose. NICE has issued guidance for Dapagliflozin (Technology Appraisal 597) and Sotagliflozin (TA 622) approving their use in patients who have inadequate glycaemic control despite having completed a structured education programme such as DAFNE; who have a BMI ≥27 kg/m²; and who have a daily insulin dose of ≥0.5 units/kg body weight/day. If there is no improvement in glycaemic control after 6 months the treatment should be discontinued. There is a >3 fold increased risk of DKA, however, and NICE also recommends the provision of blood ketone monitoring for all patients on combination therapy. These two agents have also received approval in Europe, and Dapagliflozin in Japan, but at the time of writing none have been approved by the FDA in the USA.

It is unclear whether the cardiorenal benefits seen with these agents in people with type 2 diabetes will also occur in those with type1. It is also uncertain whether the benefits in terms of glycaemic control will be sustained long-term.

CASE HISTORY

A 40-year-old manager with type 1 diabetes had noticed a gradual deterioration in his glycaemic control. He developed diabetes aged 25 when working offshore and had to change career. He was managed on a twice-daily regimen of soluble and lente insulins. His doses of insulin had increased such that he was taking >120 units/day (~1.4 units/kg bodyweight) and he periodically experienced severe hypoglycaemia with little warning. His HbA1c was 66 mmol/mol (8.2%). He exercised regularly but was finding this more difficult because of general fatigue and hypoglycaemia. Investigations showed normal thyroid function and negative insulin antibodies.

He was commenced on CSII using human insulin and his total daily dose fell to 60 units. His fatigue and hypoglycaemic episodes disappeared and his HbA1c improved to 52 mmol/mol (6.9%). He has now been on CSII for 20 years and remains in stable control with minimal retinopathy..

Comment: Lente insulins could be associated with unpredictable hypoglycaemia. Part of the problem is the excess zinc in these preparations and the potential for this to accumulate under the skin. The cause of the fatigue was probably a combination of poor glycaemic control and hyperinsulinaemia. Insulin doses often fall on CSII, on average 15%, so the 50% reduction in this case is exceptional. It is also noteworthy that hypoglycaemia rates diminished despite a reduction in HbA1c. This man was converted to CSII pre glargine. He declined a trial of this analogue although current NICE guidance now suggests such a trial prior to commencing CSII.

LANDMARK CLINICAL TRIAL

DCCT Research Group. The effect of intensive treatment of diabetes on the development and progression of long-term complications in insulin-dependent diabetes mellitus. N Engl J Med 1993; 329: 977–986.

This study is often regarded as the landmark in type 1 diabetes research: 1441 patients in 29 centres in North America were allocated randomly to either 'conventional' therapy (one or two daily insulin injections, 3-monthly clinic visits, no insulin dosage adjustments according to self-monitored glucose data) or to 'intensive' therapy (three or more daily insulin injections or insulin pump therapy, monthly clinic visits, and weekly telephone calls, frequent blood glucose self-monitoring with insulin dosage adjustment, and a diet and exercise programme). Throughout the 9-year study, there was markedly better glycaemic control in the intensively treated group. After a mean of 6.5 years follow-up, the intensive treatment arm had an HbA1c of 7.4% versus 9.1% (56 versus 76 mmol/mol) in the conventionally treated patients. However, less than 5% in the intensive arm had an average HbA1c consistently within the normal range.

In the primary prevention arm there was a 76% risk reduction in retinopathy development, and a 54% risk reduction of retinopathy progression in the secondary prevention arm (63% risk reduction for both arms combined). Moreover, the link between increasing severity of hyperglycaemia and risk of retinopathy progression was confirmed conclusively in the conventional arm.

This study, together with the UKPDS in type 2 diabetes, showed conclusively that good glycaemic control matters in terms of the prevention of complications (it may seem extraordinary to us now but until these studies there was still huge debate about the importance of tight blood glucose control). The DCCT follow-up (Epidemiology of Diabetes Interventions and Complications (EDIC) has shown the long-term benefits of early tight glycaemic control and created the concept of 'metabolic memory' (Chapter 14).

KEY WEBSITES

- National Institute for Health and Clinical Excellence: www.nice.org.uk (NG 17 Type 1 diabetes in adults; NG 18 diabetes in children and young people; TA151 Continuous subcutaneous insulin infusion for the treatment of diabetes mellitus)
- American Diabetes Association www.diabetes.org
- Diabetes UK Care www.diabetes.org.uk
- Collaborative Islet Transplant Registry: www2.niddk.nih.gov/Research/ScientificAreas/Pancreas/EndocrinePancreas/CITR.htm
- SIGN Guidelines: www.SIGN.ac.uk
- NHS Audit https://files.digital.nhs.uk/E0/030707/NationalDiabetesInsulinPumpAudit%2017-18Reportv2.pdf
- ABCD Diabetes Technology Network abcd.care/dtn Best Practice guidelines for CSII and CGM https://www.sps.nhs.uk/wp-content/uploads/2018/05/Insulin-pump-table-May-2018.pdf Comparison of insulin pumps available in the UK in 2018
- www.carbsandcals.com Useful website for carbohydrate counting

FURTHER READING

American Diabetes Association. Standards of medical care in diabetes – 2020. Diabetes Care 2020; 43(Suppl 1): S66–76.

Beck RW, Bergenstal RM, Laffel LM, et al Advances in technology for management of type 1 diabetes. Lancet 2019; dx.doi.org/10.1016/ S0140-6736(19)31142-0

Foster NC, Beck RW, Miller KM et al. State of type 1 diabetes management and outcomes from the T!D exchange in 2016-2018. Diabetes Tech Ther 2019; 21: 66–72

Fullerton B, Jeitler K, Seitz M, et al. Intensive glucose control versus conventional glucose control for type 1 diabetes mellitus. Cochrane Database Syst Rev 2014, Issue 2. Art. No.: CD009122. DOI: 10.1002/14651858.CD009122.pub2.

Fullerton B, Siebenhofer A, Jeitler K et al. Short acting insulin analogues versus regular human insulin in patients with diabetes mellitus. Cochrane Database Syst Rev 2016; doi.org/10.1002/ 14651858/CD012161

Pickup JC. Is insulin pump therapy effective in type 1 diabetes? Diabetic Med 2019; 36: 269–78

Pickup JC, Sutton AJ. Severe hypoglycaemia and glycaemic control in type 1 diabetes: meta-analysis of multiple daily insulin injections versus continuous subcutaneous insulin infusion. Diabetic Med 2008; 25: 765–774.

Richter B, Neises G. 'Human' insulin versus animal insulin in people with diabetes. Cochrane Database Syst Rev 2004; 3: CD003816.

Roze S, Smith-Palmer J, Valentine W et al. Cost effectiveness of continuous subcutaneous insulin infusion versus multiple daily injections of insulin in Type 1 diabetes: a systematic review. Diabetic Med 2015; 32: 1415-24

Rossetti P, Ampudia-Blasco FJ, Ascaso JF. Old and new basal insulin formulations: understanding pharmacodynamics is still relevant in clinical practice. Diabetes Obesity & Metabolism 2014; 16: 695–706

Management of type 2 diabetes

The starting points and mainstays of treatment for type 2 diabetes are diet and other modifications of lifestyle, such as increasing exercise and stopping smoking (Figure 11.1). The major aims are to reduce the weight of obese patients and improve glycaemic control, but also to reduce risk factors for cardiovascular disease (CVD), such as hyperlipdaemia and hypertension, which account for 70–80% of deaths in type 2 diabetes.

Weight loss is achieved by decreasing total energy intake and/or increasing physical activity and thus energy expenditure. Gradual weight loss is preferred – not more than 0.5–1 kg/week. For the effective weight loss and improvement in glycaemic control, the amount of energy restriction is more important than dietary composition, though compliance may be greater with high monounsaturated fat diets (Figure 11.2). Weight loss of as little as 4kg will often ameliorate hyperglycaemia. Reduced-calorie diets result in clinically significant weight loss regardless of which macronutrients they emphasize.

Anti-obesity drugs currently play a minor part in the management of the obese patients with diabetes. This is because of the increased availabilities of novel antidiabetic agents with concurrent weight reducing effects such as glucagon like peptide-1 (GLP-1) analogue and the sodium glucose

co-transporter-2 (SGLT-2) inhibitor. One such anti-obesity drug is Orlistat. This agent acts locally in the gastrointestinal tract, where it blocks enzymatic digestion of triglyceride by inhibiting pancreatic lipase, inhibiting the absorption of up to 30% of ingested fat (Figure 11.3). Gastrointestinal side effects are common, including flatulence, steatorrhoea, and, occasionally, faecal incontinence. A diet rich in fruit and vegetables is needed to avoid fat-soluble vitamin deficiency.

Another anti-obesity drug is Mysimba. This contains 8 mg naltrexone hydrochloride (equivalent to 7.2 mg of naltrexone)/90 mg bupropion hydrochloride (equivalent to 78 mg of bupropion. It is currently indicated, as an adjunct to a reduced calorie diet and increased physical activity, for the management of weight in adult patients (≥18 years) with an initial Body Mass Index (BMI) of ≥30 kg/m² (obese) or ≥27 kg/m² (overweight) in the presence of one or more weight-related co-morbidities (e.g. type 2 diabetes, dyslipidaemia or controlled hypertension) (Figure 11.4).

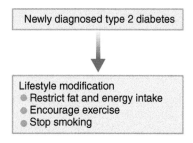

FIGURE 11.1 Management of type 2 diabetes: the initial measures.

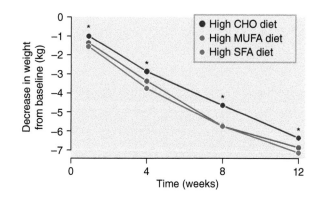

FIGURE 11.2 Change in weight during energy restriction is similar with high carbohydrate diet (CHO), high monounsaturated fatty acid (MUFA) diet and high saturated fatty acid (SFA) diet. From Heilbronn et al. Diabetes Care 1999; 22: 889 – 895.

Handbook of Diabetes, Fifth Edition. Rudy Bilous, Richard Donnelly, and Iskandar Idris.
© 2021 John Wiley & Sons Ltd. Published 2021 by John Wiley & Sons Ltd.

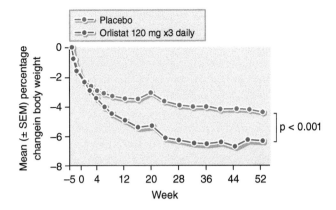

FIGURE 11.3 Effect of Orlistat in obese patients with type 2 diabetic. From Hollander et al. Diabetes Care 1998; 21: 1288 – 1294.

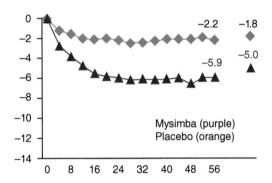

Figure 11.4 Effect of Mysimba in obese patients with type 2 diabetes. Redrawn from Hollander P. et al. *Diabetes Care*. 2013; 36: 4022–4029.

Practical food recommendations for patients with diabetes

- Quench thirst with water or other sugar- free drinks
- Eat regular meals, avoiding fried and very sugary foods
- Eat plenty of vegetables
- Have high-fibre and low glycaemic index foods, including whole grains, legumes or brown rice as the main part of each meal
- Limit consumption of high glycaemic index starchy foods, such as mashed potatoes and white bread
- Eat plenty of whole fruit
- Limit consumption of animal products with high amounts of cholesterol and saturated fat, such as red meat, eggs, liver and high-fat dairy products, and substitute them with lean meat, fish, poultry (without skin) and low-fat dairy products
- For snacks between meals, avoid convenience foods such as biscuits, cake or confectionery (which are high in saturated and trans-fats and salt); use nuts and fruits for snacks instead
- Use natural liquid vegetable oils for cooking, baking and frying instead of vegetable shortenings (solid vegetable fat, high in saturates and trans- fatty acids)
- Use trans-fat-free or soft margarine instead of stick (hardened) margarine or butter
- Be aware of the portion size of a meal, especially when eating in a restaurant. Do not overeat
- If blood glucose control is satisfactory, light to moderate drinking of alcohol (1 unit per day for women and 1–2 for men) is fine, but drink alcoholic beverages with a meal

FIGURE 11.5 Practical food recommendations for patients with diabetes.

The dietary recommendations are essentially the same for type 1 and type 2 diabetes – and, indeed, follow a healthy eating plan suitable for the entire population (Figure 11.5). Saturated fat should be reduced and replaced with mono-unsaturated fat such as olive oil or polyunsaturated fats. n-6 polyunsaturated fat, found in vegetable oils, is also beneficial for cholesterol lowering and improving glycaemic control. Dietary cholesterol may be more detrimental in diabetics than in the general population. Fish oils are rich in n-3 fatty acids and have lower triglyceride levels, and there is evidence that higher fish intake is associated with less CVD in diabetes; accordingly, 2–3 servings of fish per week are recommended. Carbohydrate consumption should be moderate and ideally should mainly come from fruit, vegetables, whole grains and pulses. The actual amount of carbohydrate that you need to eat will depend of your age, activity levels, and goals you are trying to achieve. However, the total amount of carbohydrate eaten will have the biggest effect on your glucose levels after eating, so carbohydrate awareness is important in managing blood glucose levels in people with diabetes. Simple dietary guidelines in the form of recommended foods are normally best for patients, and are better understood than measures of fat, carbohydrate, or protein. 'Diabetic' foods that contain sorbitol or fructose as sweetener are not necessary. Sucrose need be significantly restricted from the diabetic diet, and a moderate amount for sweetening is acceptable. The focus of dietary plans should be on balancing energy intake to energy expenditure and the quality of fat and carbohydrate, rather than the quantity alone. Foods that normally improve glycaemic control and CVD risk are whole grains (brown rice, whole-wheat breads, oats) and high-fibre foods (grains, cereals, fruits, vegetables, and nuts).

Several programmes have been developed in Europe and North America to educate patients about diabetes. An example in the UK for patients with type 2 diabetes is the diabetes education and self management for ongoing and newly diagnosed (DESMOND) structured education programme. Clinical studies have shown that structured education programmes focused on behaviour change can successfully engage those with newly diagnosed type 2 diabetes in starting effective lifestyle changes that are sustainable. Benefits of DESMOND include improvements in illness beliefs, weight loss, physical activity, smoking status, and depression.

Exercise should be tailored to the individual patient, according to physical condition and lifestyle, but simple advice might include moderate exercise as part of the daily schedule, such as walking for 30–60 minutes per day (preferably an extra 30–60 minutes). Current guidelines suggest that people with diabetes should accumulate a minimum of 150 minutes of moderate to vigorous intensity aerobic exercise each week, spread over at least 3 days of the week, with no more than 2 consecutive days without exercise. In addition, people with diabetes (including elderly people) should perform resistance exercise at least twice a week, and preferably 3 times per week in addition to aerobic exercise. In people with type 1 diabetes, evidence suggests that undertaking anaerobic exercise therapy first followed by aerobic exercise will reduce the risk of developing hypoglycaemia. Regular exercise has been shown to reduce long-term mortality by 50–60% in people with type 2 diabetes compared with patients with poor cardiorespiratory fitness.

There is a progressive decline in β-cell function and insulin sensitivity in type 2 diabetes, which results in deteriorating glycaemic control and the constant need to revise and intensify treatment. Diet and exercise are sufficient to achieve adequate glycaemic control in <10% of type 2 patients; when control worsens, an oral hypoglycaemic agent is generally introduced (Figure 11.6).

The particular drug treatment used in an individual patient with type 2 diabetes is decided on the basis of clinical judgement about the individual need of the patients, balance of β-cell impairment and insulin resistance, risk of hypoglycaemia, need to lose weight, patients symptoms, and optimal glucose control in that particular case. More recently, evidence has emerged regarding the efficacy of certain glucose lowering therapies to improve clinical outcomes in patients with atherosclerotic cardiovascular disease (ASCVD), heart failure or diabetic kidney disease. Accordingly, recent consensus guideline have recommended the use of selected therapies in preference of others according to presence of co-morbidities. Metformin therapy remains as the first line treatment option (Figures 11.7 and 11.8).

Metformin is a derivative of guanidine, the active ingredient of goat's rue (Galega officianalis) – used as a treatment for diabetes in medieval Europe. Metformin increases insulin action (the exact mechanism is unclear), lowering glucose mainly by decreasing hepatic glucose output. Unlike sulfonylureas, it does not cause hypoglycaemia or weight gain and, indeed, has some appetite-suppressing activity that may encourage weight loss. A typical starting dose of metformin is 500 mg daily or twice daily, rising to 850 mg thrice daily. Major side effects are nausea, anorexia, or diarrhoea, which affect about one-third of patients. Lactic acidosis is a rare but serious side-effect that carries high mortality. It can be avoided by not giving metformin to patients with renal, hepatic, cardiac, or respiratory failure or those with a history of alcohol abuse.

Sulfonylureas stimulate insulin secretion by binding to sulfonylurea (SUR-1) receptors on the β-cell plasma membrane, which leads to closure of the ATP-sensitive K+ channel (Kir6.2), membrane depolarization, opening of calcium channels, calcium influx and exocytosis of insulin granules (Figure 11.9). The most serious side effect is hypoglycaemia, which is more likely to occur with glibenclamide, especially in older patients and those with renal impairment. Modest weight gain may also accompany sulfonylurea use.

The thiazolidinediones ('glitazones') are insulin sensitizers that enter the cell and bind to the peroxisome proliferator-activated receptor-γ (PPARγ), a nuclear receptor found predominantly in adipocytes, but also in the muscle and liver (Figure 11.10). PPARγ forms a complex with the retinoid X receptor (RXR), and binding of a TZD leads to enhanced expression of certain insulin-sensitive genes, such as GLUT4, lipoprotein lipase, fatty acid transporter protein, and fatty acyl CoA synthase. This increases glucose uptake and utilisation, increases adipocyte lipogenesis and decreases circulating fatty acid levels. There is also decreased production of the cytokine tumour necrosis factor-alpha (TNF-α) and of resistin.

The first TZD, troglitazone, was associated with serious hepato-toxicity and withdrawn. Rosiglitazone and pioglitazone do not have adverse effects on the liver – in fact, they may reverse fatty infiltration of the liver and improve liver function in some patients – but they are associated

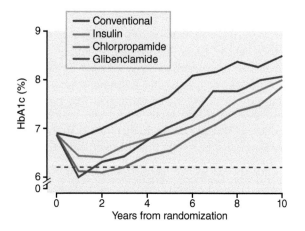

FIGURE 11.6 The progressive rise in median HbA1c with time in the conventionally treated and intensively treated groups in the United Kingdom Prospective Diabetes Study. HbA1c deteriorated in both groups, despite escalating therapy. A continued decline in β-cell function, following the diagnosis of type 2 diabetes, is likely to account for this deterioration in HbA1c over time, illustrating that type 2 diabetes is a progressive disorder. From Al-Delaimy et al. *Diabetes Care* 2001; 24: 2043 – 2048.

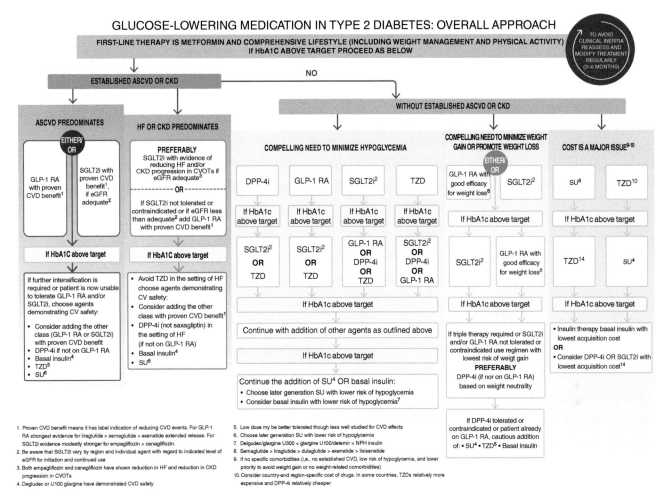

Figure 11.7 Pharmacologic Approaches to Glycemic Treatment in type 2 diabetes. Consensus statement from the American Diabetes Association (ADA) and the European Association for the Study of Diabetes (EASD). Davies MJ. *Diabetes Care* 2018; 41(12): 2669–2701.

with fluid retention, weight gain, and oedema. More importantly, some patients may develop features of heart failure. Recent data also suggest an increased risk of vertebral fracture risk associated with TZD therapy. Because PPARγ receptors are widely expressed in the vasculature, there has been considerable interest in the cardiovascular effects of these drugs. In one trial (the PROACTIVE study) pioglitazone as add-on therapy (vs placebo) was associated with significant reductions in fatal and nonfatal myocardial infarction (MI) and stroke (secondary endpoints in the trial), meanwhile a meta-analysis of studies concluded that, relative to other antidiabetic agents, rosiglitazone was associated with a two- to threefold increased risk of MI. As a result of this, rosiglitazone is no longer available for clinical use especially in Europe. Differential effects on LDL-cholesterol might explain the different effects of pioglitazone and rosiglitazone on cardiovascular outcomes.

DPP-IV inhibitors are orally active and generally well tolerated. As add-on therapy to metformin, they lower HbA1c

to the same extent as sulfonylureas but have a lower incidence of hypoglycaemia because GLP-1 effects on pancreatic β- and α-cells are dependent upon glucose. Several DPP-IV inhibitors are available, namely Sitagliptin. Saxagliptin, Alogliptin, Linagliptin and Vildagliptin. DPP-IV inhibitors are weight neutral. Evidence from randomized controlled trial suggests neutral effect on cardiovascular outcome and mortality, but in the Saxagliptin Assessment of Vascular Outcomes Recorded in Patients with Diabetes Mellitus–Thrombolysis in Myocardial Infarction 53 (SAVOR-TIMI 53), patients randomly assigned to saxagliptin unexpectedly had a significantly higher risk of hospitalisation for heart failure. The reason for this is unclear, and some suggest that this was a chance finding, since other studies including observation studies have not observed similar findings.

A new class of oral glucose lowering therapy is the sodium glucose co-transporter 2 (SGLT-2) inhibitor. Glucose from the circulation is normally filtered into the renal tubule. The normal renal glucose handling reabsorbs back into the

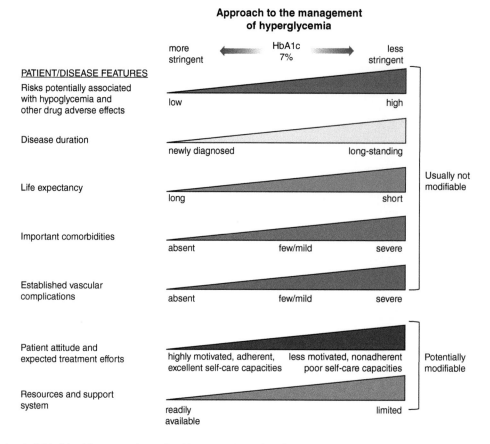

Approach to the management of hyperglycemia

Figure 11.8 Approach to individualising Hba1c target in people with type 2. Adapted from Silvio E. Inzucchi et al. *Diabetes Care* 2015; 38:140–149.

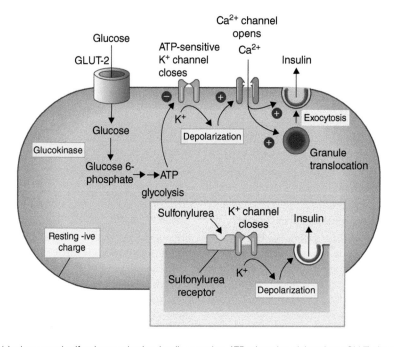

Figure 11.9 Mechanism by which glucose and sulfonylureas stimulate insulin secretion. ATP, adenosine triphosphate; GLUT, glucose transporter.

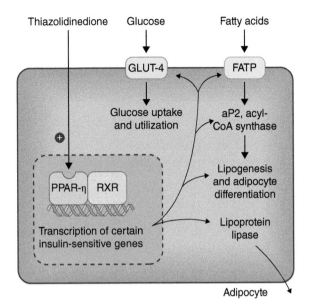

Thiazolidinedione Glucose Fatty acids

Figure 11.10 Mechanism of action of TZDs. These agents stimulate the peroxisome proliferator-activated receptor-γ (PPARγ) in the cell nucleus, mainly in the adipocyte. In conjunction with the retinoid X receptor (RXR), this promotes transcription of certain genes and increased expression of glucose transporter 4 (GLUT-4), fatty acid transporter protein (FATP), adipocyte fatty acid-binding protein (aP2), fatty acyl coenzyme A (CoA) synthase, and other enzymes involved in lipogenesis.

circulation, 90% of filtered glucose in the proximal tubule via the SGLT2 receptors. The remaining 10% of filtered glucose is reabsorbed back into the circulation via the SGLT1 receptor. The SGLT2 inhibitor therapy works by inhibiting the reabsorption of glucose back into the circulation, such that at maximum circulating hyperglycaemia, a large amount of glucose (>60g) is excreted into the urine. The net effect is the reduction of circulating glucose, concurrent energy (calorie) loss and lowering of blood pressure. Because of the mechanism of action, SGLT2 inhibitor is recommended to be initiated only in patients with preserved renal function (i.e. estimated glomerular filtration rate, eGFR of >60; or if declining eGFR, to continue until eGFR is <45. However, clinical trial evidence have shown the benefits of this therapy to improve cardiovascular and renal outcomes persists even in patients with lower eGFR, with normal HbA1c levels or even in the absence of type 2 diabetes. Therefore, clinical evaluation on risk benefits of this therapy needs to be considered when prescribing for patients with co-morbidities such as heart failure of chronic kidney disease. Important side-effects of this class of therapy include increase risk of genital tract infection, volume depletion, and a small risk of developing diabetic ketoacidosis (DKA), even with normal blood sugar levels (euglycaemic DKA). To avoid DKA, patients are advice to stop this therapy in event of volume depletion (diarrhoea or vomiting), during acute severe illness or when admitted to hospital (Figure 11.11).

In addition to Hba1c, weight and blood pressure reduction, recent studies have shown that this class of therapy was associated with a significant reduction in cardiovascular events, reduction in hospitalisation for heart failure and improvement in renal outcomes. The first of these studies was the **Empa-Reg** study which showed that Empagliflozin was associated with a lower rate of the primary composite cardiovascular outcome and of death from any cause when the study drug was added to standard care. A subsequent study known as the **CANVAS** study showed that Canagliflozin had a lower risk of cardiovascular events than those who received placebo but unexpectedly a greater risk of amputation, primarily at the level of the toe or metatarsal. The later observation on amputation risk with canagliflozin was mainly seen in patients with a history of previous amputation and peripheral vascular disease and have not been reported in any other Canagliflozin related studies. Another SGLT2 inhibitor, Dapagliflozin was shown in **DECLARE** study to not result in a higher or lower rate of Major Adverse Cardiovascular Event (MACE) than placebo but did result in a lower rate of cardiovascular death or hospitalisation for heart failure. The mechanism for the benefits of SGLT2 inhibitor is unclear, although reduction in blood pressure, heart failure progression or switch in fuel/substrate utilisation have been suggested as the potential mechanism for the observed cardiovascular benefits. Interestingly, subanalysis of all these studies have consistently shown significant benefits on heart failure and renal related endpoints. The **CREDENCE** study meanwhile investigated the specific effects of Canaglflozin on renal endpoints – the primary outcome was a composite of end-stage kidney disease (dialysis, transplantation, or a sustained estimated GFR of <15 ml per minute per 1.73 m²), a doubling of the serum creatinine level, or death from renal or cardiovascular causes. This showed that in patients with type 2 diabetes and kidney disease, the risk of kidney failure and cardiovascular events was lower in the canagliflozin group than in the placebo group.

Glucagon like peptide-1 (GLP-1) analogue is an injectable therapy available for the treatment of type 2 diabetes. Increased circulating levels of GLP-1 confers beneficial effects on glucose metabolism and energy expenditure by increasing beta cell insulin production, supressing glucagon production for the pancreatic alpha cells, delay in gastric emptying and reduction of appetite. They are licensed as add-on to metformin, SU or TZD, and as triple therapy. Currently available GLP-1 analogues include exenatide, liraglutide, lixisenatide, Exenatide (Slow release), Dulaglutide, Albiglutide and Semaglutide. They are administered by fixed-dose subcutaneous injection, once daily (Liraglutide or Lixisenatide) or once weekly (Exenatide slow release, Dulaglutide, Semaglutide and Albiglutide), and are best suited to obese patients (BMI>30) who have inadequate HbA1c control despite combination oral therapy. These drugs are associated

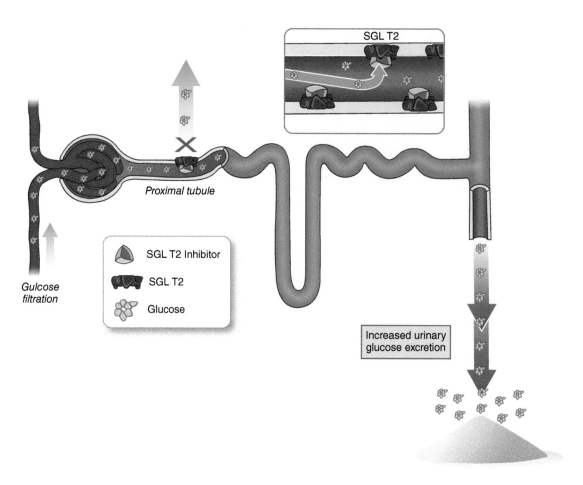

Figure 11.11 Mechanism of action of SGLT- 2 inhibitor.

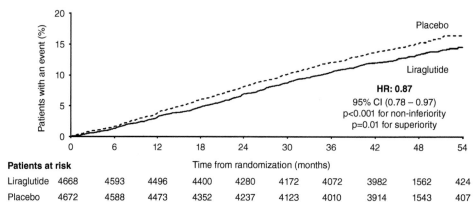

Primary outcome

CV death, non-fatal myocardial infarction, or non-fatal stroke

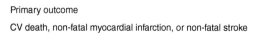

The primary composite outcome in the time-to-event analysis was the first occurrence of death from cardiovascular causes, non-fatal myocardial infarction, or non-fatal stroke. The cumulative incidences were estimated with the use of the Kaplan–Meier method, and the hazard ratios with the use of the Cox proportional-hazard regression model. The data analyses are truncated at 54 months, because less than 10% of the patients had an observation time beyond 54 months. CI: confidence interval; CV: cardiovascular; HR: hazard radio.

Presented at the American Diabetes Association 76th Scientific Sessions, Session 3-CT-SY24. June 13 2016, New Orleans, LA, USA.

Figure 11.12 LEADER STUDY. (available free online from https://tracs.unc.edu/index.php/leader?download=1925:leader-results-20160613).

with significant and progressive weight loss (more than any other class of glucose lowering therapies), but 20–30% of patients may experience nausea or sickness. Similar to SGLT 2 inhibitor, recent data have shown beneficial effects of Liraglutide, Semaglutide, Dulaglutide and Albiglutide in reducing cardiovascular event. However, unlike SGLT2 inhibitor, consistent benefits on renal or heart failure related endpoints have not been seen (Figures 11.12 and 11.13).

In recent years, significant interest has emerged considering the role of very low calorie diets (VLCD) for managing

Intervention	Mechanism of action	Expected HbA1c change (%)	Glucose	Weight	BP[a]	Lipid profile	Advantages	Associated Risks
Step 1: Initial therapy **Lifestyle modification**	– Reduce weight – Increase activity –Quit smoking/alcohol	1.0–2.0	↓↓	↓	↓	↓	– Natural – No known side–effect	– Inability to sustain glycaemic control in many after one year
Metformin	– Decreases hepatic glucose output – Increases insulin sensitivity and lowers fasting glycaemia[44, 80]	1.0–2.0	↓↓	↔	↔	↓LDL ↔HDL ↓Trigly[b]	– Weight stability or moderate weight loss – No hypos – ↓Cardiac events	– GI side effects – Contraindicated in renal problems – Lactic acidosis (in the presence of renal failure and hypovolaemia). – CKD, Hypoxia
Second line **Sulfonylureas** • Chlorpropamide • Glibenclamide • Gliclazide • Glimepiride • Glipizide • Glyburide	– Enhance insulin secretion	1.0–2.0	↓↓	↑↑↑	↔	↓LDL ↔LDL ↓Trigly	– Rapidly effective – ↓Microvascular risk	– Weight gain – Hypoglycaemia – Blunting of myocardial ischaemic preconditioning – Low durability
Thiazolidinediones • Pioglitazone • Rosiglitazone	– Reduces peripheral insulin resistance – ↑Insulin sensitivity	0.5–1.4	↓↓	↑↑↑	↑	↑LDL ↑HDL Trigly ↑(Rosi) ↓(Pio)	– Improves insulin sensitivity – Improves lipid profile – No hypos – ↑Durability – ?↓CVD events	– Fluid retention, CHF – Weight gain, bone fractures – Risk of bladder cancer – ?↑risk of MI
GLP–1RA[c] agonists • Exenatide • Liraglutide • Lixisenatide • Dulaglutide • Albiglutide • Semaglutide	– Bind and activate glucagon–like peptide (GLP–1 RA) receptors to • Suppress glucagon secretion, • Increase insulin secretion and • Slow gastric emptying • Reduce appetite	0.5–1.0	↓↓	↓↓	↓	↓LDL ↔HDL ↓Trigly	– Prevent weight gain or promote loss – No hypos – Reduce cardiovascular events with selected GLP1RA – Reduce postprandial glucose excursions	– GI side effects – High cost – ?Acute pancreatitis – Subcutaneous injection
SGLT2[d] inhibitors • Canagliflozin • Dapagliflozin • Empagliflozin • Ertugliflozin • Ipragliflozin	– Reversibly inhibit SGLT2 in the proximal convoluted tubules of the nephrons causing... • Decrease in glucose absorption • Increase in urinary glucose excretion[80]	0.7–1.3	↓	↓	↓	↑LDL ↑HDL ↔Trigly	– Reduce body weight – Lowers Systolic blood pressure – No hypos – Effective at all stages of T2DM – Reduce cardiovascular events – Improve heart failure and renal outcomes	– Genitourinary infections – Polyuria – Volume depletion, hypotension and dizziness – Transient ↑ in creatinine – Diabetic ketoacidosis

Figure 11.13 Summary of glucose lowering therapy in type 2 diabetes. Adapted Silvio E. Inzucchi et al. *Diabetes Care* 2015; 38(1): 140–149; Alvarez et al. (2015); Nathan et al. (2009).

DPP-4 Inhibitors[e] • Linagliptin • Saxagliptin • Sitagliptin • Vildagliptin • Alogliptin	– Inhibits DPP-4 activity – ↑postprandial active incretin – ↑Insulin secretion – ↓ production of glucagon	0.6–0.9	↓	↔	↔	↔LDL ↔HDL ↓Trigly	– Weight neutral – No hypos – Well tolerated	– Can interfere with immune function – Increased upper respiratory infection – Angioedema/urticaria
α-Glucosidase Inhibitors • Acarbose • Miglitol	• ↓ rate of digestion of polysaccharides • Inhibits intestinal α-Glucosidase • Lowers post-prandial glucose	0.5–0.8	↓↓	↔	↔	↔	– No hypos – ↓post-prandial glucose – ↓CVD events – Non-systemic	– Increased intestinal gas production – GI symptoms – Frequent dosing schedule
Amylin mimetics • Pramlintide	Synthetic analogue of amylin (β-cell hormone). Similar actions to GLP-1RA	0.5–0.7	↓↓	↓↓	↓	↓LDL ↔HDL ↓Trigly	– Weight loss (approx. 1–1.5kg over 6 months) – Decreases post prandial glucose excursion	– GI side effects – Hypoglycaemia – Frequent dosing – Difficulty injecting it – Reluctance by patients
Meglitinides (glinides) • Repaglinide • Nateglinide	– Closes K-channels – ↑insulin secretions	unknown	↓↓	↑↑	↔	↔	– ↓postprandial glucose excursion – Flexibility in dosing	– Hypoglycaemia – ↑weight – Frequent dosing schedule

[a]BP: Blood Pressure. [b]Tgly: Triglyceride. [c]GLP-1RA: Glucagon-like Peptide 1 agonist. [d]SGLT2: Sodium-glucose co-transporter 2. [e]DPP-4i: Dipeptidyl peptidase-4 Inhibitors

Figure 11.13 (Continued)

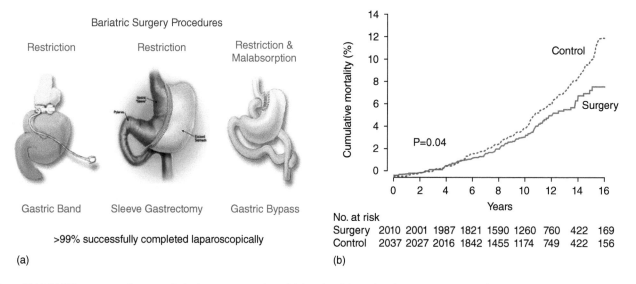

Bariatric Surgery Procedures

Restriction   Restriction   Restriction & Malabsorption

Gastric Band   Sleeve Gastrectomy   Gastric Bypass

>99% successfully completed laparoscopically

(a)

(b)

Figure 11.14 (a) Different types of common bariatric surgery procedures **(b)** there is evidence that obese patients undergoing bariatric surgery survive longer. Sjostrom et al. N Engl. J. Med. 2004; 351: 2683–2693.

overweight and obese people patients with T2D. This interest was primarily driven by a widely cited study, providing mechanistic evidence of a 600 kCal/day VLCD causing remission from T2D by reduction in pancreatic and liver triacylglycerol (a main constituent of body fat) content and recovery of pancreatic beta cell to produce insulin. Further studies have confirmed the beneficial effects of these interventions to maintain remission of type 2 diabetes in routine clinical practice. DiRECT study aimed to establish whether a structured programme, delivered by primary care nurses or dietitians, could achieve and maintain remission of type 2 diabetes. Remission

(off all anti-diabetic drugs) occurred in 46% of participants after 12 months and 36% after 24 months. Unlike previous smaller, non-randomised studies from specialist centres, the findings from DiRECT provide hard evidence of efficacy to inform decisions about provision of health care. Eligibility for this study, and subsequent roll out to patients in clinical practice in the United Kingdom are: duration of type 2 diabetes of <6 years, not taking insulin treatment and overweight – with a body mass index of 27–45 kg/m². No previous randomised trial in primary care has been specifically powered for remission of type 2 diabetes as its primary outcome. In clinical terms, VLCD is defined as a diet of <800kcal/d (<3347KJ/d) with a modified macronutrient composition to maximise weight reduction while minimising losses of lean body mass. The United Kingdom National Institute for Health and Clinical Excellence (NICE) supports the use of this approach for up to three months in a supervised setting for patients who fail to achieve a target weight loss with standard low-fat, reduced-energy approaches.

For very obese patients with type 2 diabetes (BMI>35), bariatric surgery is an increasingly recognised treatment option. Results with laparascopic adjustable gastric banding, sleeve gastrectomy, or Roux-Y-gastric bypass have demonstrated significant durable weight loss (often >20 kg), improved glycaemic control, and increased rate of remission of type 2 diabetes. Bariatric surgery has also been shown to improve obesity related comorbidities such as obstructive sleep apnoea, non-alcohol fatty liver disease (NAFLD), hypertension or hyperlipdaemia. Due to possible acute complications related to surgery and anaesthesia, as well as long-term side effects such as malabsorption, dumping syndrome, maladaptive eating behaviour, psycho-social problems, or weight regain, careful patient assessment and selection is important. Patients will also require life-long follow-up by specialist teams and/or primary care physicians to ensure that patients are receiving adequate long-term mineral and vitamin replacements (Figure 11.4).

CASE HISTORY

A 54-year-old man with a 5 year history of type 2 diabetes presents to his GP for annual review. This shows BMI 32, BP 156/94 mmHg and HbA1c 7.8% using a maximum-tolerated dose of metformin 1g bid and gliclazide 80mg bid. He has background retinopathy and a history of previous myocardial infarction. He takes some exercise, but is limited by arthritis. There have been no significant hypos, LDL-cholesterol is 3.1mmol/L using a statin. He has some symptoms of tiredness and nocturia.

Comment: If there is no further scope to improve his compliance with diet and exercise this man will require additional therapy in view of his established complications. Options would include adding basal insulin, GLP-1 analogue, pioglitazone, SGLT2 inhibitors, or a DPP-IV inhibitor. Treatment needs to be individualised according to patients' phenotype and presence of comorbidities. In view of his excess weight, consideration needs to be made on using agents which may induce weight loss like an SGLT2 inhibitor or GLP-1 analogue. These two classes of drugs have also been shown in a randomised controlled trial to reduce cardiovascular mortality in patients with a high risk of cardiovascular disease. Pioglitazone is an effective insulin sensitiser but may worsen his obesity. A DPP-IV inhibitor is also an option, either instead of SU (if hypos were a problem) or as an add-on therapy. DPP-IV inhibitor also has the advantage of being weight neutral and is generally very well tolerated.

LANDMARK CLINICAL TRIALS

Look AHEAD Research Group. Reduction in weight and cardiovascular disease risk factors in individuals with type 2 diabetes: one year results of the Look AHEAD trial. Diabetes Care 2007; 30: 1374–83.

The ACCORD study group. Effects of intensive glucose lowering in type 2 diabetes. N. Engl. J. Med. 2008; 358: 2545–59.

Marso SP, Daniels GH, Brown-Frandsen K, et al. Liraglutide and Cardiovascular Outcomes in Type 2 Diabetes. New England Journal of Medicine 2016; 375(4): 311–22.

Turnbull FM, Abraira C, Anderson RJ, et al. Intensive glucose control and macrovascular outcomes in type 2 diabetes. Diabetologia 2009; 52(11): 2288–98.

The ADVANCE Collaborative Group.Intensive Blood Glucose Control and Vascular Outcomes in Patients with Type 2 Diabetes. New England Journal of Medicine 2008; 358(24): 2560–72.

UK Prospective Diabetes Study (UKPDS) Group. Intensive blood-glucose control with sulfonylureas or insulin compared with conventional treatment and risk of complications in patients with type 2 diabetes (UKPDS 33). The Lancet 1998; 352(9131): 837–53.

Zinman B, Wanner C, Lachin JM et al., for the EMPA-REG OUTCOME Investigators Empagliflozin, Cardiovascular Outcomes, and Mortality in Type 2 Diabetes NEJM 2015; 373: 2117–2128 November 26, 2015 DOI: 10.1056/NEJMoa1504720

Perkovic V, Jardine MJ, Neal B et al. Canagliflozin and renal outcomes in type 2 diabetes and nephropathy. NEJM 2019; 380: 2295–2306

Wiviott SD, Raz I, Bonaca MP et al. Dapagliflozin and cardiovascular outcomes in type 2 diabetes. NEJM 2019; 380: 347–357

Marso SP, McGuire DK, Zinman B, et al. Efficacy and Safety of Degludec versus Glargine in Type 2 Diabetes. New England Journal of Medicine 2017; 377: 723–732 August 24, 2017 DOI: 10.1056/NEJMoa1615692l.

Lean MEJ, Leslie WS, Barnes AC et al. Primary care-led weight management for remission of type 2 diabetes (DiRECT): an open-label, cluster-randomised trial. Lancet. 2017; 391: 541–551

KEY WEBSITES

- www.nice.org.uk/guidance/cg87/chapter/1-Guidance
- http://www.who.int/diabetes/facts/world_figures/en/
- www.idf.org/diabetesatlas;

FURTHER READING

Davies MJ Diabetes Care Consensus statement from the American Diabetes Association (ADA) and the European Association for the Study of Diabetes (EASD) 2018 Diabetes Dec; 41(12): 2669–2701

Inzucchi SE, Bergenstal RM, Buse JB, et al. Management of Hyperglycemia in Type 2 Diabetes, 2015: A Patient-Centered Approach: Update to a Position Statement of the American Diabetes Association and the European Association for the Study of Diabetes. Diabetes Care 2015; 38(1): 140–9.

Riddle MC, Ambrosius WT, Brillon DJ, et al. Epidemiologic relationships between A1C and all-cause mortality during a median 3.4-year follow-up of glycemic treatment in the ACCORD trial. Diabetes Care 2010; 33(5): 983–90.

Diabetic ketoacidosis (DKA), hyperglycaemic hyperosmolar state (HHS) and lactic acidosis

KEY POINTS

- Diabetic ketoacidosis (DKA) is a state of severe uncontrolled diabetes characterized by hyperglycaemia, hyperketonaemia and metabolic acidosis in the context of absolute insulin deficiency.
- Frequency of DKA at diagnosis may be increasing, especially in children. In 2014 the incidence of admission for DKA in the USA was 7.7/1000 people with diabetes. Reported adult prevalence is between 50–100/1000 with type 1 diabetes.
- Reported mortality rates range from 0.7–5.0% but have declined from 4.2/10,000 people with diabetes in the USA in 1990 to 1.5/10,000 in 2010. DKA accounts for 54–76% of deaths in people with type 1 diabetes under 30 years of age.
- Treatment requires fluid and electrolyte infusions with careful potassium replacement, and insulin by either intravenous infusion or intramuscular or subcutaneous injection (in milder cases).

- Hyperosmolar hyperglycaemic state (HHS) used to be called HONK. It is characterized by extreme hyperglycaemia and dehydration without acidosis. Treatment is similar to that for DKA with the notable difference that insulin is commenced after rehydration. Mortality is higher as a reflection of its occurrence in the older population and the severity of the underlying precipitating causes.
- Lactic acidosis is a rare but serious metabolic crisis that may be more frequent in people with diabetes. Treatment requires intravenous bicarbonate infusion in addition to rehydration, and mortality is high.

Diabetic ketoacidosis (DKA) is a state of severe uncontrolled diabetes caused by insulin deficiency. It is characterised by hyperglycaemia, hyperketonaemia, and metabolic acidosis. There is no universal consensus on the diagnostic criteria or the grading of severity, but in the USA, DKA has been somewhat arbitrarily divided into mild, moderate, and severe based upon biochemical and clinical features (Table 12.1).

The frequency of DKA increased by 35% in the USA in the decade 1996–2006. There were 188 965 hospital admissions in 2014 costing over 5.1 billion US dollars. Incidence rates of 1–5% have been reported worldwide and are higher in younger type 1 patients and in females. In the UK there were 12 326 emergency admissions coded as DKA in the 12 months to March 2007. Estimated cost per admission was £2064 from a 2014 audit. Admission rates for children <15 years of age in the UK range between 0.05 and 0.38 per patient-year; and internationally, DKA is the mode of presentation of between 12.8% (Sweden) and 80.0% (Middle East) of all children with newly diagnosed type 1 diabetes. Overall mortality in developed countries is reportedly low (<5%) but much higher in older patients, probably as a result of the underlying cause (often cardiovascular disease) (Figure 12.1). Deaths from hyperglycaemic emergencies (including DKA and HHS) declined in the USA from 4.2/10,000 people with diabetes in 1990 to 1.5/10,000 in 2010. For DKA specifically, mortality declined from 0.51 in 2003 to 0.30% in 2014. However, DKA accounts for more than 50% of all deaths in people with type 1 diabetes <24 years of age in the USA; and in Scotland, it is the recorded cause of death in people with diabetes in 29.4% of men and 21.7% of women aged <50 years.

Although DKA mainly occurs in type 1 patients, it can occur in African American and Hispanic people who subsequently can be managed without insulin and thus behave as

Handbook of Diabetes, Fifth Edition. Rudy Bilous, Richard Donnelly, and Iskandar Idris.
© 2021 John Wiley & Sons Ltd. Published 2021 by John Wiley & Sons Ltd.

Table 12.1 UK and US Diagnostic criteria for DKA and HHS.

	DKA	US Mild	US Moderate	US Severe	HHS	
	UK				UK	US
Plasma glucose (mmol/L)	≥ 11.0 or known diabetes	≥ 13.9 (250 mg/dL)	≥ 13.9 (250 mg/dL)	≥ 13.9 (250 mg/dL)	≥ 30.0	≥ 33.3 (600 mg/dL)
pH	≤ 7.30	7.25 – 7.30	7.00 - 7.24	≤ 7.00	≥ 7.30	≥ 7.30
Plasma bicarbonate (mmol/L)	≤ 15	15 – 18	10 – 15	≤ 10	≥ 15	≥ 20
Blood ketones (mmol/L)	≥ 3.0	Positive	Positive	Positive	< 3.0	< 3.0
Urine ketones	NA	Positive (≥2+)	Positive (≥2+)	Positive (≥2+)	≤2+	Low
Anion gap	NA	≥ 10	≥ 12	≥ 12	NA	Variable
Osmolality (mOsmol/kg)	Variable	Variable	Variable	Variable	≥ 320	≥ 320

Anion gap = [plasma sodium] – [plasma chloride + plasma bicarbonate]. Normal varies by laboratory but usually 8 – 14.
Osmolality = 2[plasma sodium] + plasma glucose + plasma urea in UK; 2[plasma sodium] + plasma glucose in USA.
NB approximately 10% of DKA can present with near normoglycaemia (especially in pregnancy) Mental state alterations are almost invariable in HHS and an ominous development in DKA.
Adapted from Kitabchi et al. *Diabetes Care* 2009; 32: 1335–1343.

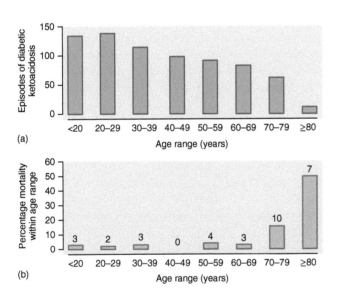

(a)
(b)

Box 12.1 Features of ketosis-prone type 2 diabetes mellitus

- Acute presentation
- Mean age >40 years
- Male preponderance
- BMI ≥28 (for African American, less for Hispanic and Taiwanese)
- Mostly newly diagnosed with diabetes
- Strong family history of type 2 diabetes
- HbA1c at presentation >12% (>108 mmol/mol)
- Autoimmune markers for type 1 diabetes negative
- Fasting C-peptide detectable
- Most do not require long-term insulin therapy

Figure 12.1 (a) Age distribution of 746 episodes of diabetic ketoacidosis (excluding paediatric cases). (b) Age distribution of deaths related to diabetic ketoacidosis (*n* = 32). Numbers of deaths in each age range are also shown. Data based upon 746 consecutive cases of DKA from Birmingham General Hospital 1971 – 85. Latest update from 2000–2009 revealed overall mortality was 1.8% of 137 patients. Courtesy of Dr M Nattrass.

Table 12.2 Precipitating causes of DKA.

Cause	Reported frequency
Infection	14–58%
Insulin error/omission	13–60%
Newly diagnosed	3–24%
Cardiovascular (myocardial infarction, stroke)	
Pancreatitis	
Pulmonary embolism	<10%
Alcohol excess	
Steroid use	

type 2 diabetes. This phenomenon is now termed 'ketosis-prone type 2 diabetes'; it can account for 25–50% of African American or Hispanic cases of DKA. Their clinical characteristics are shown in Box 12.1.

Precipitating factors for diabetic ketoacidosis

The most common precipitating factor is poor adherence to therapy (13–60% in internationally reported surveys). Intercurrent infection is also common (14–58%), but it is

important to remember that a polymorphonucleocytosis is common in DKA, probably secondary to physiological stress, and does not necessarily imply sepsis. Other causes of DKA and their range of frequency from reported series are shown in Table 12.2. The frequency of cause will vary according to age and ethnicity. Not infrequently, no obvious cause is found.

Some people with diabetes experience recurrent episodes of DKA. In a recent national audit in the UK of 5 sequential cases of DKA in 72 hospitals, over one third of the five had a previous admission in the preceding 12 months. In the Chicago area in the USA, out of 3615 patients with a recorded hospital admission for DKA between 2006–2012, 211 had had > 4 episodes. The patients in both countries had shared characteristics : they were more likely to be female, have been diagnosed at an early age and be younger than those with isolated admissions. They also tended to have poorer glycaemic control and had a poor record of clinic attendance. Many also had a history of psychological problems, with > 50% having received a prescription for antidepressants at some time in one UK series, and they tend to have poorer socio-economic backgrounds and lower educational achievement. Lack of health insurance is a factor in the USA. The concern is that 'out of hospital' mortality in this group is worryingly high, 13.6% in the US series and 23.4% over a follow up of 2–3.8 years in the UK. There is an urgent need to find strategies to re-engage these vulnerable young people with diabetes care services.

Pathophysiology

Relative or absolute insulin deficiency in the presence of catabolic counter-regulatory stress hormones (particularly glucagon and catecholamines, but also growth hormone and cortisol) leads to hepatic overproduction of glucose and ketones. Lack of insulin combined with excess stress hormones promotes lipolysis, with the release of NEFAs from adipose tissue into the circulation. In the liver, fatty acids are partially oxidised to the ketone bodies acetoacetic acid and β-hydroxybutyric acid which contribute to the acidosis, and acetone (formed by the non-enzymatic decarboxylation of acetoacetate) (Figure 12.2). The latter is volatile and excreted via the lungs.

Hyperglycaemia results from four main mechanisms : (i) increased glycogenolysis secondary to glucagon excess; (ii) gluconeogenesis as a result of increased lipolysis and proteolysis; (iii) diminished peripheral uptake of glucose due to absent insulin stimulated uptake; and (iv) utilisation of alternative fuels such as NEFA and ketone bodies in preference to glucose.

Hyperglycaemia causes an osmotic diuresis that leads to dehydration and loss of electrolytes. Sodium depletion is worsened because of diminished renal sodium reabsorption due to insulin deficiency. Metabolic acidosis leads to the loss of intracellular potassium in exchange for hydrogen ions, and insulin deficiency also results in potassium loss from cells. These processes can result in relatively high circulating plasma potassium which masks an underlying total body insufficiency.

The symptoms of DKA include increasing polyuria and thirst, weight loss, weakness, drowsiness, and eventually coma (in about 10% of cases) (Box 12.2). Abdominal pain can occur, particularly in the young, and should resolve

Box 12.2 Clinical features of diabetic ketoacidosis.

- Polyuria and nocturia; thirst
- Weight loss
- Weakness
- Blurred vision
- Acidotic (Kussmaul) respiration
- Abdominal pain, especially in children
- Leg cramps
- Nausea and vomiting
- Confusion and drowsiness
- Coma (10% of cases)

within 24 hours. If not, alternative causes should be looked for. Physical signs include dehydration, hypotension, tachycardia, and hypothermia. Acidosis stimulates the respiratory centre, which results in deep and rapid (Kussmaul) respirations. The smell of acetone on the patient's breath (similar to nail-varnish remover) may be obvious to some, but many people are unable to detect it.

The mechanism by which DKA induces coma is obscure, but impaired consciousness generally correlates with plasma glucose concentration and osmolality; coma at presentation is associated with a worse prognosis. This is because the unconscious brain stops utilising circulating ketone bodies which therefore accumulate more rapidly and result in a worsening metabolic acidosis. Co-existing causes of coma, such as stroke, head injury, meningitis, and drug overdose, should always be considered and excluded if clinical signs suggest one of these diagnoses. Cerebral oedema should be suspected when the conscious level declines during treatment (see below).

Treatment

Diabetic ketoacidosis is a medical emergency (Figures 12.3 and 12.4). A rapid history, physical examination, and bedside blood and urine tests should allow a provisional diagnosis in the emergency department and avoid treatment delays (Figure 12.3). Immediate bedside investigations should include blood glucose concentration and a test for the presence of urine or blood ketones with reagent strips, followed by laboratory measurements of blood glucose, urea, Na$^+$, K$^+$, Cl$^-$, bicarbonate (for calculation of the anion gap), magnesium, phosphate, venous blood pH, blood count, and blood and urine cultures. Arterial blood gas estimation may be indicated if the precipitating cause is respiratory (e.g. pneumonia) or an assessment of oxygenation is required (e.g. in coma). An understanding of likely fluid and electrolyte deficiencies is important to guide treatment (Table 12.3).

Fluid replacement

Initial treatment involves rehydration with 0.9% sodium chloride (normal or isotonic saline). There are concerns

Table 12.3 Water and electrolyte deficiencies in DKA and HHS.

	DKA	HHS
Water mL/kg bodyweight	Approximately 100	100–220
Sodium mmol/kg bodyweight	7–10	5–13
Potassium mmol/kg bodyweight	3–5	4–6
Phosphate mmol/kg bodyweight	1–1.5	1–2
Magnesium mmol/kg bodyweight	1–2	1–2

that prolonged 0.9% sodium chloride infusion may produce a hyperchloraemic acidosis that might affect measures of response to therapy such as blood pH and bicarbonate. Trials comparing 0.9% sodium chloride with Hartmann's solution have shown no advantage of the latter, so current guidance recommends isotonic saline as the fluid of choice.

Potassium

Although initial serum potassium levels may be normal or even high, there will be an overall deficiency (Table 12.3), and replacement should commence more or less immediately at 40 mmol/L unless there is significant renal impairment (acute or chronic), or hyperkalaemia >5.5 mmol/L. Serum potassium will fall with treatment as a result of correction of acidosis and insulin administration, both of which increase cellular uptake. Careful and regular monitoring of serum potassium is essential as treatment-induced hypokalaemia is a significant cause of cardiac dysrhythmia and even death.

Ketone monitoring

The ready availability of bedside monitoring devices for capillary blood ketone concentrations has led to their adoption in management protocols for DKA in the UK. There are sound scientific reasons for this as they measure β-hydroxybutyrate which is the main ketone body produced. The urine Ketostix only measure aceto-acetate which is present in concentrations up to 10 times lower. Moreover, aceto-acetate levels paradoxically rise as a result of insulin therapy which inhibits the β-hydroxybutyrate dehydrogenase enzyme (Figure 12.2). However, the strips are much less accurate at

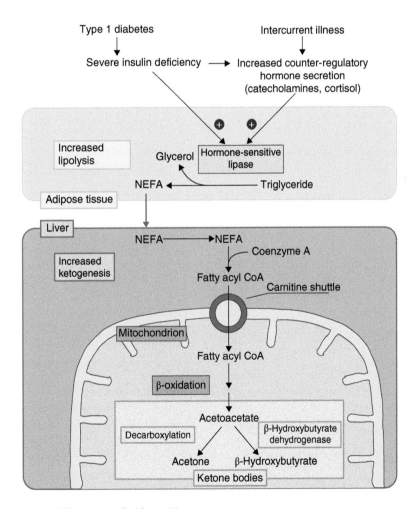

Figure 12.2 Mechanisms of ketacidosis. NEFA, non-esterified fatty acids.

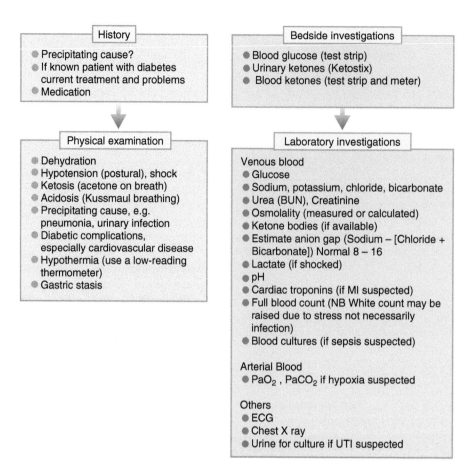

Figure 12.3 Flowchart for the investigation of diabetic ketoacidosis.

blood concentrations >3 mmol/L and so should not be used solely to assess severity of DKA. This inaccuracy also means that they should be used cautiously in the evaluation of the rate of improvement of DKA which needs to be assessed using a combination of measures including clinical condition, and blood pH, glucose, and bicarbonate. Despite these caveats, use of capillary blood ketone monitoring has been shown to shorten hospital stay, and to help to detect early ketoacidosis in the community and prevent hospital admission. All people with type 1 diabetes ideally should have access to blood ketone monitoring to help manage intercurrent infections and identify incipient DKA.

Insulin

Regular/soluble insulin is usually given by continuous infusion; UK and US guidelines suggest a dose of 0.1 unit/kg bodyweight/hour for adults and 0.05 unit/kg bodyweight/hour for children. Alternatively, insulin can be given by hourly IM injection if there is no infusion pump available. Regular SC injection of short-acting insulin analogues in a dose of 0.2 unit/kg bodyweight every 2 hours has been shown to be as effective as IV infusion

in mild to moderate DKA. The overall treatment goal is a reduction in blood glucose of no more than 3–5 mmol/L/h, blood β-hydroxybutyrate 0.5 mmol/L/h, and osmolality by 3 mOsm/kg/h.

Bicarbonate

The role of intravenous bicarbonate is controversial. There is no proven benefit in patients with an arterial pH ≥6.9. There are good theoretical reasons why IV bicarbonate should not be given and its' use has been associated with the development of cerebral oedema. The American Diabetes Association guidelines suggest 100 mmol diluted and given over 2 hours in patients with a pH <6.9 or in whom the acidosis is felt to be contributing to their clinical status.

Other electrolytes

Although phosphate and magnesium depletion are also present (Table 12.3), there is no evidence that routine replacement is of benefit. However, serum phosphate levels <0.35 mmol/L can cause muscle weakness and myocardial dysfunction and need correction. Similarly, serum magnesium levels <0.7 mmol/L should also be treated.

Adult Diabetic Ketoacidosis Emergency Care Pathway

DKA pathway: Guidance for use

Initial results and guidance for use of the pathway:

ADDRESSOGRAPH
LABEL

ESSENTIAL INITIAL RESULTS, ALL MUST BE DOCUMENTED
Blood ketones _____mmol/L   Blood glucose _____mmol/L
Venous bicarbonate _____mmol/L   Venous (or arterial) pH_____
Potassium _____mmol/L [Beware initial low K+, if low (<3.5 mmol/L) call for senior immediately]
Creatinine _____ μmol/L

EARLY MANAGEMENT – 1st hour fluids / potassium / insulin	

Intravenous fluid	• If systolic BP < 90mmHg:
	  • Give 1 litre of 0.9% sodium chloride solution over 15 minutes
	  • If systolic BP remains < 90mmHg repeat and call senior medical colleague for advice
	  • Consider septic shock / heart failure as a potential cause
	  • Consider calling the critical care outreach team from HDU/ITU
	  Do NOT use plasma expanders
	
	• If the systolic BP is > 90mmHg
	
	The rate of fluid replacement depends on the age / fitness / dehydration of the patient. Plan fluid replacement and use clinical judgment
	
	Typically though:
	  • 0.9% sodium chloride 1L with potassium chloride over next 2 hours
	  • 0.9% sodium chloride 1L with potassium chloride over next 2 hours
	  • 0.9% sodium chloride 1L with potassium chloride over next 4 hours
	
	  • Add 10% glucose given at 125ml/hr if the blood glucose falls below 14mmol/L
	
	More cautious fluid replacement should be considered in young people aged 18-25 years, elderly, pregnant, heart or renal failure. (Consider HDU and/or central line)
	
	Reduce the rate of fluid replacement in the elderly / cardiac disease / mild DKA (bicarbonate >10mmol/L). More rapid infusion increases risk of respiratory distress syndrome and cerebral oedema

Potassium
 	
NB: Low potassium KILLS
	Serum potassium is often normal or high initially but total body potassium is low
	  • Add potassium using pre-prepared bags only as follows:
	    o >5.5mmol/L - none
	    o 3.5 - 5.5mmol/L - 20mmol in each 500ml (i.e. 40mmol/L)
	    o <3.5mmol/L - senior advice is required and possible pharmacy involvement.
	      In addition the patient MUST be looked after in a High Care Area
	Anticipate a fall in potassium and replace, once the first plasma potassium result is known SEE APPENDIX 1

Figure 12.4 Guide to the initial treatment of diabetic ketacidosis in adults. Reproduced with permission from the Joint British Diabetes Societies Inpatient Care Group - Management of Diabetic Ketoacidosis in Adults; Second Edition 2013.

Adult Diabetic Ketoacidosis Emergency Care Pathway

ADDRESSOGRAPH
LABEL

Insulin	DO NOT STOP subcutaneous NPH insulin (Insulatard®, Humulin I®, Insuman Basal®), or analogue (Lantus®, Levemir® or Tresiba®).
	DO disconnect Continuous Subcutaneous Insulin Infusion (CSII) pump and DO NOT attempt to use it without diabetes specialist team input under any circumstances.
	A Fixed Rate Intravenous Insulin Infusion (FRIVII) is to be used at 0.1 U/Kg of patient weight
	Add 50 units of soluble insulin made up to 50ml with 0.9% sodium chloride solution in a 50ml syringe
	Weigh or estimate patient weight in Kg, if pregnant, use their current pregnant weight
	Infuse intravenous insulin using Trust–approved syringe driver
	Paradigm / ethos is to drive ketones down aggressively by at least 0.5mmol/L per hour. A variable rate intravenous insulin infusion is NOT to be used until blood ketones are < 0.6mmol/L.
Other Important Notes and Measures	Call the diabetes specialist team or diabetes inpatient specialist nurse as soon as possible
	If ketone and / or glucose levels do not fall as expected, call for senior advice
	High Care Area (HDU or dedicated beds) care is needed if:
	• Hypokalaemia is present on admission (K+ <3.5mmol/L)
	• Young (18 - 25 years old)
	• regnant. Call for urgent senior obstetric involvement. KETONES KILL BABIES, NOT GLUCOSE
	• GCS <12
	• Shocked: pulse >100bpm or systolic BP <90mmHg
	Consider urinary catheter if no urine passed after 2 hours or incontinent
	Consider naso-gastric tube and aspiration if the patient does not respond to commands (NB protect airway)
	Consider thromboprophylaxis with low-molecular weight heparin in elderly or high risk patients unless it is contraindicated. If the patient is in a "hyperosmolar" state, fully anticoagulate with low-molecular weight heparin unless contraindications exist; see BNF and consider referring to the National Guideline on the Management of HHS
	Screen for infection and give antibiotics if clinical evidence of infection (NB The WBC is not helpful because it may be markedly raised from DKA alone)
	Continue the FRIII and fluids until the acidosis is reversed and the VRIII until the patient is ready to eat and drink
	Discontinue the VRIII 30-60 minutes after the subcutaneous insulin has been given
Bicarbonate administration	In most cases bicarbonate is **NOT** helpful and is potentially dangerous
	If bicarbonate is being considered, the patient should be in a level 2 (HDU / ITU) environment
	Only consider after discussion with the consultant in charge of the patient's care
Re-starting subcutaneous Insulin	If you are confident enough, re-start subcutaneous insulin without diabetes specialist team input as follows (firstly ensure that the long acting analogue, if the patient was previously on it, was not stopped):
	• Allow the patient to eat
	• If no sickness, inject normal meal time insulin and stop intravenous insulin 30-60 minutes later
	Otherwise await the input of the diabetes specialist team

Figure 12.4 (Continued)

Euglycaemic ketoacidosis

DKA at relatively low or even normal blood glucose levels has been described, especially in the context of pregnancy (see case history). It is also important to recognise that capillary blood glucose strips are not as accurate in the acidaemic patient. In the UK audit of hospital cases in 2014, 3.5% occurred in patients whose presenting blood glucose was said to be <12 mmol/L (220 mg/dL). It is partly for this reason that blood glucose concentration should not be used as the sole measure of metabolic decompensation in people with diabetes who are unwell.

Complications of diabetic ketoacidosis

These include cerebral oedema which is a particular problem for children. This can cause 'coning', in which swelling of the brain within the enclosed space of the cranium forces the medulla and brainstem to herniate through the foramen magnum, leading to cardiorespiratory arrest. Cerebral oedema is often fatal, and accounts for 50% of deaths in newly presenting DKA in children. The cellular mechanisms responsible for cerebral oedema in DKA are uncertain, but clinically it is associated with rapid rehydration, a higher serum urea and lower arterial CO_2 tension at presentation and, in some cases, with IV bicarbonate replacement. Because of this, more cautious fluid replacement is now recommended (see NICE National Guidance NG18).

Cerebral oedema presents as a decline in conscious level, rapidly progressing to coma. The diagnosis should be confirmed by computed tomography or magnetic resonance scanning of the brain. A reasonable treatment approach includes slowing the rate of IV fluid infusion, avoidance of hypotonic fluids, decreasing the insulin delivery rate and giving intravenous mannitol (0.2 g/kg over 30 minutes, repeated hourly if there is no improvement, or a single dose of 1 g/kg). Mechanical ventilation to remove carbon dioxide and improve acidosis has also been advocated.

Adult respiratory distress syndrome occasionally occurs in DKA, mostly in those under 50 years of age. The features include breathlessness, tachypnoea, central cyanosis, and arterial hypoxia. Chest X-rays show bilateral infiltrates which resemble pulmonary oedema. Management involves mechanical ventilation and avoidance of fluid overload.

Thromboembolism is a further potentially fatal complication usually associated with severe dehydration, increased blood viscosity and hypercoagulability. Prophylactic anticoagulation in DKA is not recommended routinely, but patients at high risk should be considered for heparin therapy.

Hyperosmolar hyperglycaemic state

Hyperosmolar hyperglycaemic state (HHS) used to be called hyperosmolar non-ketotic hyperglycaemic coma, or HONK, but is now termed HHS because mild ketosis can be present and because not all patients are comatose. It used to be seen in older adults with diabetes, but is now recognised

in teenagers and young adults. Around 20% of cases occur in people who were not previously known to have diabetes. There are no universally agreed diagnostic criteria, but all patients are very unwell presenting with high osmolality, very high blood glucose concentrations, and severe dehydration. The diagnostic biochemical criteria are contrasted with DKA in Table 12.1 and the fluid and electrolyte deficiencies in Table 12.3. It tends to occur gradually and is often associated with medications (notably thiazide and loop diuretics, β-blockers, steroids, and atypical anti-psychotic agents). Because of its gradual onset with thirst, many patients inadvertently compound the problem by drinking fruit juices or fluids high in glucose. Precisely why ketosis is not a feature in HHS is not known, but because there is only a relative deficiency of insulin and generally lower levels of glucagon than in DKA, portal venous concentrations of insulin may be enough to prevent hepatic ketogenesis, but peripheral insulin levels are insufficient to stimulate glucose uptake.

Around 25% of patients with HHS have newly diagnosed diabetes. However, HHS is unusual, accounting for <1% of hospital admissions due to diabetes in the UK. Mortality is high (5–20%), partly because of age and underlying cause – often cardiovascular disease or serious infection. In addition, thromboembolic complications may occur secondary to the marked hyperosmolality and UK guidelines recommend prophylactic heparinisation.

The first objective of treatment is to correct the hyperosmolality, but this must be done cautiously to avoid rapid fluid shifts and circulatory collapse. The latest UK Guidelines suggest correction of 50% of the estimated fluid deficit within the first 12 hours using 0.9% sodium chloride. The target reduction in osmolality is 3–8 mOsmol/kg/h. In itself this should correct the hyperglycaemia without the immediate need for IV insulin, and the suggested rate of decline of plasma glucose is 4–6 mmol/L/h. As glucose falls then plasma sodium is likely to rise as water moves into cells. This is not a problem unless the effective plasma osmolality also begins to rise. This situation is the only indication for hypotonic 0.45% sodium chloride and great care must be taken to avoid a fall in plasma sodium of >10 mmol/L in the first 24 hours. (This is an area of difference in guidance in the USA where 0.45% sodium chloride solution is recommended if the patient is hypernatraemic and after initial 0.9% resuscitation). Once plasma glucose remains stable then insulin can be commenced at a dose of 0.05 u/kg/h, but the target should be 10–15 mmol/L not normoglycemia. Around 20% of patients may have associated ketoacidosis in which case insulin will need to be started earlier.

Potassium replacement is as for DKA, but total losses are less in HHS and, as many elderly patients will have chronic kidney disease, care must be taken not to cause hyperkalaemia. There is no evidence for routine phosphate replacement, but many patients may be malnourished and cachectic and thus be prone to refeeding syndrome and hypophosphataemia once insulin is started. Many patients can be managed ultimately without insulin once they are metabolically stable.

Lactic acidosis

This is a rare but very serious and life-threatening metabolic crisis that is said to occur more frequently in people with diabetes. There are two types (type A-anaerobic and type B-aerobic) and their causes are listed in Table 12.4.

Whereas there is good evidence for a causative role of the biguanide phenformin which is no longer available, there is considerable debate as to whether metformin use *per se* is associated with lactic acidosis. A Cochrane systematic review of all reported trials found no episodes in 59,321 patient-years of metformin therapy or in 51,627 patient-years in diabetic patients not on metformin. Most reported cases in people with diabetes (on metformin or not) are in those with one of the serious underlying conditions listed in the table.

Most patients present with a profound metabolic acidosis with a massive anion gap. Treatment is of the underlying condition (which often determines outcome) and large volumes of IV bicarbonate are recommended if the arterial pH is ≤7.15. The evidence base for this recommendation is weak and there are no animal or human data to support it. There are several metabolic reasons why giving bicarbonate may be harmful but in the absence of any controlled data the recommendation stands. The role of dialysis or ultrafiltration is likewise unsubstantiated with evidence but is often carried out in extreme cases. Most patients require ITU monitoring and care, and the outcome is dependent upon the underlying cause.

Table 12.4 Causes of lactic acidosis.

Type A (Anaerobic)		Type B (Aerobic)	
Shock	Cardiogenic	Systemic disease	Diabetes
	Endotoxic		Neoplasia
	Hypovolaemic		Hepatic failure
			Renal failure
Heart failure		Drugs	Phenformin (possibly metformin)
Asphyxia			Ethanol/methanol/ ethylene glycol
Carbon monoxide poisoning			Salicylate/paracetamol overdose
			Inborn errors of metabolism

where she was found to be slightly breathless and mildly febrile (37.9°C), and urinalysis showed 3+ ketones, trace proteinuria and glycosuria 55 mmol/L (990 mg/dL). Her capillary blood glucose was 11.9 mmol/L (214 mg/dL). A diagnosis of urinary tract infection was made, she was commenced on oral cefalexin and discharged.

Twelve hours later she was brought to the accident and emergency department severely breathless and vomiting with severe abdominal pain. She was tachycardic (pulse 120/min, regular), hypotensive (BP 90/50 mmHg lying, 70/40 mmHg sitting), dehydrated and unwell. Laboratory plasma glucose was 35.6 mmol/L (641 mg/dL), blood β-hydroxybutyrate was 8.1 mmol/L. Arterial pH was 7.0.

She was commenced on IV 0.9% sodium chloride and insulin. She made a rapid recovery over the next 24 hours. Her abdominal pain settled, foetal ultrasound was normal. She was delivered by elective Caesarean section at 36 weeks gestation.

Comment: Pregnancy is considered to be a proketotic state. Serum bicarbonate routinely falls in normal pregnancy; the normal range is 16–19 mmol/L. This means that DKA can occur at a relatively low blood glucose and numerous cases of normoglycaemic DKA have been described. The clues in this patient were the heavy ketonuria and her breathlessness at initial presentation. After this case, new guidelines were drawn up that mandated serum electrolyte samples and whole-blood ketone tests in all diabetic women presenting with ketonuria to the obstetric unit, irrespective of the blood glucose result.

Urinary tract infection rarely occurs without either positive urinary nitrite or leucocytes; proteinuria alone is not diagnostic.

KEY WEBSITES

- www.diabetes.org.uk Diabetes UK website for DKA guidelines
- www.nice.org.uk NG17 Type 1 diabetes in adults and NG18 Type 1 diabetes in children
- https://www.bsped.org.uk/media/1745/bsped-dka-guidelines-no-dka-link.pdf Paediatric DKA and HHS guidelines
- https://www.cdc.gov/diabetes/data/index.html Centers for Disease Control website on Diabetes in the USA
- www.diabetologists-abcd.org.uk/JBDS/JBDS_IP_HHS_Adults.pdf UK guidelines for HHS

FURTHER READING

Angus VC, Waugh N. Hospital admission patterns subsequent to diagnosis of type 1 diabetes in children: a systematic review. BMC Health Serv Res 2007; 7: 199. Available from: www.biomedcentral.com/1472-6963/7/199.

Desai D, Mehta D, Mathias P, Menon G, Schubert UK. Health care utilisation and burden of diabetic ketoacidosis in the U.S. over the past decade: a nationwide analysis. Diabetes Care 2018: https://doi.org/10.2337/dc17-1379

Dhatariya KK, Nunney I, Higgins K, Sampson MJ, Iceton G. National survey of the management of diabetic ketoacidosis in the UK in 2014. Diabetic Med 2016; 33: 252–60 doi 10.1111/dme.12875

Dhatariya KK, Vellanki P. Treatment of diabetic ketoacidosis (DKA) / hyperglycemic hyperosmolar state (HHS): novel advances in the management of hyperglycaemic crises (UK versus USA). Current Diabetes Rep 2017; 17: 33 doi 10.1007/s11892-017-0857-4

English P, Williams G. Hyperglycaemic crises and lactic acidosis in diabetes mellitus. Postgrad Med J 2004; 80: 253–261.

Farsani SF, Brodovicz K,Soleymanlu N, Marquard J, Wissinger E, Maiese BA. Incidence and prevalence of diabetic ketoacidosis (DKA) among adults with type 1 diabetes (T1D): a systematic literature review. BMJ Open 2017; 7: e016587. doi: 10.1136/bmjopen-2017-016587

Gibb F, Toen WL, Graham J, Lockman KA. Risk of death following admission to a UK hospital with diabetic ketoacidosis. Diabetologia 2016; 59: 2082–87 doi 10.1007/s00126-016-4034-0

Gregg EW, Li Y, Wang J, Burrows NR, Ali MK, Rolka D, Williams DE, Geiss L. Changes in diabetes complications in the United States, 1990–2010. NEJM 2014; 370: 1514–23 doi 10.1056/NEJMoa1310799

Joint British Diabetes Societies Inpatient Care Group. The management of diabetic ketoacidosis in adults. Second Edition. Available at: www.diabetologists-abcd.org.uk/JBDS/JBDS.htm and at www.diabetes.org.uk. Accessed May 2020

Kitabchi AE, Miles JM, Umpierrez GE, Fisher JW. Hyperglycaemic crises in adult patients with diabetes. Diabetes Care 2009; 32: 1335–1343.

Misra S & Oliver NS. Utility of ketone measurement in the prevention, diagnosis and management of diabetic ketoacidosis. Diabetic Med 2015; 32: 14–23 doi 10.1111/dme.12604

Scott AR on behalf of the Joint British Diabetes Societies (JBDS). Management of hyperglycaemic hyperosmolar state in adults with diabetes. Diabetic Med 2015; 32: 714–24 doi 10.1111/dme.12757

Umpierrez GE, Smiley D, Kitabchi AE. Narrative review: ketosis prone type 2 diabetes mellitus: Ann Intern Med 2006; 144: 350–357.

Chapter 13

Hypoglycaemia

Hypoglycaemia is a common side effect of treatment with insulin and sulfonylureas therapy and is a major factor preventing patients with type 1 and 2 diabetes from achieving near normoglycaemia. For practical purpose, it is defined as finger prick blood glucose of less than 3.9 mmol/l during which patients will need to take action to avoid further drop of blood glucose values. For patients who are monitoring blood glucose using sensors, they will need to double check their glucose values with a fingerstick reading if their sensor suggests that they are hypoglycaemic or becoming hypoglycaemic. The brain is dependent on a continuous supply of glucose, and its interruption for more than a few minutes leads to central nervous system dysfunction, impaired cognition, and eventually coma. The brain cannot synthesise glucose or store more than 5 minutes supply as glycogen. Hypoglycaemia is more common in young children and may be responsible for the cognitive impairment and lowered academic achievement in children diagnosed with diabetes under the age of 5 years – the developing brain is especially sensitive to hypoglycaemia.

Iatrogenic hypoglycaemia often causes physical and psychosocial morbidity and sometimes causes death (the 'dead-in bed' syndrome may be due to cardiac arrythmias secondary to nocturnal hypoglycaemia) (Figure 13.1).

In the non-diabetic person, hypoglycaemia is limited in part by inhibition of insulin release from the pancreatic β-cells and stimulation of glucagon from the α-cells. The major physiological responses to hypoglycaemia occur as a result of activation of neurones in the ventromedial region of the hypothalamus and elsewhere in the brain; these neurones sense the lowered plasma glucose levels, activate the autonomic nervous system and stimulate

Some consequences of hypoglycaemia in diabetes
• Obstacle to achieving normoglycaemia
• Disabling symptoms
• Sudden death syndrome
• Cognitive impairment in children
• Major source of anxiety in patients

Figure 13.1 Some consequences of hypoglycaemia in diabetes.

pituitary counter-regulatory hormone release (Figure 13.2). Glucagon and epinephrine (adrenaline) release are probably the main factors that limit hypoglycaemia and ensure glucose recovery in normal subjects.

The physiological responses to a falling plasma glucose level produce a range of symptoms that help individuals to recognise hypoglycaemia and take corrective action. Hypoglycaemic symptoms can be classified as 'autonomic', caused by the activation of the sympathetic or parasympathetic nervous system (e.g. tremor, palpitations, or sweating), or 'neuroglycopenic', caused by the effects of glucose deprivation on the brain (e.g. drowsiness, confusion, and loss of consciousness). Headache and nausea are probably non-specific symptoms of malaise. Autonomic symptoms are prominent in subjects with a short duration of diabetes, but diminish with increasing duration of diabetes (Figure 13.3).

In patients with type 1 diabetes, episodes of asymptomatic hypoglycaemia can be common. Typically, 2–5% of night will have prolonged hypoglycaemia. In a previous study from Denmark, patients with good awareness of hypoglycaemia

Handbook of Diabetes, Fifth Edition. Rudy Bilous, Richard Donnelly, and Iskandar Idris.
© 2021 John Wiley & Sons Ltd. Published 2021 by John Wiley & Sons Ltd.

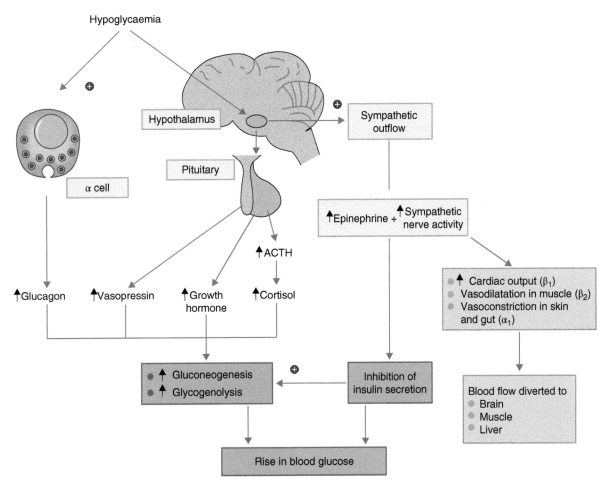

Figure 13.2 Major components of the counter-regulatory and sympathetic nervous system responses to hypoglycaemia. Vasopressin has weak counter-regulatory effects on its own, but acts synergistically with the other hormones.

were shown to be unaware of almost two thirds of hypoglycaemic episodes captured on blinded continuous glucose monitoring (CGM). However, with the development of modern sensor technologies, % of time below range (TbR) can easily be detected, such that the treatment regimen can be individualised in order to reduce % of TbR. Generally, a TbR of >10% is considered to be the excessive amount of hypoglycaemia which is associated with increased risks of harm. Patients should work towards reducing time spent <70mg/dl (<3.9mmol/L) to less than 1 hour (4%) per day, and time spent <54mg/dl (<3mmol/L) to be less than 15 minutes ((1%) per day. Previous data suggest that 2–4% of deaths among people with type 1 diabetes are attributed to hypoglycaemia. Hypoglycaemia causes unpleasant symptoms, e.g anxiety, palpitations, sweating, and the neurological consequences include behavioural changes, cognitive dysfunction, seizures, and coma (Figure 13.4).

The frequency of iatrogenic hypoglycaemia is much lower in patients with type 2 diabetes. For example, published rates of severe hypoglycaemia among patients with type 1

diabetes who are treated aggressively with an insulin range from 60–170 episodes per 100 patient–years. Corresponding rates for insulin-treated type 2 diabetic patients range from 3–70 per 100 patient–years. Severe hypoglycaemia rates in type 2 diabetes are only 10% of those in type 1 diabetes, even during aggressive insulin therapy. During 6-years of follow-up in the UKPDS, only 2.4% of metformin-treated patients, 3.3% of sulfonylurea-treated patients and 11.2% of those on insulin reported a major hypoglycaemia episode (requiring third party assistance). Modern therapies, including long-acting insulin analogues and third generation sulfonylureas, are associated with less hypoglycaemia (Figure 13.5).

Hypoglycaemia in diabetes is caused by absolute or relative insulin excess, but the integrity of glucose counter-regulatory mechanisms has an important effect on the clinical outcomes. Thus, compromised glucose counter-regulation is well recognised in type 1 diabetes and probably also occurs in advanced type 2 diabetes. Risk factors for compromised glucose counter-regulation include: (1) insulin deficiency states;

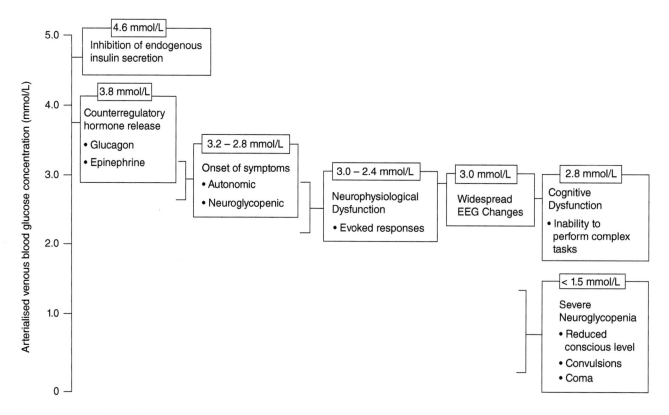

Figure 13.3 Glycemic thresholds for secretion of counterregulatory hormones and onset of physiological, symptomatic, and cognitive changes in response to hypoglycemia in the nondiabetic human. Reproduced from Zammitt and Frier. *Diabetes Care* 2005; 28: 2948–2961.

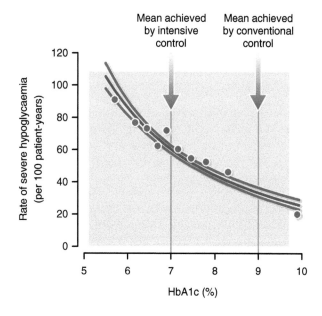

Figure 13.4 In the Diabetes Control and Complications Trial (DCCT, a landmark trial that compared the effects of 'intensive' and 'conventional' glycaemic control on vascular complications in patients with type 1 diabetes), the risk of hypoglycaemia increased in proportion to the reduction in HbA1c. At lower levels of HbA1c (e.g <7%), tighter glycaemic control may confer only small additional benefits in terms of preventing retinopathy but carry a significant increased risk of life-threatening hypoglycaemia. From Diabetes Control and Complications Trial. *N Engl J Med* 1993; 329: 977–986.

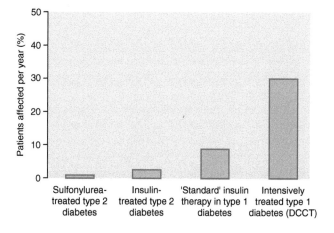

Figure 13.5 Risks of severe hypoglycaemia associated with different diabetes treatments.

(2) history of severe hypoglycaemia, hypoglycaemia unawareness or both; and (3) aggressive antidiabetic therapy, as shown by lower HbA1c (Table 13.1).

The initial response to hypoglycaemia is the acute release of counter-regulatory hormones (in particular, glucagon and epinephrine) which occurs at a plasma glucose concentration of about 3.6–3.8 mmol/L (65–68 mg/dL). Autonomic symptoms develop at about 3.2 mmol/L (58 mg/dL), before cognitive function starts to deteriorate at

Table 13.1 Factors that precipitate or predispose to hypoglycaemia in patients with diabetes.

Excessive insulin levels		Enhanced insulin effect		
Excessive dosage	Increased insulin bio-availability	Increased insulin Sensitivity	Inadequate carbohydrate Intake	Other factors
Error by patient, doctor or pharmacist	Accelerated absorption • Exercise • Injection into abdomen • Change to human Insulin	Counter-regulatory hormone deficiencies • Addison's disease • Hypopituitarism	Missed, small or delayed Meals	Exercise • Acute: accelerated absorption • Late: repletion of muscle Glycogen
Poor matching to patient's needs or lifestyle needs	Insulin antibodies (release of bound insulin)	Weight loss	Slimming diets	Alcohol (inhibits hepatic glucose production)
Deliberate overdose (fictitious hypoglycaemia)	Renal failure (reduced insulin clearance)	Physical training	Anorexia nervosa	Drugs • Enhance sulfonylurea action (salicylates, sulphonamides) • Block counter-regulation (non-selective b-blockers)
	'Honeymoon period' (partial b cell recovery) in type 1 diabetes	Postpartum	Vomiting, including Gastroparesis	
		Menstrual cycle variation	Breastfeeding Failure to cover exercise (early or delayed hypoglycaemia)	

around 3 mmol/l (54 mg/dL) (Figure 13.6). Those patients who retain awareness of hypoglycaemia are thus alerted before significant cerebral dysfunction occurs. However, the inability to recognize symptoms of impending hypogly-caemia, known as 'hypoglycaemia unawareness', is a major clinical problem in those with insulin-treated diabetes. Hypoglycaemic unawareness affects about 25% of patients with type 1 diabetes. In these patients, sympatho-adrenal activation occurs at a lower plasma glucose level than for cognitive impairment. The risk of a severe episode of hypo-glycaemia increases 6–7 fold in patients with hypoglycae-mia unawareness.

Nearly all people with insulin-treated diabetes have some defect in the mechanisms that protect them against hypo-glycaemia, although the impairment is mild in type 2 dia-betes. The glucagon response to hypoglycaemia begins to fail within 1–2 years of type 1 diabetes, probably because of disruption to paracrine mechanisms of cross-talk within the islet, as endogenous insulin production declines. A reduced sympatho-adrenal response is common in type 1 diabetes of long duration; those who exhibit both gluca-gon and epinephrine impairment are particularly suscep-tible to hypoglycaemia, because of both impaired glucose counter-regulation and impaired hypoglycaemia awareness (Figure 13.7). Autonomic neuropathy is a major cause of hypoglycaemia unawareness.

The incretin hormone GLP-1, released by the gut in response to food intake, acts on β- and α-cells in the

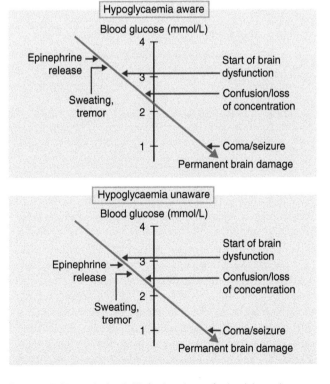

Figure 13.6 Glycaemic thresholds for the release of epinephrine and activation of autonomic symptoms and for neuroglycopenic effects in diabetic subjects who are aware or unaware of hypoglycaemia. Note that in those who are unaware of hypoglycaemia, activation of autonomic symptoms occurs at a glycaemic threshold below that for cognitive impairment.

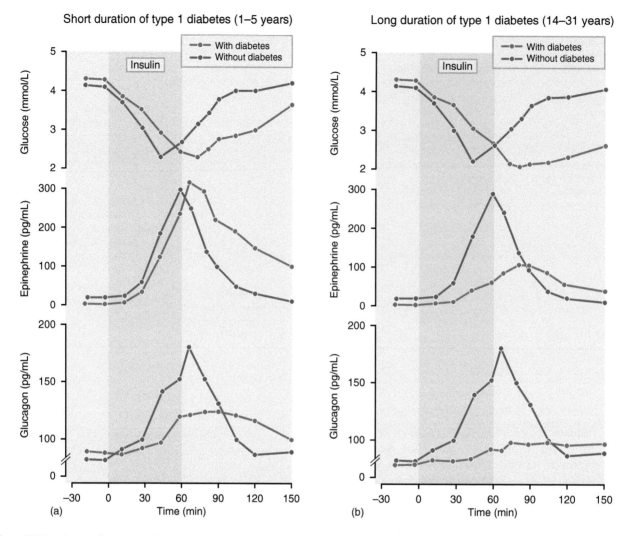

Figure 13.7 Impairment of counter-regulatory responses in type 1 diabetes. (a) After 1–5 years of type 1 diabetes, the mean glucagon response (lower panel) is blunted, but the rise in epinephrine secretion is preserved (middle panel) and glycaemic recovery is delayed (upper panel). (b) With long-standing type 2 diabetes, both glucagon and epinephrine responses are impaired severely and glycaemic recovery is markedly delayed and slowed. From Boli et al. *Diabetes* 1983; 32: 134–141.

pancreatic islets to increase insulin secretion and decrease glucagon secretion, respectively. But the glucose-lowering effects of GLP-1 are glucose-dependent. This means that GLP-1 effects are attenuated at low plasma glucose concentrations. Thus, GLP-1 analogues and the DPP-IV inhibitors which lower glucose levels by GLP-1-mediated effects, appear to have a very low incidence of hypoglycaemia in clinical trials. Similarly, urinary glucose excretion facilitated by the SGLT2 inhibitor therapy is dependent on glucose filtrated via the glomerulus, which in turn is dependent in circulating plasma glucose. Thus, avoidance of hypoglycaemia, especially in comparison with sulfonylureas and insulin, is likely to be the major advantage of these newer treatments for type 2 diabetes.

Tight glycaemic control is a risk factor for impaired glucose counter-regulation and hypoglycaemia unawareness – lower levels of HbA1c result in a resetting of thresholds for the counter-regulatory and symptomatic responses to hypoglycaemia at lower glucose concentrations. In addition, recurrent hypoglycaemia exacerbates the defective responses to subsequent hypoglycaemia, thus leading to a vicious circle of reduced awareness, increased vulnerability and further episodes of hypoglycaemia. It is likely that the neurones that initiate the autonomic response adapt to chronic hypoglycaemia by increasing glucose transporter expression and glucose uptake. Subsequent hypoglycaemia then fails to produce sufficient intracellular glycopenia and therefore no longer elicits a response. There is also evidence that cortisol (released during the counter-regulatory response to hypoglycaemia) dampens the hypothalamic sensing of glucose (Figure 13.8).

Recent evidence from a large scale randomised controlled trial investigating the cardiovascular outcomes between tight control versus more tight glucose control has reinvigorated the interests in the potential adverse cardiovascular outcomes induced by hypoglycaemia (Figure 13.9).

Most episodes of hypoglycaemia can be self-treated by ingestion of glucose tablets, jelly babies, or carbohydrate in the form of juice, crackers, or a meal. If patients experience symptoms of hypoglycaemia but are not yet hypoglycaemic, patients should consider taking 5–10g of carbs (1–2 jelly babies or dextrose tablets). If blood glucose is less than 3.5 mmol/L: patients should take 15–20g of rapid acting carbohydrate (150ml of lucozade, orange juice or 3–4 dextrose tablets) and to recheck in 15 minutes. Parenteral therapy is needed when a hypoglycaemic patient is unable or unwilling (because of neuroglycopenia) to take carbohydrate orally. Intramuscular glucagon is used by family members or carers of patients with type 1 diabetes; glucagon is less useful in type 2 diabetes because it stimulates insulin secretion as well as glycogenolysis. Continuous subcutaneous insulin infusion (CSII, see Chapter 10) is associated with a lower frequency of hypoglycaemia than multiple insulin injection therapy and should be considered as a therapeutic option in those type 1 diabetic patients with frequent, unpredictable hypoglycaemia. Newer long acting insulin analogues with flatter insulin profiles such as Insulin Degludec or Toujeo may also decrease the risk of hypoglycaemia (Box 13.1).

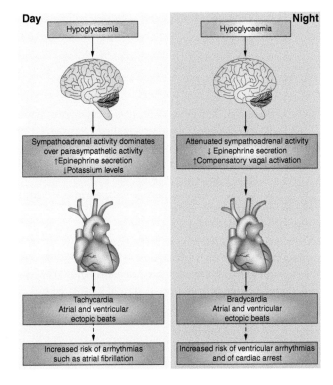

Figure 13.9 Proposed mechanism of linking hypoglycaemia and arrhythmias in patients with type 2 diabetes mellitus during the day and during the night. Adapted from Frier. *Nat Reviews Endo*, 2014).

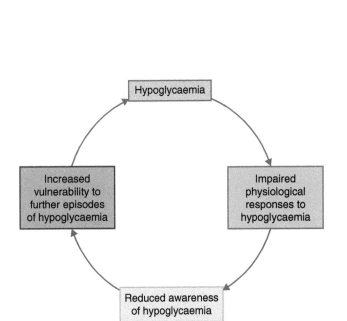

Figure 13.8 The vicious circle of repeated hypoglycaemia.

Box 13.1 General principles for optimizing glycaemic control and minimizing the risk of hypoglycaemia in patients with troubling hypoglycaemia.

- Structured patient education and empowerment
- Assessing hypoglycaemia awareness using the GOLD score or CLARKE score
- Use of sensor technologies to derive ambulatory glucose profiles to highlight times at risk and % of Times below range
- Identify cause of hypoglycaemia (e.g. inadequate reduction of basal insulin for exercise/alcohol; over correction of a high glucose, overestimation of carbs, too frequentrapid acting insulin corrections)
- Flexible insulin regimen, use of insulin pump therapy, use of continuous glucose monitoring with alarms or sensor augmented insulin pump therapy
- Individualization of glycaemic targets
- Ongoing professional advice and support

- Structured patient education and empowerment.
- Assessing hypoglycaemia awareness using the GOLD score or CLARKE score.
- Use of sensor technologies to derive ambulatory glucose profiles to highlight times at risk and % of Times below range.
- Identify cause of hypoglycaemia (e.g. inadequate reduction of basal insulin for exercise/alcohol; over correction of a high glucose, overestimation of carbs, too frequent rapid acting insulin corrections).
- Flexible insulin regimen, use of insulin pump therapy, use of continuous glucose monitoring with alarms or sensor augmented insulin pump therapy.
- Individualization of glycaemic targets.
- Ongoing professional advice and support.

Suspected severe hypoglycaemia (e.g. in a patient with diabetes and impaired consciousness or coma) should be confirmed by blood glucose testing. It should be treated immediately with oral glucose, or if the patient is unconscious or unable to swallow safely, with intravenous glucose or intramuscular or subcutaneous glucagon injection (Figures 13.10 and Box 13.2). Patients usually recover within minutes.

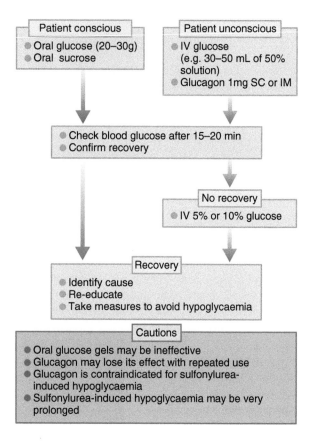

Figure 13.10 Algorithm for treating acute hypoglycaemia in patients with diabetes. Some important cautions are also indicated.

Box 13.2 Management of hypoglycaemia unawareness.

- Refer to the specialist diabetes team if the person is not already under specialist care
- Review the insulin regimen aiming for 50%of the total daily dose (TDD) as basal insulin and the rest as prandial insulin.
- Review insulin technique (including injection sites)
- Recommend structured type 1 diabetes education if this has not already been accessed
- Offer specific hypoglycaemia avoidance training if structured education has already been provided (frequent contact e.g monthly for 6months has been shown to be effective).
- Advise maintaining the fasting blood glucose above 5mmol/L to reduce the risk of nocturnal hypoglycaemia

- Ensure regular monitoring, particularly when driving
- Make person aware of National Driving regulations regarding major hypoglycaemia (requiring assistance from a third party)
- Offer CSII
- Consider real-time Continuous Glucose Monitoring (CGM)
- If all of the above measures are ineffective in resolving the problem, consider a tertiary referral for the possibility of islet transplant where available.

Adapted from The Association of British Clinical Diabetologists (ABCD) Standards of care for management of adults with type 1 diabetes.

CASE HISTORY

A 36-year-old woman with a 25+ year history of type 1 diabetes presents with recurrent severe hypoglycaemia, often in the early hours of the morning. She has multiple microangiopathic complications, including proliferative retinopathy (treated by laser photocoagulation), painful neuropathy, microalbuminuria, and gastroparesis. HbA1c is 8.4% using a basal-bolus insulin regimen. She has considerable anxiety about hypoglycaemia, having embarrassed herself at work with odd behaviour associated with a hypo. She has mostly lost her awareness of hypoglycaemic symptoms, and is reluctant to modify her insulin doses (in order to improve HbA1c) because of the risk of hypos. On admission to hospital, she reports at least six severe hypos in the past year requiring third party assistance.

Comment: Hypoglycaemia unawareness is common among patients with long-duration type 1 diabetes, especially when autonomic dysfunction is present. Fear of severe hypoglycaemia, associated with behavioural disturbance and altered cognition, is an understandable barrier to improving glycaemic control, yet because of advanced microvascular complications this woman would benefit from lower HbA1c levels in the long term. This is a complex management problem. She should undergo a structured diabetes education, would be a candidate for continuous subcutaneous insulin infusion (CSII) using a pump, ideally with sensor device.

LANDMARK CLINICAL TRIALS

Pickup JC, et al. Severe hypoglycaemia and glycaemic control in type 1 diabetes: meta-analysis of multiple daily insulin injections compared with continuous subcutaneous insulin infusion. Diabetic Med. 2008; 25: 765–774.

Amiel SA et al. Defective glucose counterregulation after strict glycemic control of insulin-dependent diabetes mellitus. N Engl J Med. 1987 May 28; 316(22): 1376–83

The ADVANCE Collaborative Group. Intensive blood glucose control and vascular outcomes in patients with type 2 diabetes. N. Engl. J. Med. 2008; 358: 2560–72.

Riddle MC et al.Action to Control Cardiovascular Risk in Diabetes Investigators. Epidemiologic relationships between A1C and all-cause mortality during a median 3.4-year follow-up of glycaemic treatment in the ACCORD trial. Diabetes Care. 2010; 33(5): 983–990

van Beers CA et al. Continuous glucose monitoring for patients with type 1 diabetes and impaired awareness of hypoglycaemia (IN CONTROL): a randomised, open-label, crossover trial. Lancet Diabetes Endocrinol. 2016 Nov;4(11): 893–902. doi: 10.1016/S2213–8587(16)30193–0

Bolinder J. et al. Novel glucose-sensing technology and hypoglycaemia in type 1 diabetes: a multicentre, non-masked, randomised controlled trial. Lancet. 2016; 388(10057): 2254–2263.

KEY WEBSITES

- http://www.diabetes.co.uk/Diabetes-and-Hypoglycaemia.html
- http://www.gpnotebook.co.uk/simplepage.cfm?ID=-19922936
- https://www.niddk.nih.gov/health-information/diabetes/overview/preventing-problems/low-blood-glucose-hypoglycemia
- http://www.diabetes.org/type-1-diabetes/hypoglycemia.jsp

FURTHER READING

Seaquist ER et al. Hypoglycemia and diabetes: a report of a workgroup of the American Diabetes Association and the Endocrine Society. Diabetes Care. 2013; 36(5): 1384–95.

Cryer PE, et al. Hypoglycaemia in diabetes. Diabetes Care 2003; 26: 1902–1912.

Cryer PE. The barrier of hypoglycaemia in diabetes. Diabetes 2008; 57: 3169–76.

Hoe FM. Hypoglycaemia in infants and children. Adv. Paediatr. 2008; 55: 367–84.

Gough SC. A review of human and analogue insulin trials. Diab. Res. Clin. Pract. 2007; 77: 1–15.

Goto A. et al. Severe hypoglycaemia and cardiovascular disease: systematic review and meta-analysis with bias analysis BMJ. 2013 Jul 29; 347: f4533

Villani M et al. Emergency treatment of hypoglycaemia: a guideline and evidence review. Diabetic Medicine. 2017; doi:10.1111/dme.13379

Eldridge CL et al. Prevalence and Incidence of Hypoglycaemia in 532,542 People with Type 2 Diabetes on Oral Therapies and Insulin: A Systematic Review and Meta-Analysis of Population Based Studies. PLoS One. 2015; 10(6): e0126427. doi: 10.1371/journal.pone.0126427. eCollection 2015. Review.

Rodband D. Continuous glucose monitoring; a review of recent studies demonstrating improved glycaemic outcomes. Diabetes, Technol Ther 2017; 19(S3): S25–37

Causes of complications

Much of the impact of chronic diabetes results from the development of tissue complications, mainly microvascular (retinopathy, nephropathy, and neuropathy) and macrovascular disease (atherosclerosis). Microangiopathy is characterised by progressive occlusion of the capillary lumen with subsequent impaired tissue perfusion, increased vascular permeability and increased production of extracellular material by perivascular cells, resulting in basement membrane thickening. Macrovascular disease in diabetes has been characterised as an accelerated atherosclerosis and has few diabetes specific pathological features. Both metabolic and haemodynamic factors play a role in the aetiopathogenesis of diabetes complications (Figure 14.1). This chapter will discuss these factors and outline the cellular processes that lead to tissue damage in diabetes.

Hyperglycaemia
Microvascular complications

There is strong evidence that microvascular disease is related to the duration and severity of hyperglycaemia in both type 1 and type 2 diabetes. A classic observational study by Pirart demonstrated this link in 4400 type 1 and 2 patients followed for up to 25 years (Figure 14.2). As diabetes duration increased, the prevalence of retinopathy, nephropathy, and neuropathy was greatest in those with the worst glycaemic control and least in those with the best control.

Many other epidemiological studies have supported this relationship. In the Wisconsin Epidemiologic Study of Diabetic Retinopathy (WESDR), the incidence and progression of retinopathy in subjects with type 1 ('younger onset') and type 2 ('older onset') diabetes were clearly related to glycaemic status (Figure 14.3).

Convincing proof that good glycaemic control could prevent complications in type 1 diabetes came with the Diabetes Control and Complications Trial (DCCT), which reported in 1993. This study is often regarded as a landmark in diabetes research: 1441 patients in 29 centres in North America were allocated randomly to either 'conventional' therapy (one or two daily insulin injections, 3-monthly clinic visits, no insulin dosage adjustments according to self-monitored glucose data) or to 'intensive' therapy (three or more daily insulin injections or insulin pump therapy, monthly clinic visits and

Handbook of Diabetes, Fifth Edition. Rudy Bilous, Richard Donnelly, and Iskandar Idris.
© 2021 John Wiley & Sons Ltd. Published 2021 by John Wiley & Sons Ltd.

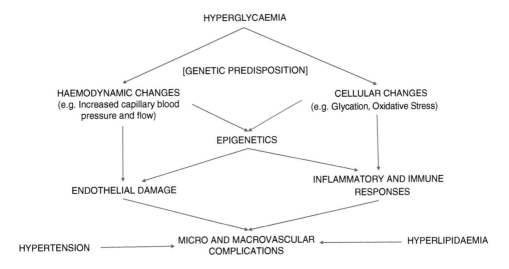

Figure 14.1 Schematic showing interaction of haemodynamic and cellular factors in aetiopathogenesis of diabetic complications.

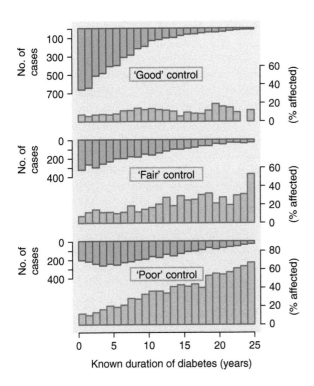

Figure 14.2 Prevalence of diabetic neuropathy as a function of duration of diabetes in patients with 'good', 'fair' and 'poor' control. From Pirart. Diabetes Care 1978; 1: 168–188, 262–261.

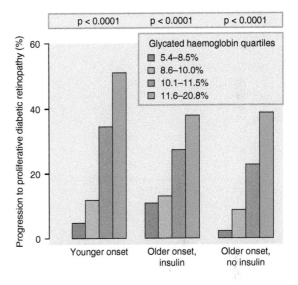

Figure 14.3 Progression of proliferative retinopathy is related to glycated haemoglobin percentage in the Wisconsin Eye Study. From Klein et al. Ann Intern Med 1996; 124: 90–96.

weekly telephone calls, frequent blood glucose self-monitoring with insulin dosage adjustment, and a diet and exercise programme). Throughout the 9-year study, there was markedly better glycaemic control in the intensively treated group. After a mean of 6.5 years follow-up, the intensive treatment arm had an HbA1c of 7.4% versus 9.1% (56 versus 76 mmol/mol) in the conventionally treated patients.

However, less than 5% in the intensive arm had an average HbA1c consistently within the normal range.

Patients were divided into those who had no evidence of retinopathy at baseline (primary prevention) and those with mild to moderate retinopathy (secondary prevention). The study was powered for retinal and not renal or neurological endpoints.

However, the study showed clinically important reductions in retinopathy, nephropathy (as defined by urinary albumin excretion) and neuropathy in the intensively treated patients. Retinopathy was assessed by seven field fundus stereophotographs and classified according to the Early Treatment

Diabetic Retinopathy Study (ETDRS) scale. A three-step change was regarded as significant (see Chapter 15).

In the primary prevention arm there was a 76% risk reduction (Figure 14.4), and a 54% risk reduction in the secondary prevention arm (63% risk reduction for both arms combined). Moreover, the link between increasing severity of hyperglycaemia and risk of retinopathy progression was confirmed conclusively in the conventional arm (Figure 14.5).

In type 2 diabetes similar evidence came from the UKPDS which reported in 1998. This was a 20-year study recruiting over 5000 patients with type 2 diabetes in 23 centres throughout the UK. In the main study, 3867 patients with newly diagnosed type 2 diabetes were allocated randomly to 'intensive' therapy (sulfonylureas, [chlorpropamide, or glibenclamide/glyburide] or to insulin) or to 'conventional' therapy, which was diet only initially, although tablets or

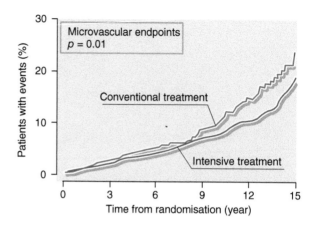

Figure 14.6 Effect of intensive blood glucose control on microvascular complications in type 2 diabetes (UKPDS). From UKPDS Group. Lancet 1998; 352: 837–854.

insulin could be added later if patients became symptomatic or developed a fasting blood glucose above 15 mmol/L.

Over 10 years those in the intensive arm had an HbA1c of 7.0% versus 7.9% (53 versus 63 mmol/mol) in the conventionally treated patients. Intensive therapy was associated with a significant 25% reduction in microvascular disease endpoints (an aggregate of vitreous haemorrhage, laser photocoagulation, renal failure, defined as a serum creatinine >250 μmol/L, or death from renal failure) (Figure 14.6). At 12 years using the ETDRS scale, there was a 21% reduction in a two-step change in retinopathy level in the intensively treated patients. The more recent ACCORD, ADVANCE, and VADT trials have also shown benefit of improved glycaemic control on microvascular complications in the eye (ACCORD), and kidney. However, most of these studies have shown a consistent effect on prevention of development or early progression of microvascular complications, but less of an impact on established or advanced disease. Part of the explanation may lie in the duration of these trials. Evidence from kidney biopsies in patients undergoing a whole organ pancreas transplant shows that an improvement in glomerulopathy is only measurable after 10 years or more of normoglycaemia.

Macrovascular disease

Epidemiological studies show a clear positive relationship between glycaemia and macrovascular disease in the general population. For example, in the European Prospective Investigation of Cancer and Nutrition (EPIC) study of 4600 men in the UK, HbA1c was continuously related to cardiovascular mortality from low normal levels <31 mmol/mol (<5%) to values >53 mmol/mol (>7%), and in people with self-reported diabetes (Figure 14.7).

In the UKPDS, however, there was no significant impact of intensive glycaemic control on macrovascular complications

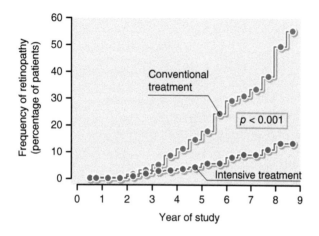

Figure 14.4 Effect of intensive treatment on the onset of retinopathy. Cumulative incidence of background retinopathy in patients with type 1 diabetes who entered the DCCT without retinopathy (primary prevention). From DCCT. N Engl J Med 1993; 329: 977–986.

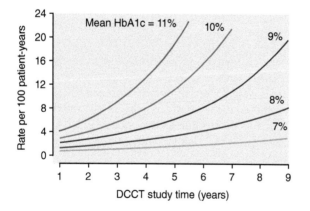

Figure 14.5 Risk of retinopathy progression and mean glycated haemoglobin in the conventional arm of the DCCT.

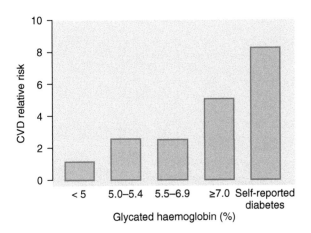

Figure 14.7 The relationship between glycated haemoglobin percentage and cardiovascular disease (CVD) in the EPIC Norfolk Study of 4662 men. From Khaw et al. BMJ 2001; 322:15–18.

although at 10 years there was a 16% reduction in relative risk for myocardial infarction which just failed to reach statistical significance (p = 0.052).

In 2008 the results from three large randomised controlled trials were reported, involving over 23,000 patients with type 2 diabetes who were allocated to a strategy of intensive versus less intensive glycaemic control and for whom the main outcome variable was macrovascular disease. These trials showed no benefit of glycaemic control on the standard combined cardiovascular endpoint of fatal and non-fatal myocardial infarction and stroke. Moreover, there was a slight increase in cardiac mortality in the intensively treated arm of the ACCORD trial although the total number of myocardial infarctions was almost identical in the intensive and less intensive arms (Table 14.1).

The reason for this discrepancy with the findings from intensive control on microvascular disease probably relates to their pathogenesis. Retinopathy, nephropathy, and neuropathy are virtually diabetes specific and therefore hyperglycaemia is the main driving force for them. On the other hand, atherosclerosis is more multifactorial and although blood glucose is important, it is only one of many factors which contribute. Moreover, many of the participants in the macrovascular outcome trials had established cardiovascular disease and, as in the DCCT and UKPDS, it may be that tight glycaemic control is more effective as a primary preventative measure for atherosclerosis.

Blood pressure

In the DCCT, patients were normotensive at entry. In the UKPDS, however, nearly one-third of patients were hypertensive at entry. Embedded within the trial was a blood pressure-lowering study in which 1148 hypertensive patients were allocated to either tight (target <150/<85 mmHg) or less tight (target <180/<105 mmHg) control (Figure 14.8). Moreover, the tight control group were further randomised to a regimen based upon either captopril or atenolol.

Using the same aggregate microvascular endpoint as for the glycaemic control study, there was a reduction of 37% in the tight control group. No difference was seen in those treated with either atenolol or captopril. Lower blood pressure was also associated with reduced macrovascular events, particularly stroke.

However, in the blood pressure arm of the ACCORD trial the intensively treated patients (target BP <120 mmHg systolic) showed no benefit in terms of retinopathy or

Table 14.1 Main features of the ACCORD (Action to Control CardiOvascular Risk in Diabetes), ADVANCE (Action in Diabetes and Vascular Disease – Preterax and Diamicron Modified Release Controlled Evaluation), and VADT (Veterans Affairs Diabetes Trials) studies.

	ACCORD	ADVANCE	VADT
Patient characteristics n (male %)	10,251 (39%)	11,140 (42%)	1791 (97%)
Mean age (years)	62	66	60
Known duration of diabetes (years)	10	8	11.5
History of cardiovascular disease (%)	35	32	40
BMI kg/m²	32	28	31
Median baseline HbA1c (%)	8.1	7.2	9.4
Target HbA1c (%)	<6.0 vs 7.0–7.9	<6.5	<6.0 vs planned separation of 1.5
Study characteristics			
Median duration of follow-up (years)	3.5	5.0	5.6
Achieved median HbA1c (%)*	6.4 vs 7.5	6.3 vs 7.0	6.9 vs 8.5
Weight change (kg)*	+3.5 vs +0.4	–0.1 vs –1.0	+7.8 vs +3.4
Participants with one or more severe hypoglycaemic reactions (%)*	16.2 vs 5.1	2.7 vs 1.5	21.2 vs 9.9
Hazard ratio for primary macrovascular outcome (95% CI)	0.90 (0.78–1.04)	0.94 (0.84–1.06)	0.88 (0.74–1.05)

* Intensive versus less intensive arms. Adapted from Skyler et al. Diabetes Care 2009; 32: 187–192.

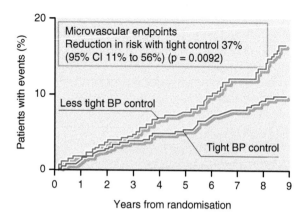

Figure 14.8 Kaplan–Meier plots of proportions of patients who developed microvascular endpoints (mostly retinal photocoagulation) during tight or less tight BP control (UKPDS). From UKPDS Group. BMJ 1998; 317: 703–713.

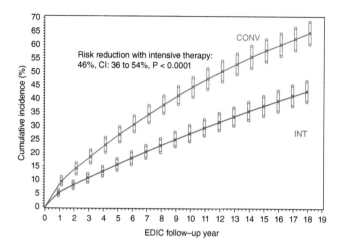

Figure 14.9 Cumulative incidence of a three-step change in ETDRS retinopathy severity in the DCCT/EDIC cohort 18 years after the completion of the original trial. The individuals in the conventional arm (CONV) continue to show an increase in cumulative incidence of retinopathy in follow-up compared to the intensive arm (INT) despite having a near identical HbA1c during the follow up period. Reproduced from DCCT/EDIC Research Group. Diabetes 2015;64:631–642 with permission.

myocardial infarction. There was a reduction in stroke but only at the expense of increased side effects.

There is evidence that agents that block the renin angiotensin system may have benefits in terms of prevention of progression of retinopathy and nephropathy over and above their blood pressure lowering action (see Chapters 15 and 16). For more details on blood pressure see Chapter 19.

Metabolic memory

The DCCT and UKPDS have published follow-up of the patients who took part in the original studies. At the end of the respective trials, patients were followed but no longer randomised to differing standards of glycaemic control.

Most of the DCCT patients took part in the Epidemiology of Diabetes Interventions and Complications (EDIC) Study. Eight years after the end of the DCCT, the relative risk for development of new microalbuminuria was 49% (95% CI 32–62%) for intensive control and for clinical or overt nephropathy (severe albuminuria) 85% (68–92%). For retinopathy, the risk reduction with intensive therapy at 18 years was 46% (95% CI 36–54) (Figure 14.9). This was despite the fact that the HbA1c levels in the original intensive and conventional groups had almost merged at 64 versus 67 mmol/mol (8.0 versus 8.2%) respectively. The benefits of intensive therapy on retinopathy were still present in the 18 year EDIC follow up, although the year on year incidence was similar in both the intensive and conventional groups, largely as a result of a reduction in incidence rates in the originally conventionally treated patients.

Similarly, in the UKPDS, a 10-year follow-up at the end of the trial revealed that glycaemia was almost identical in the intensive and conventional groups (HbA1c approximately 7.8%; 62 mmol/mol) but there was a remaining relative risk of 0.76 (95% CI 0.64–0.89) for the combined microvascular disease endpoint in the intensive arm.

Interestingly, for myocardial infarction there was a significantly lower relative risk of 0.85 (0.74–0.97) for the intensively treated group in the UKPDS, and the DCCT/EDIC study also showed a benefit in terms of cardiovascular events in the intensively treated group eight years after the close of the original study (risk reduction 42%; 9–68%), although numbers of events were very small (46 versus 98). During 30 years combined follow-up in the DCCT/EDIC there were 149 cardiovascular events in 82 subjects in the intensive arm, and 217 events in 102 subjects in the conventional arm.

The long-term benefit of intensive control despite the fact that there is no long-term glycaemic separation remains unexplained. It is not clear whether there is merely a delay in the intensively treated patients and that ultimately, they will catch up or whether this is of long-term clinical benefit. It is also possible that a period of hyperglycaemia induces both structural (such as glycation of matrix proteins such as collagen), and functional changes (such as epigenetic) that are likely to continue even after glycaemic correction. As the DCCT participants had relatively short duration of diabetes, and the UKPDS involved patients with newly diagnosed type 2 diabetes, the message is that the better the glycaemic control in the early stages of diabetes, the better the long-term outlook in terms of both micro- and macrovascular complications.

How does hyperglycaemia cause tissue complications?

Microvascular and macrovascular complications occur in cells and tissues which are unable to limit glucose transport in the face of hyperglycaemia (particularly the retina, the

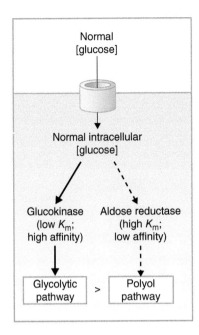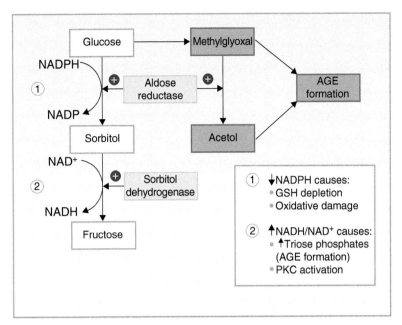

Figure 14.10 The polyol pathway. (*Left*) The pathway is normally inactive, but becomes active when intracellular glucose levels rise. (*Right*) Consequences of increased glucose flux through the polyol pathway include the generation of powerful glycating sugars (methylglyoxal, acetol and triose phosphates), enhanced oxidative damage and protein kinase C (PKC) activation. AGE, advanced glycation end-products; GSH, reduced glutathione; NAD, nicotinamide adenine dinucleotide.

mesangium in the kidney, Schwann cells, and endothelial cells). The resulting increase in intracellular glucose initiates a range of changes which initiate or up regulate various metabolic pathways which lead to vascular complications. Many of these pathways are closely related and thus abnormal activity in one is facilitated by others. This means that blockade of an individual process is much less likely to be effective in preventing damage as others will still be active. It must also be noted that much of our understanding has come from experimental diabetes or from gene knockout rodents. So far, and disappointingly, these approaches have not led to any major therapeutic advances although several experimental treatments have been explored in Phase 2 trials. Nonetheless, an understanding of these mechanisms is critical for our understanding of aetiopathogenesis of diabetic complications.

Polyol pathway

In this pathway, the rate-limiting enzyme, aldose reductase, reduces glucose to its sugar alcohol, sorbitol. This is then oxidised by sorbitol dehydrogenase into fructose. Aldose reductase is a ubiquitous enzyme found in many tissues but specifically nerve cells, retinal cells, the glomerulus and kidney tubule, and vascular cells. It can also use alternative substrates to glucose such as glycolytic metabolites, e.g. glyceraldehyde-3-phosphate. The pathway is normally inactive but in the presence of hyperglycaemia there is increased flux leading to accumulation of intracellular glucose and

glucose-derived substances, such as methylglyoxal and acetol, which can rapidly glycate proteins (see Figure 14.10). Sorbitol does not diffuse easily across cell membranes and damage may occur because of osmotic stress (currently thought to be less likely except in the lens of the eye in the formation of cataract). More likely, the decrease in levels of nicotinamide adenine dinucleotide phosphate hydrogen (NADPH) leads to impaired regeneration of reduced glutathione (GSH) which is an important scavenger of reactive oxygen species (ROS). There are also increases in nicotinamide adenine dinucleotide plus hydrogen (NADH) production from sorbitol dehydrogenase action. The result of both these changes is increased oxidative stress (see below).

Advanced glycation endproducts

Advanced glycation endproducts (AGEs) are formed by the non-enzymatic reaction of glucose, and other glycating compounds, such as glyoxal, methylglyoxal, and 3-deoxyglucosone, with proteins (an analagous process to the formation of glycated haemoglobin), and other long-lived molecules, such as nucleic acids. Early glycation products are reversible, but eventually they undergo irreversible change through cross-linking (Figure 14.11).

AGEs can cause damage and ultimately complications of diabetes in three ways; firstly, as a result of cross-linkage of matrix proteins, such as collagen and laminin, leading to thickening and stiffening of blood vessels which can affect permeability and elasticity. These matrix alterations also

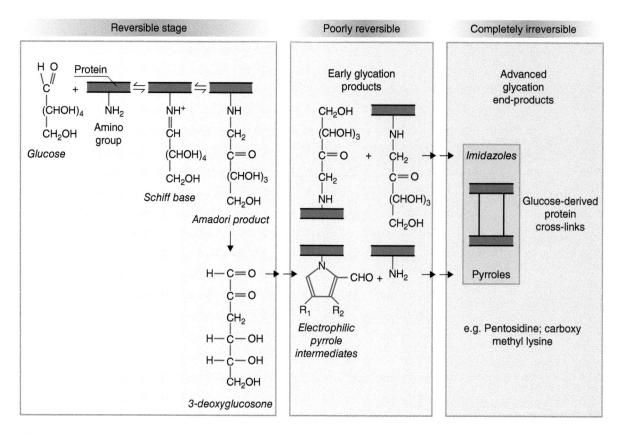

Figure 14.11 Formation of reversible, early, non-enzymatic glycation products, and of irreversible advanced glycation end-products (AGEs). Through a complex series of chemical reactions, Amadori products can form families of imidazole-based and pyrrole-based glucose-derived cross-links.

affect reactions with receptors such as integrins. Secondly, AGE modification of intracellular proteins changes their function. Finally, AGE-modified circulating proteins bind to specific receptors (RAGEs – three subtypes have now been described) on several types of cell, including monocyte/macrophages, glomerular mesangial cells, retinal pericytes and endothelial cells (Figure 14.12). This binding leads to the generation of reactive oxygen species; activation of secondary messengers such as protein kinase C (PKC); release of transcription factor NFκB leading to overproduction of vasoactive proteins such as endothelins; and stimulation of cytokine and growth factor production, which, in turn, can result in inflammatory cell adhesion (via increased VCAM-1), procoagulant protein expression, and increased vascular permeability (via VEGF) (Figure 14.12).

Recently a circulating soluble RAGE has been identified which appears to mop up AGEs; reduced levels of this scavenger have been linked with increased atherosclerosis.

Several experimental agents that either reduce AGE formation or break cross-links have been tested in animals and humans, but they have proven to be too toxic or have limited benefit. RAGE antagonists have also been used experimentally and shown benefit in animal models.

Extrinsic AGEs are found in tobacco smoke and processed foods (notably roasted meats and some soft drinks). High levels of dietary AGEs have been associated with accelerated atherosclerosis in animals but their role in human disease is uncertain.

Protein Kinase C (PKC)

Protein kinase C is an enzyme that phosphorylates several target proteins (Figure 14.13). It exists in 10 isoforms and is activated by diacylglycerol which is a direct product of increased glucose flux and increased glycolysis. Overactivity of PKC α, β and δ have been implicated in human diabetes and lead to increased vascular permeability and blood flow by increasing VEGF production, particularly in the retina. PKC activation also leads to increased mitogen-activated protein kinase (MAPK) in retinal pericytes leading to apoptosis. Other consequences include a reduction in endogenous nitric oxide synthase (eNOS) which acts as an anti-atherogenic enzyme; an increase in the transcription factor NFκB in endothelial and vascular smooth muscle cells; a possible increase in matrix protein production via TGF-β; and an increase in the plasminogen activation inhibitor PAI-1 (which inhibits fibrinolysis).

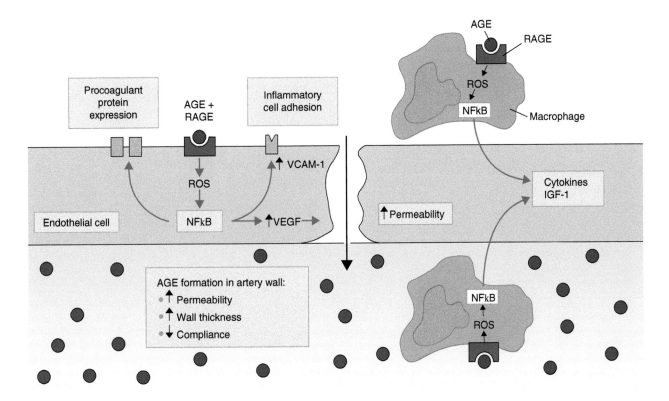

Figure 14.12 Possible mechanisms of cell damage by interactions of advanced glycation end-products (AGEs) with their receptor (RAGE) in endothelial cells and macrophages. IGF, insulin-like growth factor; NFκB, nuclear factor kappa B; ROS, reactive oxygen species; VCAM-1, vascular cell adhesion molecule-1; VEGF, vascular endothelium-derived growth factor.

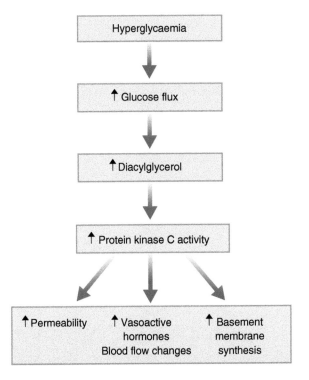

Figure 14.13 Activation of protein kinase C by *de novo* synthesis of diacylglycerol, following increased glucose utilisation.

Interest in this pathway has been stimulated by the development of a PKC β inhibitor, ruboxistaurin, which was shown in experimental animals to reduce the development of retinopathy. Trials in humans initially showed some benefit in advanced eye disease, but no effect on nephropathy. These disappointing results may have been a reflection of the narrow focus of PKC inhibition, agents which block several isoforms may be prove to be more effective.

Hexosamine pathway

An increased flux of glucose and oxidised fatty acids can result in activation of the hexosamine pathway (Figure 14.14). Fructose-6-phosphate is diverted from glycolysis to form UDP-*N*-acetylglucosamine, which is used in the synthesis of glycoproteins. The rate-limiting step in the conversion of glucose to glucosamine is regulated by glutamine:fructose-6-phosphate amidotransferase (GFAT). It is thought that glycation of transcription factors by *N*-acetylglucosamine increases the activity of many genes. Amongst these are TGF-β (a key profibrogenic cytokine), acetyl CoA carboxylase (the rate-limiting enzyme for fatty acid synthesis and which might increase insulin resistance) and PAI-1 which inhibits fibrinolysis.

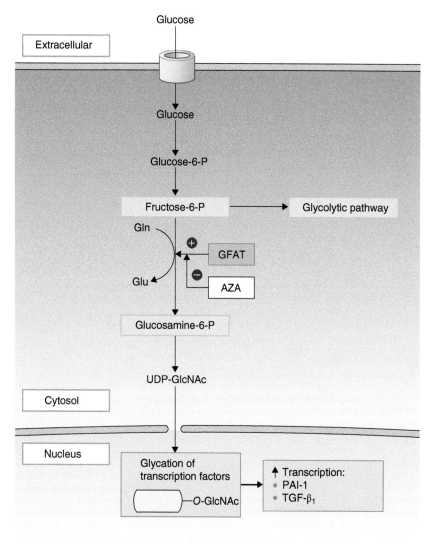

Figure 14.14 The hexosamine pathway. Glucosamine-6-phosphate, generated from fructose-6-phosphate and glutamine (Gln), is converted into UDP-N-acetylglucosamine (UDP-GlcNAc), which can glycate transcription factors and thus enhance transcription of genes including plasminogen activator inhibitor (PAI)-1 and transforming growth factor-β1 (TGF-β1). Glutamine:fructose-6-phosphate amidotransferase (GFAT), the rate-limiting enzyme, is inhibited by azaserine (AZA). Glu, glutamic acid.

Oxidative stress

Increased intracellular glucose in response to hyperglycaemia in vulnerable cells leads to mitochondrial superoxide overproduction following changes in the proton gradient and alterations in the electron transfer process (Figure 14.15). Another rich source of reactive oxygen species (ROS) are the NOX family of NADPH oxidases which are stimulated by activation of the PKC and polyol pathways. Some researchers think that mitochondrial overproduction of ROS is the initiating step in the development of complications, whereas others feel it is the final result of the activation of the polyol, AGE, PKC and hexosamine pathways. Either way, excess ROS is a common finding in experimental diabetes and initiates a range of potentially damaging processes.

Epigenetics

Post translational modifications of histones by methylation can lead to altered gene expression which does not involve

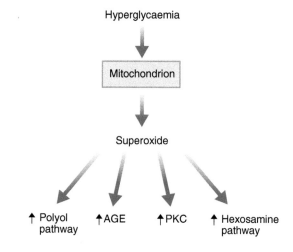

Figure 14.15 Superoxide links glucose and diabetic complications.

changing the DNA sequence. This process has been called epigenetics and is thought to be a possible explanation for metabolic memory. For example, oxidative stress can promote DNA strand breaks which activates the enzyme poly (ADP ribose) polymerase (PARP) which results in changes in the proximal promoter of the transcription factor NFκB subunit in endothelial cells. This leads to an increased expression of pro inflammatory genes and this effect persists for up to six days in tissue culture and six months in experimental animals. Thus, short term hyperglycaemia could initiate a long term change that would take many months of normoglycemia to correct.

Other mechanisms

In normoglycemic individuals, the highest quintile of insulin resistance (corrected for blood pressure, obesity, LDL and HDL cholesterol, and smoking) was associated with a twofold increased risk for cardiovascular disease than the lowest quintile. Impaired insulin function also down regulates prostacyclin synthase and eNOS which are both anti atherogenic. Insulin resistance (IR) results in higher peripheral circulating insulin concentrations and this probably explains the observed association between fasting insulin levels and cardiovascular disease risk in some studies. IR also leads to free fatty acid release and increased lipid oxidation which can activate the hexosamine pathway, and lipid peroxidation can alter cell membrane structure and function.

There is increasing interest in the role of endoplasmic reticulum stress in mediating IR with obesity. The ER is responsible for protein folding and redox homeostasis. The overproduction of ROS in diabetes disrupts these functions which can initiate cell signalling pathways that result in apoptosis.

Angiotensin II production is increased in diabetes, often at the cellular and tissue level rather than systemically. This affects microvascular haemodynamics in the eye and kidney as well as increasing the production of profibrogenic messengers such as TGFβ and pro inflammatory cytokines such as TNFα and IL-6 (see Chapters 16 and 19).

CASE HISTORY

A 65-year-old man with type 1 diabetes for over 50 years attended for annual review. He had few tissue complications apart from minor cheiroarthropathy, minimal background retinopathy, and mild angina, well-controlled medically. His control had always been excellent with HbA1c levels never above 7.5% (58 mmol/mol). He had noticed hypoglycaemic unawareness, however, and because of this he was commenced on CSII 2 years previously.

He is remarkable in other ways. He and his wife had their own family, but they have also fostered over 20 children and have a consequently very large and globally dispersed extended family. He says he was always too active and busy not to look after his diet and diabetes.

Cohorts of people with long duration of type 1 diabetes and minimal complications have been studied both in the UK and the USA. Extensive search for genetic or other factors has failed to identify the reasons for their complication free longevity. Many have had long periods of good glycaemic control which may have resulted in a legacy of a favourable 'metabolic memory'.

LANDMARK CLINICAL TRIAL

Pirart J. Diabetes mellitus and its degenerative complications: a prospective study of 4,400 patients observed between 1947 and 1973. Diabetes Care 1978; 1: 168–188.

This report was initially published in French in *Diabete et Metabolisme* in three parts in 1977 but was felt to be so important that the editor of the new journal *Diabetes Care* had it translated into English to reach a wider audience. It is a remarkable analysis of 4398 patients (2795 since diagnosis) cared for by one physician and his small team since 1947. About 21,000 annual examinations for microvascular complications were correlated with a long-term estimate of glycaemic control (remember, this was before computer spreadsheets and databases). Patients were categorised as having good, fair, or poor control based upon home urinalysis, clinic fasting and postprandial blood glucose levels and episodes of DKA. As shown in Figure 14.1, a clear relationship was found between numbers developing microvascular complications in the eye, kidney and nerve and level of control. This study is an exceptional example of how meticulous observation and record keeping can establish a crucial clinical concept.

FURTHER READING

Barrett, EJ, Liu Z, Khamaisi M et al. Diabetic microvascular disease: an endocrine society statement. JClin Endocrinol Metab 2017; 102: 4343–4410

Cooper ME, El-Osta A, Allen TJ et al. Metabolic karma- the atherogenic legacy of diabetes: the 2017 Edwin Bierman award lecture. Diabetes 2018; 67: 785–90

DCCT Research Group. The effect of intensive treatment of diabetes on the development and progression of long term complications in insulin-dependent diabetes mellitus. N Engl J Med 1993; 329: 977–986.

DCCT/EDIC Research Group. Effect of intensive therapy on the microvascular complications of type 1 diabetes mellitus. JAMA 2002; 287: 2563–2569.

DCCT/EDIC Research Group. Sustained effective intensive treatment of type 1 diabetes mellitus on development and progression of diabetic nephropathy. JAMA 2003; 290: 2159–2167.

DCCT/EDIC Research Group. Effect of intensive diabetes therapy on the progression of diabetic retinopathy in patients with type 1 diabetes: 18 years of follow-up in the DCCT/EDIC. Diabetes 2015; 64: 631–42

Giacco F, Brownlee M. Oxidative stress and diabetic complications. Circulation Research 2010; 107: 1058–70

Holman RR, Paul SK, Bethel MA, Matthews DR, Neil HAW. 10-year follow-up of intensive glucose control in type 2 diabetes. N Engl J Med 2008; 359: 1577–1589.

Khaw K-T, Wareham N, Luben R, et al. Glycated haemoglobin, diabetes and mortality in men in the Norfolk cohort of the European Prospective Investigation of Cancer and Nutrition (EPIC-Norfolk). BMJ 2001; 322: 1–6.

Rask-Madsen C, King GL. Vascular complications of diabetes: mechanisms of injury and protective factors. Cell Metab 2013; 17: 20–33

Skyler JS, Bergenstal R, Bonow RO, et al. Intensive glycaemic control and the prevention of cardiovascular events: implications of the ACCORD, ADVANCE and VA Diabetes Trials. Diabetes Care 2009; 32: 187–192.

Sun J, Wang YCUI W et al. Role of epigenetic histone modifications in diabetic kidney disease involving renal fibrosis. J Diabetes Res 2017; doi: 10.1155/2017/7242384

Yan L-J. Redox imbalance stress in diabetes mellitus: role of the polyol pathway. Animal Models and Experimental Medicine 2018; 1: 7–13

Stratton IM, Cull CA, Adler AI, Matthews DR, Neil HAW, Holman RR. Additive effects of glycaemia and blood pressure exposure on risk of complications in type 2 diabetes: a prospective observational study (UKPDS 75). Diabetologia 2006; 49: 1761–1769.

UK Prospective Diabetes Study (UKPDS) Group. Intensive blood-glucose control with sulphonylureas or insulin compared with conventional treatment and risk of complications in patients with type II diabetes (UKPDS 33). Lancet 1998; 352: 837–853.

Diabetic eye disease

Diabetic eye disease primarily affects the retinal vasculature, but the iris and lens can also be involved. Most people with diabetes will show signs of retinopathy after 25 years duration, but only a minority (around 10%) develop sight threatening disease. Proliferative retinopathy is the commonest sight threatening lesion in type 1 diabetes, whilst for type 2 diabetes it is macular oedema. Progression rates over four years have declined significantly from 40% in 1979 to 10% in 2010, but remain more rapid in those with more severe lesions. The majority (75%) of significant visual loss associated with diabetes is accounted for by macular oedema. Even with anti-VEGF therapy, about one third of patients do not completely respond, and diabetes still remains a significant cause of visual loss in the working-age population in the UK. Adults with diabetes in the USA have 1.85 times the risk of having a non-correctable reduction in visual acuity compared to age matched controls. The Global Burden of Disease report for 2015 reveals that 34.7% of people with diabetes have recorded visual loss, which is an increase of 5% over the preceding 10 years. The same study estimates a global total of over 300,000 years living with visual disability due to diabetes. However, even though diabetes is no longer the commonest cause of blindness in the working age population in the UK and USA, it still accounts for 14.4% of annual registrations in the UK. Newer therapies are proving more effective in preventing visual loss, but more research is needed to determine their optimum sequence and for the development of less invasive and cheaper treatment options.

Pathology and clinical appearances
Retinopathy

Essentially, diabetic retinopathy can be classified as non-proliferative (now often split into background and pre-proliferative) and proliferative.

The earliest pathological features are thickening of the retinal capillary basement membrane, loss of tight junctions in the retinal endothelium, and loss of pericytes which are the contractile cells enveloping the capillaries and which control vessel calibre and thus perfusion (Figure 15.1). Physiologically, an increase in retinal blood flow is an early feature of diabetes and it is possible that this creates mechanical stress that leads to endothelial separation and pericyte loss. Ultimately, endothelial cell loss leads to acellular capillaries which are prone to thrombosis, leading to retinal ischaemia.

Handbook of Diabetes, Fifth Edition. Rudy Bilous, Richard Donnelly, and Iskandar Idris.
© 2021 John Wiley & Sons Ltd. Published 2021 by John Wiley & Sons Ltd.

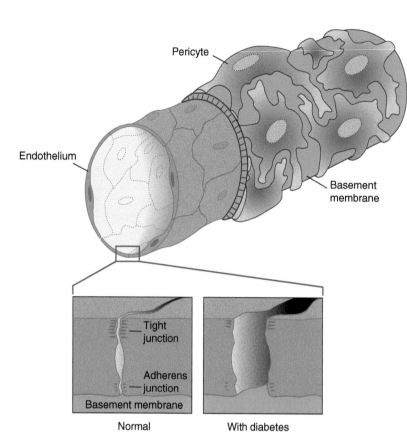

Figure 15.1 Structure of the retinal microvasculature. The endothelial cells are normally joined by tight junctions, which constitute much of the blood–retinal barrier; these separate in diabetes, causing increased vascular permeability. Other abnormalities in diabetes include thickening of the basement membrane and fall-out of both the endothelial cells and the contractile pericytes.

Much of the nutrient supply to the photoreceptors comes via the choroidal circulation, which has a circulatory flow rate up to 10 times that of the retina. Unlike the retinal circulation, these vessels are under autonomic nervous system control and are therefore vulnerable to neuropathic damage due to diabetes. Choroidal thickness is also reduced in people with early retinopathy, and blood oxygen levels are lower during hyperglycaemia. The precise consequences of these observations for the development and progression of retinopathy are unclear.

The first noticeable lesions on ophthalmoscopy are microaneurysms, which appear as small red dots varying in size from 20 to 200 μm in diameter (Figures 15.2, 15.3). They are blind pouches arising from capillaries, probably from weakened endothelial cell junctions adjacent to an area of pericyte loss. Microaneurysms are rarely sight threatening (unless occurring in the macula) and can seem to disappear although this is probably a result of thrombosis within the aneurysm or closure of the feeding capillary. Capillary closure is a feature of advancing retinopathy and the resultant ischaemia is a driver for subsequent proliferation.

Haemorrhages can occur superficially when they tend to be flame shaped (limited by nerve fibres) or deep (blot or round shaped and indicative of underlying ischaemia) (Figure 15.4).

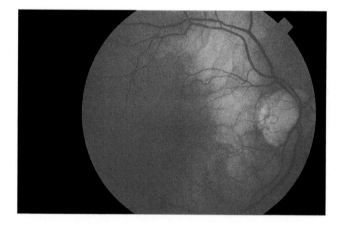

Figure 15.2 Microaneurysms, the earliest sign of diabetic retinopathy appearing as small red dots above and around the macula. This is a myopic eye with a pale fundus.

Hard exudates are the result of leakage of lipid rich proteins into the retina (Figure 15.5). They appear as discrete yellow-creamy white patches which are often ring-shaped or circinate around a central area of ischaemia and capillary leakage.

Capillary closure causes microinfarcts in the nerve fibre layer and these appear as indistinct white patches and are termed cotton wool spots (previously known as soft

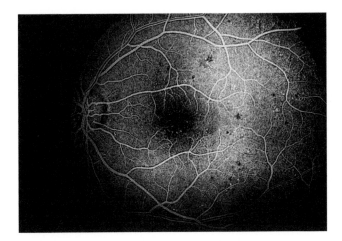

Figure 15.3 Fluorescein angiogram, showing microaneurysms as small white dots and haemorrhages as larger black spots. These lesions are more easily demonstrated by angiography.

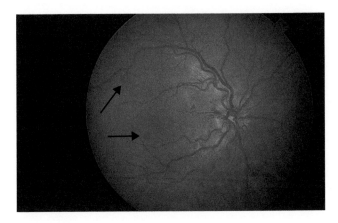

Figure 15.4 Retinal haemorrhages: red 'blots'.

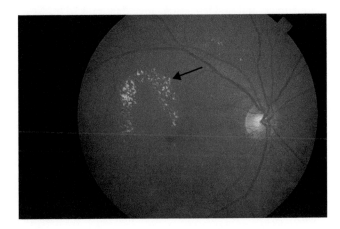

Figure 15.5 Focal diabetic maculopathy with circinate (ring-shaped) exudate. Laser treatment is applied to the leaking microaneurysms at the centre of the circinate exudates.

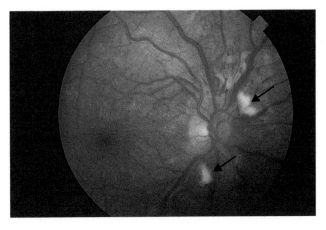

Figure 15.6 Cotton wool spots around the optic disc. Note also flame and blot shaped haemorrhages above the optic disc.

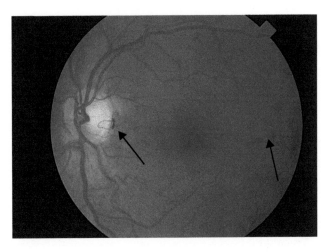

Figure 15.7 Intraretinal microvascular abnormalities (IRMAs) appearing as a fine mesh of vessels.

exudates) (Figure 15.6). More advanced ischaemia results in the development of intraretinal microvascular abnormalities (IRMAs) (Figure 15.7), which are clumps of small irregularly branching vessels within the retina. There is often concomitant venous dilatation, beading (segmental dilatation resembling a string of sausages) (Figure 15.8), loops, and reduplication; sometimes into patterns resembling a four-leafed clover.

New vessel growth or neovascularisation is the hallmark of proliferative retinopathy and results from the local release of growth factors (such as vascular endothelium-derived growth factor – (VEGF), although others are also produced such as angiopoietins, platelet derived growth factor, fibroblast growth factor and connective tissue growth factor) in response to ischaemia (Figures 15.9, 15.10). These vessels are fragile, fine outgrowths from retinal veins and grow forward into the vitreous. Because of this, they are prone to shear stress and rupture, resulting in preretinal or vitreous

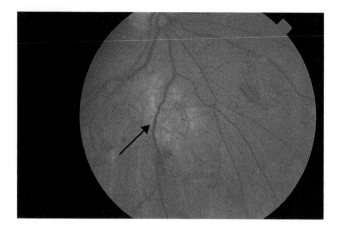

Figure 15.8 Venous irregularity or 'beading' (centre of field) and new vessels with associated haemorrhage in the top right field.

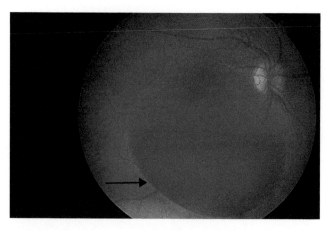

Figure 15.11 Preretinal haemorrhage. Note the settling of the uncoagulated blood. Courtesy of Dr PJ Barry, Royal Victoria Eye and Ear Hospital, Belfast, UK.

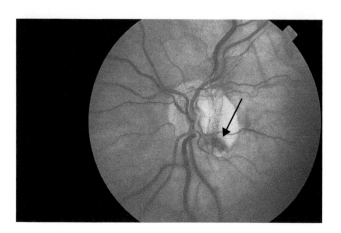

Figure 15.9 More extensive new vessels on the disc, occupying more than half the disc diameter.

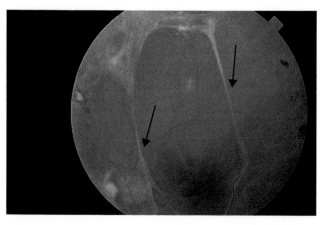

Figure 15.12 Fibrous bands that are exerting traction on the retina. The retinal scars (dark patches in the periphery) result from previous xenon laser treatment.

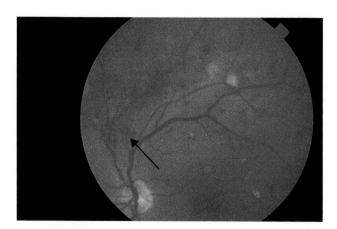

Figure 15.10 Extensive neovascularisation above the disc, with widespread signs of retinal ischaemia.

haemorrhage and sudden visual loss (Figure 15.11). New vessels are associated with fibrous bands that can cause traction retinal detachment or tearing of vessels, leading to further haemorrhage (Figure 15.12). Sometimes the haemorrhage remains encapsulated between these fibrous bands, the retina, and the vitreous, leading to a fluid level and a flat-topped (boat-shaped) appearance.

Tractional detachment results in 'tenting' or folding of the retina with grey-white bands and occasional tears (Figure 15.13). Ophthalmic ultrasound is often helpful at detecting detachment, particularly if the retina is obscured by haemorrhage (Figure 15.14).

The most common cause of visual loss, however, is maculopathy which results from ischaemia and subsequent oedema of the central retina. Focal maculopathy is usually associated with areas of circinate or star-shaped exudate within one optic disc diameter of the macula (Figure 15.15).

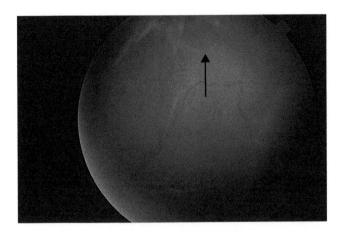

Figure 15.13 Rhegmatogenous retinal detachment: a large retinal tear (red lesion; arrow) is present at the top, and the detached retina appears grey and folded.

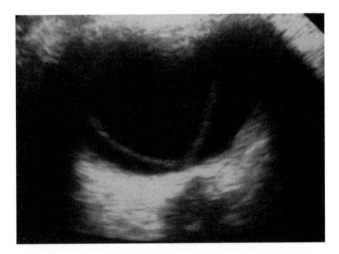

Figure 15.14 B-scan ultrasound image of the eye, showing a retinal detachment that was invisible behind a dense vitreous haemorrhage.

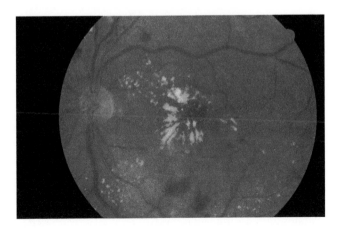

Figure 15.15 Diffuse macular oedema, with a macular 'star'. This requires laser photocoagulation. Courtesy of Professor Simon Harding, Liverpool.

Diffuse macular oedema results from ischaemia and causes thickening of the retina. It is harder to detect clinically and needs either stereo ophthalmoscopy or optical coherence tomography (OCT) which can generate clear images of the retina and accurate estimates of thickness (Figure 15.16).

Iris

New vessel growth on the iris (rubeosis iridis – also in response to ischaemia) (Figure 15.17) can close the drainage angle and cause acute glaucoma. This condition is called rubeotic glaucoma, it is acutely painful and can occasionally occur following cataract surgery or vitrectomy if there is underlying active proliferative retinopathy. Treatment is unsatisfactory and the end result is often a painful blind eye.

Lens

Cataract is common in diabetes and can occur acutely and diffusely with newly diagnosed diabetes (so-called snowstorm cataract) or, more commonly, posterior subcapsular and cortical cataracts which occur after several years' duration (Figure 15.18). The 10-year cumulative incidence of cataract surgery in the WESDR study was 8% and 25% for patients with type 1 and type 2 diabetes respectively. The underlying cause for snowstorm cataract is probably acute fluid shift due to hyperglycaemia and hyperosmolality. Linear or central cataract probably results from non-enzymatic glycation and subsequent cross-linkage of lens crystallins. Sorbitol accumulation secondary to activation of the polyol pathway may also contribute. Extraction and replacement with a plastic implant is the treatment of choice. The results are generally good but active proliferative retinopathy should be treated first.

Optic disc

Anterior ischaemic optic neuropathy is caused by microvascular disease of the anterior optic nerve. Patients present with painless loss of vision usually upon wakening. The condition often remains stable but there is no known effective treatment.

A related problem of acute disc oedema and moderate visual loss can occur and is termed diabetic papillopathy. This usually improves spontaneously but it may take up to 12 months and it can be confused with papilloedema.

Other optic conditions

It is important to bear in mind that non-diabetes associated ophthalmic conditions may contribute to visual problems in people with diabetes. Glaucoma is now not thought to be more common in people with diabetes, although there may be ethnic differences in this regard. It still needs to be considered in older people or those from susceptible ethnic minorities (such as Afro-Caribbean and Hispanic) who have higher prevalences of the condition. Refractive changes are common in diabetes, notably during acute hyperglycaemia or in those with newly diagnosed type 1. There is also some

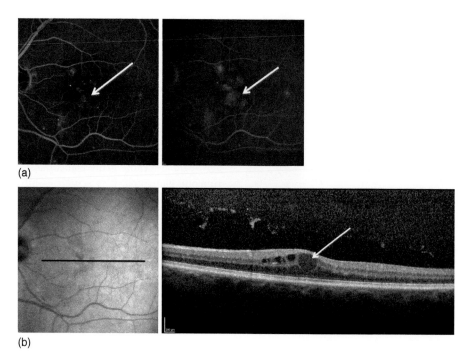

(a)

(b)

Figure 15.16 Left eye of a patient with diffuse diabetic macular oedema. (a) Mid (*left*) and late (*right*) phase fluorescein angiogram image showing leaking microaneurysms and pooling of dye in intraretinal spaces (*arrows*). (b) Red free image (*left*) showing location of single line scan on Spectralis OCT (optical coherence tomography). OCT (*right*) shows mixed reflectivity intraretinal cysts with thickening of the retina and a detached hyaloid face (*arrow*). Courtesy of Professor Simon Harding, Liverpool.

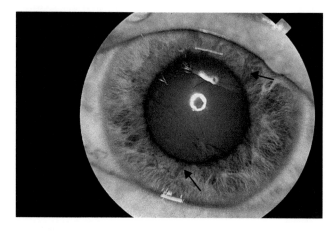

Figure 15.17 New vessels (arrows) on the iris (rubeosis iridis). There is also loss of the red reflex indicating a vitreous haemorrhage and linear lens cataract.

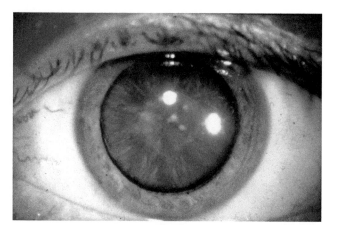

Figure 15.18 Diabetic cataract appearing as pale opacification of the lens.

evidence that presbyopia may occur at an earlier age in people with type 1 diabetes. See Box 15.1.

Factors associated with the development of retinopathy

Many of these have been identified from epidemiological studies and are therefore associations (Box 15.2), but most have been confirmed from intervention trials such as the DCCT, UKPDS, ACCORD, and ADVANCE.

Some of these factors are co-related, for example hyperglycaemia (as estimated from HbA1c levels and thus severity of protein glycation) and duration of diabetes (being a measure of exposure to the hyperglycaemic insult). Other factors are less intuitive; in pregnancy, many women rapidly improve glycaemic control in order to minimise foetal risk of malformation. This can precipitate worsening of retinopathy, perhaps by reducing blood flow through an already ischaemic retina and causing a sudden release of growth factors. This phenomenon can also occur with too rapid correction of glycaemia in non-pregnant patients (e.g. commencing CSII). Careful retinal surveillance is needed in these situations (see below). Heritability estimates for proliferative retinopathy range from 25–50% but the genetic basis has not been identified. Experimental studies have demonstrated a number of epigenetic effects induced in retinal cells by growth factors, oxidative stress, and hypoxia.

Classification of retinopathy

The clinical categories of non-proliferative and proliferative, although clinically useful, have proven too broad for research purposes. Moreover, the nomenclature 'background' implies a somewhat benign condition which nonetheless represents pathological damage and can progress.

The Early Treatment Diabetic Retinopathy Study (ETDRS) devised a modified scale based upon the Airlie House classification and this has become the gold standard for all intervention trials such as the DCCT and UKPDS (Box 15.3). A two- or three-step change in combined eye score is positively associated with progression to proliferative retinopathy and visual loss. Moreover, in the UKPDS, 30% of patients with a level of ≥35 in both eyes required photocoagulation after 9 years.

However, this grading is complex and was based upon seven-field stereo fundus photographs which are both time consuming and expensive, as well as being uncomfortable for the patient. Moreover, the classification is hard to apply without expert training and experience. The UK National Screening Committee has proposed a simpler classification that feeds into a treatment algorithm with referral targets, and forms the basis of the Diabetic Retinopathy Screening Programme in the UK (Box 15.4).

Treatment of retinopathy
Glycaemic control

Both the DCCT in type 1 and the UKPDS in type 2 diabetes demonstrated the benefit of glycaemic control for the primary prevention of new retinopathy, and secondary prevention of progression of existing retinopathy. Neither the ACCORD nor ADVANCE studies showed a consistent benefit of improved glycaemic control on a range of retinopathy end points, but a meta-analysis of these and other studies showed a relative risk reduction of 20% (95% CI 6,33; p = 0.009) on retinopathy severity as assessed using the ETDRS scale (Box 15.3). The 8-year follow-up of the ACCORD trial continued to show improvement in retinopathy in the tight glycaemic control cohort with 5.8% vs. 12.7% progressing by 3 or more levels on the ETDRS scale, but there was no impact on preservation of visual acuity. There are, however, other potential long-term benefits of glycaemic control in terms of prevention of complications (see Chapter 14).

As previously mentioned, rapid improvement in glycaemia can result in an early worsening of retinopathy, but most of the trials in which this was noticed (DCCT, Kroc, Stockholm and Oslo Studies) found that in the long-term, patients on intensive insulin regimens still had better retinal outcomes than their conventionally treated controls, despite the early deterioration.

Blood pressure control

Embedded within the UKPDS was a trial of tight (target <150/<85 mmHg) or less tight (target <180/<105 mmHg) blood pressure control in 1148 hypertensive, newly diagnosed, type 2 diabetic patients. There was a 34% (99% CI

Box 15.3 Modified Airlie House Classification of Retinopathy (Early Treatment Diabetic Retinopathy Study [ETDRS] Scale) and annual rates of progression.

ETDRS Retinopathy Severity scale	ETDRS Grading	Lesions	Risk of progression to PDR in 1 year
No apparent retinopathy	10	Nil	
Mild NPDR	20	1 or more microaneurysms only	
Mild NPDR	35	Microaneurysms and haemorrhages and/or hard exudates and/or cotton wool spots	Grade 30 = 6.2%
Moderate NPDR	43	As above plus severe haemorrhages or IRMA	Grade 41 = 11.3%
Moderately severe NPDR	47	As 35 plus severe haemorrhages and IRMA and/or venous beading	Grade 45 = 20.7%
Severe NPDR	53	Severe haemorrhages and IRMA and venous beading and cotton wool spots	Grade 51 = 41.2% Grade 55 = 54.8%
PDR	61+	Proliferative diabetic retinopathy	

IRMA = intra retinal microvascular abnormalities; NPDR = non proliferative diabetic retinopathy; PDR = proliferative diabetic retinopathy.
Adapted from Scanlon PH Acta Diabetologica 2017 DOI: 10.1007/s00592-017-0974-1.

11–50%) risk reduction in progression (two-step ETDRS change), and 35% risk reduction in the need for laser photocoagulation. *Post hoc* analysis suggested a 13% decrease in the aggregate microvascular endpoint (combination of retinopathy requiring photocoagulation, vitreous haemorrhage and/or fatal or non-fatal renal failure) for every 10 mmHg reduction in blood pressure.

Similar results were found in the normotensive (but not hypertensive) patients in the Appropriate Blood Pressure Control in Diabetes (ABCD) trial, and the ADVANCE study also failed to demonstrate a benefit on retinopathy progression of a mean reduction in blood pressure of 5.6/2.2 mmHg in 11,140 mainly hypertensive type 2 patients. The ACCORD study assigned patients to a target systolic blood pressure of either <120 or <140 mmHg and found no benefit of the lower target on retinopathy progression. The reasons for these disparities between normo- and hypertensive patients are not clear. The magnitude of the blood pressure reduction was greater in the two positive studies, and the ascertainment of effect was most precise in the UKPDS. A Cochrane review of 15 trials in type 1 and 2 diabetes suggested an overall benefit of blood pressure lowering on retinopathy development, but not progression.

There are no data on the effect of blood pressure lowering on retinopathy in type 1 diabetes.

Renin angiotensin system (RAS) blockade
The EURODIAB Controlled Trial of Lisinopril in Insulin-Dependent Diabetes Mellitus (EUCLID) found a benefit of lisinopril on retinopathy progression over 2 years, but statistical significance was lost when results were corrected for HbA1c.

The much larger and longer DIRECT study (DIabetic REtinopathy Candesartan Trial) looked at the effect of a median 4.7 years of candesartan 32 mg per day on development and progression of retinopathy in 3326 normotensive type 1 and 1905 normotensive or well-controlled hypertensive patients with type 2 diabetes. There was a 35% relative risk reduction in a three-step ETDRS change in incidence of retinopathy in type 1 diabetes, and a 34% increase in the chance of regression (three steps for 1 year or two steps for 2 or more years) in type 2 diabetes. No significant effect was seen on three-step progression of existing retinopathy in patients with type 1 or type 2 diabetes, although candesartan use was uniformly and statistically significantly associated with less retinopathy progression (one-step change).

A meta-analysis of 21 trials with 13,823 participants showed reductions in both development and progression of diabetic retinopathy associated with RAS blocking agents, and the magnitude of effect was greater in normotensive patients.

PKC β inhibition
Ruboxistaurin was shown to reduce visual loss in patients with moderately severe non-proliferative retinopathy and macular oedema, but no further studies with this agent have been reported and no license for its use in people with retinopathy has been granted.

Lipid-lowering agents
The Fenofibrate Intervention and Event Lowering in Diabetes (FIELD) study found a significant reduction in the need for laser therapy (5.2% versus 3.6%: p = 0.0003) in

Box 15.4 UK National Screening Committee Grading of Retinopathy and US Grading [in brackets].

NSC	International Term	Symptoms	Features	Action
R0	No DR	None	Normal retina. [Grade 0 (US)]	annual rescreen
RI	Mild non-proliferative (mild pre-proliferative)	None	Haemorrhages & microaneurysms only Very minor IRMAs [Grade 1 (US)]	Inform diabetes team
R2	Moderate non-proliferative, moderate pre-proliferative	None	Previously termed mild pre-proliferative. Extensive Microaneurysm, intraretinal haemorrhage, and hard exudates. [Grade 2 (US)]	refer HES
R2	Severe non-proliferative severe pre-proliferative	None	Previously termed severe pre-proliferative. Venous abnormalities, large blot haemorrhages, cotton wool spots (small infarcts), venous beading, venous loop, venous reduplication, IRMA [Grade 3 (US)]	urgent refer HES
R3	Proliferative retinopathy	Floaters, sudden visual loss	New vessel formation either at the disc (NVD) or elsewhere (NVE). [Grade 4a (US)]	urgent refer HES
R3	Pre-retinal fibrosis+/- tractional retinal detachment	Floaters, central loss of vision	Extensive fibrovascular proliferation, retinal detachment, pre retinal or vitreous haemorrhage, glaucoma. [Grade 4b (US)]	urgent refer HES
R3s	treated proliferative retinopathy (s = stable)		No haemorrhages or exudates or new vessels, laser ('P' added)	annual rescreen
M 0			No maculopathy	annual rescreen
M 1	Diabetic maculopathy	Blurred central vision	The macula is defined as a circle centred on the fovea, with a radius of the distance to the disc margin. If the leakage involves or is near the fovea the condition is termed clinically significant macular oedema (CSME). Exudative maculopathy presents with leakage, retinal thickening, microaneurysms, hard exudates at the macula. Ischaemic form can have a featureless macular with NVE and poor vision. Milder forms: • exudate < or = 1DD of centre of fovea • circinate or group of exudates within macula • any microaneurysm or haemorrhage < or = 1DD of centre of fovea only is associated with a best VA of < or = 6/12 retinal thickening < or = 1DD of centre of fovea (if stereos available)	refer HES
P	Photocoagulation	Reduced night vision, glare	Small retinal scars through out the peripheral retina. [Grade 4b (US)]	
OL/ BUG	Other lesion/ Un-gradable		Un-gradable is usually due to cataract, other lesions usually referred for assessment	

DR = diabetic retinopathy; DD = disc diameter; HES = Hospital Eye Services; IRMAs = intraretinal microvascular abnormalities (part of severe pre-proliferative retinopathy, vessels will not leak with angiogram, otherwise they would be 'new vessels' making the condition 'proliferative'); MA = microaneurysms; MO = macular oedema; NPDR = non-proliferative retinopathy; NVE = new vessels elsewhere.
Adapted from www. diabeticretinopathy.org.uk

9795 patients with type 2 diabetes treated for 5 years. This effect was independent of blood lipid levels. More recently, the ACCORD study also showed a positive benefit of fenofibrate on progressive retinopathy, with a reduction of progression using the ETDRS scale of one-third. As no consistent effect of statin therapy on retinopathy has been reported, it is likely that any effect of fenofibrate is independent of lipid lowering and perhaps related to its PPAR-α inhibiting effect. Fenofibrate is not licensed for use in diabetic retinopathy in the UK.

Growth hormone inhibitors

The observation of a regression in proliferative retinopathy in a woman with Sheehan's syndrome (postpartum hypopituitarism) and the subsequent clinical trials (in the days before photocoagulation) of hypophysectomy in patients with advanced eye disease, established a potential link between growth hormone and neovascularisation. Octreotide (a somatostatin analogue that blocks growth hormone release) has been shown to decrease progression of severe non-proliferative or early proliferative retinopathy, but had significant GI side effects. Clinical trials of topical somatostatin analogues are currently ongoing.

Intravitreal steroids

Triamcinolone (by injection) and fluocinolone and dexamethasone (by implant) have been shown to reduce macular oedema and improve visual acuity, but with the serious side effects of glaucoma and cataract formation. Many patients required multiple steroid injections (although these can be avoided by using implants) and some developed infections. The long-term benefits and safety of these treatments still need to be established and they have been largely superseded by VEGF inhibitors.

VEGF inhibitors

A Cochrane Review of anti-VEGF therapy for proliferative diabetic retinopathy confirmed the safety of intravitreal injection therapy, and suggested benefit in terms of preventing vitreous haemorrhage when combined with vireo-retinal surgery. More recently, aflibercept has been shown to result in better visual acuity compared to pan retinal photocoagulation at one year post randomisation. However, the cost, convenience, number of treatment visits and small risk of infection makes this treatment less acceptable to many patients, and its' routine use is not currently recommended.

For diabetes related macular oedema, the evidence of greater benefit for anti-VEGF therapy over grid laser photocoagulation is much stronger. The greatest benefit was seen in those with central retinal thickness >400µm, and NICE has approved intravitreal injection therapy for these patients. Further research is required on the long-term benefit and comparative cost effectiveness of different anti-VEGF agents and treatment regimens. Currently, monthly injections are often recommended for the first year, with less frequency thereafter, but there is a need for more research to determine the best and safest regimens. Published complication rates are very low, and concerns about potential adverse systemic side effects appear unfounded. However, around 20–40% of patients do not achieve full resolution of macular oedema, and the optimum next step is still uncertain with some recommending steroid implant and others grid laser. There also remains uncertainty over the best first line therapy for those with well-preserved visual acuity as most studies recruited subjects with a baseline visual acuity of <20/32 (<6/9.5). The documented effectiveness, lower cost, and need for fewer visits makes grid laser an attractive option for these patients. A recent review suggests a watch and wait policy for those with a visual acuity ≤20/25 (6/7.5) and intervention only if vision deteriorates.

Laser photocoagulation

Meta-analysis shows that pan-retinal laser photocoagulation (PRP) (Figure 15.19) reduces the risk of blindness in eyes with proliferative retinopathy by 61%, and this has now become the cornerstone of treatment of advanced disease. Focal laser photocoagulation can be effective for more discrete neovascularisation or ischaemia. There is no evidence that PRP confers benefit until sight-threatening proliferative retinopathy is present.

Similarly, in the ETDRS, focal grid laser photocoagulation to the macula decreased the risk of moderate visual loss due to macula oedema by 50% (95% CI 47,53%) over 3 years in 2244 patients with bilateral disease (Figure 15.20).

Photocoagulation is generally well tolerated but some patients can experience discomfort and need local anaesthetic. Up to 23% of patients experience transient or permanent visual loss following PRP; there can also be visual field constriction and night blindness which can affect eligibility for driving.

These problems emphasise the essentially destructive nature of PRP which is why prevention of retinopathy is so important, and also why there is active research into alternative medical treatments.

Vitreoretinal surgery

Surgical vitrectomy in advanced eye disease results in sustained benefit in terms of visual acuity, with 6/12 (20/40) or greater vision in at least 25% of eyes at 4 years. Improved operative technique with intraoperative imaging has greatly advanced the field and is likely to have improved outcomes.

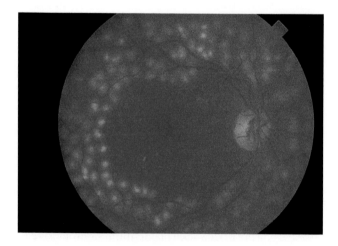

Figure 15.19 Recent panretinal (scatter) laser photocoagulation burns for treating new vessels on the disc.

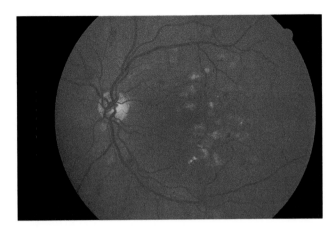

Figure 15.20 Focal laser photocoagulation scars around the macula following successful focal treatment. Note also widespread microaneurysms and blot haemorrhages around the areas of photocoagulation.

Stem cell and other therapies

The discovery of circulating endothelial progenitor cells (EPCs) and the observation of reduced numbers in people with diabetes has resulted in studies of their use in experimental animals with mixed results. No trial data are available in humans, although stem cell therapy is widely promoted on the web. The risks are unclear, the benefits uncertain and patients should be advised accordingly.

Erythropoietin levels are unregulated in the eye in early diabetic retinopathy and are thought to be protective. However, in advanced disease it may enhance the effects of VEGF and exacerbate proliferation.

Calcium dobesilate has been shown in meta analysis to reduce some of the features of retinopathy but not macular oedema. It is licensed for use in some countries but not the UK or USA.

The dark-adapted eye has a high oxygen consumption and preliminary studies of eye masks at night which expose the eye to infra-red light showed encouraging results. Unfortunately, the larger CLEOPATRA trial failed to demonstrate benefit, but others are ongoing.

Surveillance and screening

Regular retinal examination is recommended by all national guidelines. The ADA suggests expert examination within 5 years of diagnosis of all with type 1 diabetes aged >10 years because retinopathy is most unlikely to develop within that time, and as soon as possible after diagnosis of type 2 diabetes because of the significant prevalence of retinopathy in newly diagnosed patients. The best periodicity thereafter is controversial. The ADA suggests that review could be every two or more years if there are several annual assessments with no retinopathy. Studies from Liverpool in the UK suggest that there is a minimal likelihood of progression from no retinopathy to significant change requiring therapy in less than two years in patients with type 2 diabetes.

The most effective mode of surveillance has been the subject of intense research and in the UK there is general agreement that digital fundus photography is superior to both optometrist-based slit lamp ophthalmoscopy, as well as opportunistic direct ophthalmoscopy performed by diabetologists. The National Screening Committee has recommended annual two-field digital fundus photography for everyone with diabetes, and a nationally funded programme is now in place. In pregnancy, women should be screened as soon as possible after booking and also at 28 weeks' gestation. An additional review should occur at 16–20 weeks if the first one reveals any retinopathy.

Photographs are graded according to the scale in Box 15.4 and there are set referral targets based upon their score. 98% of individuals with a grade of R2 or worse, and/or M1 in the worst affected eye should be referred to a specialist clinic within 3 weeks of their screening, and ≥ 80% of those with R3a within 6 weeks. In England in 2015/16, 82.8% (2,144,007) of those invited for screening attended. 7593 were referred urgently with proliferative retinopathy, and 52 597 were referred with screen positive maculopathy or pre-proliferative retinopathy. Only 20% of those with maculopathy needed therapy, however, and in order to improve efficiency artificial intelligence systems are being developed to improve diagnostic precision. The National Screening Programme has been responsible for reducing the contribution of diabetes to rates of visual loss in the population, although there are continuing challenges to improve uptake in more socially deprived communities.

CASE HISTORY

A 29-year-old woman with type 1 diabetes and coeliac disease had a profound fear of hypoglycaemia. Consequently, she maintained high blood glucose levels and her HbA1c was consistently above 75 mmol/mol (9%). Because of developing retinopathy, she elected to try CSII. There was a dramatic improvement in blood glucose control without hypoglycaemia, and her HbA1c came down to 47 mmol/mol (6.5%) over 6 months. Regular ophthalmic assessments were scheduled but she missed two appointments. Four months later she presented with acute vitreous haemorrhage in her right eye secondary to advanced proliferative retinopathy. Extensive panretinal photocoagulation has prevented further haemorrhage and preserved vision in her left eye, but she required vitreoretinal surgery on the right for traction detachment.

Comment: This case demonstrates the potential for rapid worsening of retinopathy with glycaemic improvement. It is essential to arrange frequent eye examinations in this and similar situations (such as pregnancy) and also to impress upon the patient their importance. Panretinal photocoagulation is best carried out before neovascularisation and haemorrhage.

LANDMARK CLINICAL TRIAL

Kroc Collaborative Study Group. Blood glucose control and the evolution of diabetic retinopathy and albuminuria. A preliminary multicentre trial. N Engl J Med 1984; 311: 365–372.

This was an international, multicentre trial of improved versus conventional glycaemic control on microvascular complications in the eye and kidney. Seventy patients were randomised to either CSII or conventional insulin (CIT) for 8 months. All had non-proliferative retinopathy at baseline. Twenty-four hour average blood glucose from a seven-point profile collected at home using plastic fluoridated tubes was 11 mmol/L (198 mg/dL) and 10.4 mmol/L (187 mg/dL) at baseline in the CSII and CIT groups respectively. Baseline total HbA1c (normal range 47 – 62 mmol/mol (6.5–7.8%) was 89 mmol/mol (10.3%) and 87 mmol/mol (10.1%) respectively. During the 8-month trial glycaemia did not change in those on CIT but mean 24-hour glucose was 6.4 mmol/L (115 mg/dL) and HbA1c 65 mmol/mol (8.1%) in those on CSII. Retinopathy worsened with the appearance of IRMAs and cotton wool spots suggestive of ischaemia. Albuminuria, however, was significantly reduced in the 10 patients with baseline values >12 μg/min on CSII with no change in the 10 on CIT. The authors concluded that medium-term maintenance of glycaemic separation was possible (previously this had been extremely difficult to achieve) but that the worsening of retinopathy was a concern. They concluded: 'These preliminary observations indicate the need for longer trials (particularly of primary prevention)'.

This study set the stage for the much bigger DCCT – it could almost be considered as the pilot. The finding of acute worsening of retinopathy was confirmed by the Stockholm and Oslo studies and was seen in the secondary prevention arm of the DCCT. Later analysis of the Kroc patients showed that in the long term, eye complications were less severe in the CSII group, thus providing reassurance for the DCCT.

The study also showed that CSII was an effective, safe and practicable research tool.

The study name derived from the Kroc Family Foundation which funded the trial. Dr Robert Kroc was one of the founders of the MacDonalds hamburger chain.

KEY WEBSITES

- UKPDS: www.dtu.ox.ac.uk/ukpds/
- DCCT/EDIC: www.niddk.nih.gov/patient/edic/edic-public.htm
- UK National Screening Committee portal: www.screening.nhs.uk/
- www.NICE.org.uk
- SIGN Guidelines: www.SIGN.ac.uk
- Royal College of Ophthalmologists UK www.diabeticretinopathy.org.uk

FURTHER READING

American Diabetes Association. Standards of medical care in diabetes – 2020. Diabetes Care 2020; 43(Suppl 1): S141–S143.

Do DV, Wang X, Vedula SS, Marrone M, Sleilati G, Hawkins BS, Frank BN. Blood pressure control for diabetic retinopathy. Cochrane Database of Systematic Reviews 2015.Issue1.Art.No.: CD006127 DOI: 10.1002/14651858.CD006127.pub2

Evans JR, Michelessi M, Virgili G. Laser photocoagulation for diabetic proliferative retinopathy. Cochrane Database of Systematic Reviews 2014, Issue 11, Art.No.: CD011234 DOI: 10.1002/14651858.CD011234.pub2

Jampol LE, Glassman AR, Sun J. Evaluation and care of patients with diabetic retinopathy. N Engl J Med 2020; 382: 1629–37.

Khan A, Petropoulos IN, Ponirakis G, Malik RA. Visual complications in diabetes mellitus: beyond retinopathy. Diabetic Med 2016 DOI: 10.1111/dme13296

Martinez-Zapata MJ, Marti-Carvajal AJ, Sola I, Pijoan JI, Buil-Calvo JA, Cordero JA, Evans JR. Anti-vascular endothelial growth factor for proliferative diabetic retinopathy. Cochrane Database of Systematic Reviews 2014. Issue 11. Art.No.: CD008721 DOI: 10.1002/14651858.CD008721.pub2

Scanlon PH. The English National Screening Programme for diabetic retinopathy 2003 – 2016 Acta Diabetologica 2017; 54: 515–25 DOI: 10.1007/s00592-017-0974-1

Simo R, Hernandez C. Novel treatments for diabetic retinopathy based on recent pathogenic evidence. Progress in Retinal and Eye Research 2015; 48: 160–80.

Sivaprasad S, Vasconcelos JC, Prevost AT et al Clinical efficacy and safety of a face mask for prevention of dark adaptation in treating and preventing progression of early diabetic macular oedema at 24 months (CLEOPATRA): a multicentre, phase 3, randomised controlled trial. Lancet Diabetes and Endocrinol 2018; 6: 382–91.

Solomon SD, Chew E,Duh EJ, Sobrin L, Sun JK, Van der Beek BL, Wykoff CC, Gardner TW. Diabetic retinopathy: a position statement by the American Diabetes Association. Diabetes Care 2017; 40: 412–18 DOI: 10.2337/dc16-2641

Virgili G, Parravano M, Meschini F, Evans JR. Anti-vascular endothelial growth factor for diabetic macular oedema. Cochrane Database of Systematic Reviews 2014; Issue 10, Art.No.: CD 007419 DOI: 10.1002/14651858.CD007419.pub4

Wang B, Wang F, Zhang Y, Zhao S-H, Zhao W-J, Yan S-L, Wang Y-G. Effects of RAS inhibitors on diabetic retinopathy: a systematic review and meta analysis. Lancet Diabetes and Endocrinology 2015; 3: 263–74. DOI: http://dx.doi.org/10.1016/S2213-8587(14)70256-6

Diabetic nephropathy

KEY POINTS

- Diabetic nephropathy is a clinical diagnosis based upon the presence of albuminuria in a person with diabetes.
- Classic staging based upon albuminuria does not map clearly to the current classification of chronic kidney disease. Once patients develop severe albuminuria (urinary albumin concentration >300 mg/L or Albustix* positive), their renal function steadily declines toward end-stage renal failure, albeit at different rates in different individuals.
- Patients with nephropathy have an increased cardiovascular mortality, which increases further as proteinuria and renal function worsen.
- The pathological features are of glomerular basement membrane thickening and diffuse glomerulosclerosis, both secondary to matrix protein accumulation. Both metabolic and haemodynamic factors play a role in pathogenesis.

- Tight glycaemic control can prevent nephropathy developing but once it is established, the cornerstone of treatment is blood pressure lowering, primarily with agents that block the renin-angiotensin system. SGLT2 inhibitors appear to have a specific but non-glycaemic related benefit in patients with type 2 diabetes and established nephropathy.
- Diabetes is the biggest single cause of end-stage renal failure requiring renal replacement therapy worldwide, accounting for 46.9% of incident cases in the USA and 29.4% in the UK in 2018.
- Survival on renal replacement therapy is best for kidney transplant recipients, but is improving for all modalities. In the UK overall 5-year survival on renal replacement therapy for all modalities is around 30%

Diabetic nephropathy is a clinical diagnosis based upon the detection of proteinuria in a patient with diabetes in the absence of another obvious cause such as infection. Many of these patients will also be hypertensive, have retinopathy and, in advanced stages, renal impairment.

The original definition was based upon relatively crude tests that detected protein concentrations of around 500 mg/L. With the development of accurate dipstick urine tests, this fell to 300 mg/L (largely albumin), and it is now possible to detect much lower concentrations using laboratory and dipstick tests leading to the concept of microalbuminuria or incipient nephropathy in the 1980s. More recent classification is based upon the correction of albuminuria for urine creatinine concentration – the albumin:creatinine ratio (ACR) and the terminology has changed. Normal is defined as <3 mg/mmol, microalbuminuria (or moderately increased albuminuria) 3–70 mg/mmol, and clinical or overt nephropathy (severely increased albuminuria) ≥70 mg/mmol (Figure 16.1). In this chapter the terms moderate and severe albuminuria will be used to be consistent with the international classification. Persistent, moderate albuminuria is now widely accepted as a positive diagnosis for diabetic nephropathy (Table 16.1). National Institute of Health and Care Excellence (NICE) guidance suggests that a moderate test result for albuminuria should be confirmed with a second early morning sample before making a diagnosis of nephropathy, but that there is no need to repeat if the initial result is in the severe category. The development of estimates of glomerular filtration rate (GFR) derived from plasma creatinine concentrations has led to the recognition of the association between renal impairment and increased cardiovascular mortality, and the concept of chronic kidney disease (CKD). This has had implications for the classification and staging of diabetic nephropathy (Figure 16.1).

Natural history

Classically, patients were considered to progress relentlessly from normoalbuminuria through moderate to severe

---

Handbook of Diabetes, Fifth Edition. Rudy Bilous, Richard Donnelly, and Iskandar Idris.
© 2021 John Wiley & Sons Ltd. Published 2021 by John Wiley & Sons Ltd.

Prognosis of CKD by GFR and albuminuria category

				Persistent albuminuria categories Description and range		
Prognosis of CKD by GFR and Albuminuria Categories: KDIGO 2012				**A1** Normal to mildly increased <30 mg/g <3 mg/mmol	**A2** Moderately increased 30–300 mg/g 3–30 mg/mmol	**A3** Severely increased >300 mg/g >30 mg/mmol
GFR categories (ml/min/1.73 m²) Description and range	G1	Normal or high	≥90			
	G2	Mildly decreased	60–89			
	G3a	Mildly to moderately decreased	45–59			
	G3b	Moderately to severely decreased	30–44			
	G4	Severely decreased	15–29			
	G5	Kidney failure	<15			

Green: low risk (if no other markers of kidney disease, no CKD); Yellow: moderately increased risk; Orange: high risk; Red, very high risk.

Figure 16.1 Classification and prognosis for end stage renal disease based upon eGFR stage and albuminuria. Albuminuria category based upon urinary albumin:creatinine ratio. Reproduced with permission from Kidney Disease Improving Global Outcomes (KDIGO) CKD Work Group. KDIGO 2012 Clinical Practice Guideline for the Evaluation and Management of Chronic Kidney Disease. Kidney Int 2013; Suppl 3: 1–150

Table 16.1 Definition of diabetic nephropathy by albuminuria and test specimen.

Urine specimen	Microalbuminuria (Moderately increased)	Clinical nephropathy (Severely increased)
Timed overnight collection	20–199 µg/min	>200 µg/min
24-hour collection	30–299 mg/d	≥300 mg/d
Albumin concentration	20–300 mg/L	>300 mg/L
Albumin:creatinine ratio (Europe)	Men 2.5–30 mg/mmol Women 3.5–30 mg/mmol	>30 mg/mmol >30 mg/mmol
USA	Both 30–300 mg/g	>300 mg/g

albuminuria. It is now recognised that patients with moderate albuminuria may spontaneously revert to normoalbuminuria in up to 50% of type 1 patients. Moreover, albuminuria can increase during periods of poor glycaemic control (and then decrease with glycaemic correction), and is reduced with antihypertensive therapy (notably drugs which block the renin-angiotensin system (RAS)). Moderate albuminuria has also been found in patients with coronary artery disease and essential hypertension and who have either normal or only mildly impaired glucose tolerance. In the UKPDS, the majority of those with moderate albuminuria did not progress to renal replacement therapy and the median period spent in the moderate albuminuria range was

11 years. Thus it is not inevitable that all moderate albuminuria patients will progress to renal failure and it also means that the contribution from cardiovascular or renal disease or both to albuminuria will vary from patient to patient.

It is also increasingly recognised that some type 1 and considerably more type 2 patients have a reduced GFR in the absence of moderate albuminuria (sometimes called normoalbuminuric CKD). In the UKPDS, 60% of those developing a reduced creatinine clearance (an estimate of GFR) did not have an increased urinary albumin concentration beforehand. Part of the explanation may be in the relative infrequency of urine testing in that study, but other cohort studies have confirmed the phenomenon. Renal biopsy in these patients confirms the presence of typical diabetic glomerulosclerosis in most, but has not been able to explain the observed low levels of albuminuria. Dietary factors such as protein intake may play a part. These patients tend to have a lower annual rate of loss of GFR (see below).

GFR is often abnormally high (>135 mL/min/1.73 m²) in patients with newly diagnosed type 1, and, to a lesser extent, type 2 diabetes. This is called hyperfiltration and its relationship to subsequent nephropathy risk remains controversial. Improving glycaemic control in hyperfiltering patients reduces GFR toward normal. The advent of the SGLT2 inhibitors and their apparent effectiveness in reducing nephropathy independent of glycaemic control has improved our understanding of the aetiopathogenesis of hyperfiltration in diabetes (Figure 16.2) and has implied a greater role in the development of nephropathy than was previously realised.

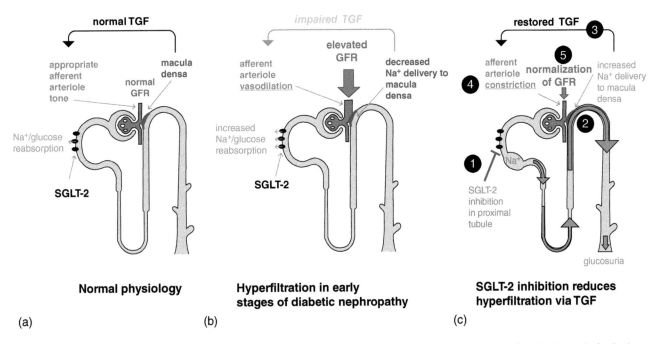

Figure 16.2 Hyperfiltration in diabetes and its correction by SGLT-2 (sodium glucose cotransporter 2) inhibition by restoration of tubular-glomerular feedback (TGF). Panel (a) shows the non-diabetic situation with normal TGF. Panel (b)–Increased glucose filtration leads to activation of SGLT2 in the proximal tubule. As a result, sodium concentration in the distal tubule is low and leads to afferent glomerular arteriolar dilatation and an increased GFR. Panel (c)-SGLT2 inhibition restores distal tubular sodium levels and reduces GFR. Reproduced with permission from Cherney DZ et al. Renal Hemodynamic Effect of Sodium-Glucose Cotransporter 2 Inhibition in Patients With Type 1 Diabetes Mellitus. Circulation 2014; 129: 5: 587-97

Over time, GFR declines and the rate of loss is greater in those with higher systemic blood pressure and greater albuminuria. In the Diabetes Control and Complications/Epidemiology of Diabetes Interventions and Complications (DCCT/EDIC) study those who developed severe albuminuria had a fifteenfold increased risk of developing an eGFR ≤ 60 mL/min/1.73 m². Historically, patients with severe albuminuria had a rate of loss of GFR of 10–12 mL/min/yr. More recent studies suggest rates of decline of <4 mL/min/yr in patients with well-controlled blood pressure. GFR declined in the DCCT/EDIC cohort by 1.2% per annum in those with low albuminuria compared to 1.8% and 5.7% in those with moderate and severe albuminuria respectively. Ultimately, GFR declines relentlessly towards end-stage renal disease (ESRD) (GFR <15 mL/min/1.73 m2) in patients with severe albuminuria, albeit at very different rates in individual patients.

The other clinical concomitant of nephropathy is blood pressure. In type 1 diabetes this is normal until moderate albuminuria starts to develop although some studies have shown that, on average, patients who go on to develop nephropathy have higher blood pressures (although still well within the normal range) when normoalbuminuric. In type 2 diabetes, many patients have hypertension at the time of diagnosis of their diabetes, and these individuals are at higher risk of developing nephropathy. Thus, hypertension

is a feature of developing nephropathy in type 1, whereas it may be an initiating factor in type 2 diabetes; it is an exacerbating factor in both.

Patients with nephropathy are at much greater risk of cardiovascular disease. In the UKPDS, annual mortality was over twice and three times higher for those with moderate or severe albuminuria respectively compared to their normoalbuminuric comparators. For those with a plasma creatinine >175 μmol/L and/or on renal replacement therapy, the mortality was 14 times greater. In the NHANES study in the USA, 10 year all-cause mortality was 7.7, 11.5 and 31.1% in those without diabetes or CKD, those with diabetes and no CKD and those with both diabetes and CKD, respectively (CKD was defined as an estimated GFR ≤ 60 mL/min/1.73 m² and/or increased albuminuria).

In type 1 diabetes, excess mortality in patients with severe albuminuria was 10–20 times higher than for their age-matched non-proteinuric comparators in a study published in1989 (Figure 16.3). This negative impact of increased albuminuria on mortality in type 1 diabetes was confirmed by more recent data from the FinnDiane Study. They showed standardised mortality ratios of 2.8, 9.2 and 18.3 for those with moderate, severe albuminuria and ESRD (eGFR ≤15 mL/min/1.73 m²) respectively compared to normoalbuminuric controls. Moreover, in their population, the presence

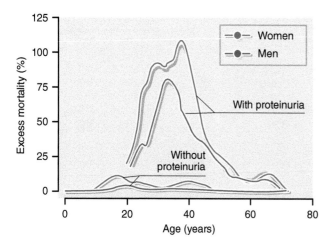

Figure 16.3 Relative mortality of patients with diabetes with and without persistent proteinuria in men and women as a function of age. Mortality is greatly increased at all ages in proteinuric patients. From Borch-Johnsen et al. Diabetologia 1989; 28: 590–596.

of albuminuria explained all of the observed excess mortality seen in type 1 diabetes.

The excess mortality associated with albuminuria and CKD explains why many patients with renal impairment do not survive to require dialysis, although with better treatment of cardiovascular risk factors many more are now doing so.

Stages of nephropathy

An international classification of CKD has now been widely adopted (Figure 16.1), but unfortunately it does not map precisely to the historical staging of diabetic nephropathy based upon albuminuria (Table 16.2). The new staging is based upon GFR as estimated (eGFR) from a plasma creatinine concentration using a formula derived from the

Modification of Diet in Renal Disease (MDRD) Study and subsequently modified (CKD-Epi).

These formulae use a serum creatinine assay aligned to an international reference method. Alternative formulae for estimating creatinine clearance (<u>not</u> GFR) exist, such as Cockroft–Gault, and for GFR using serum cystatin C. Both have their advocates but although cystatin C has advantages, it is expensive and not widely available in the UK.

The MDRD eGFR is much less accurate above 60 mL/min/1.73 m^2 and tends to underestimate true GFR below this value. The CKD-Epi equation is better at higher GFR but still has wide confidence intervals. Values below 60 mL/min/1.73 m^2 with both equations are, however, associated with an increasing cardiovascular mortality in US and UK populations, and more so in those with diabetes. An eGFR below 60 mL/min/1.73 m^2 is therefore now considered as an extra cardiovascular disease risk factor in its' own right. Estimates from plasma creatinine concentrations are often reported automatically by clinical laboratories (usually using the original MDRD equation) or can be derived from online calculators (https://www.kidney.org/professionals/kdoqi/gfr_calculator). It must be remembered that these estimates are only valid in steady state conditions (not in pregnancy or acute kidney injury), and plasma creatinine concentrations can be increased after vigorous exercise and a meat protein meal.

Despite its drawbacks as an accurate measure of kidney function, eGFR is useful in alerting the clinician (and patient) to renal impairment that would not be apparent from the serum creatinine concentration alone. It also provides a reasonable measure of rate of progression of renal impairment in the individual patient. This helps to guide therapy (therapeutic dose adjustment or drug avoidance) and also a rapidly declining eGFR should prompt referral for specialist assessment (see later).

Table 16.2 Stages of chronic kidney disease (CKD) and their mapping to historical stages of diabetic kidney disease (DKD).

Stage	Defining eGFR (mL/min/1.73 m²)	Other required features	Patients with diabetes		
			Normoalbuminuria	Moderate Albuminuria (Microalbuminuria)	Severe Albuminuria (Clinical or overt Nephropathy)
1	>90	Abnormal urinalysis and/or renal imaging	At risk for DKD	Likely DKD (type 1) Possible DKD (type 2)	DKD
2	60–89	Abnormal urinalysis and/or renal imaging	At risk for DKD	Likely DKD (type 1) Possible DKD (type 2)	DKD
3A	45–59	None	Likely DKD (type 1)	DKD (type 1)	DKD
3B	30–44		Possible DKD (type 2)	Likely DKD (type 2)	
4	15–29	None	Probable DKD	DKD	DKD
5	<15 or RRT	None	DKD	DKD	DKD

RRT = renal replacement therapy. Abnormal urinalysis = albuminuria and/or haematuria.

Epidemiology

Reported prevalence and incidence of moderate and severe albuminuria vary according to the population under study (type 1 versus type 2; age range; whether the sample is population or hospital clinic based; ethnicity; year of reporting; type of test). Historically, in population-based studies the prevalence of moderate albuminuria ranged from 12.3% to 27.2% for type 1 and 19.4% to 42.1% for type 2 diabetes. For severe albuminuria, the figures were 0.3–24% and 9.2–32.9% for type 1 and type 2 diabetes, respectively. Those with an earlier age of onset of type 2 diabetes appear to be at a particularly high risk for developing microvascular complications. This is very apparent in areas where there has been a rapid increase in type 2 diabetes and obesity such as the Middle East, South East Asia and Latin America.

The incidence of persistent moderate albuminuria is around 2% per annum for both type 1 and type 2 diabetes who are normoalbuminuric at baseline. For moderately albuminuric patients, the incidence of severe albuminuria is around 3% per annum.

Rates for ESRD are more difficult to interpret because they are not linear with time and vary according to duration of diabetes. Some of the best data come from Scandinavia where there is a tradition of national disease registries for both diabetes and renal disease. For type 1 diabetes, the latest Finnish National Data reported rates of 2.2% at 20 years' and 7.8% at 30 years' duration in 2005, and in Norway 4.6% at 30 years in 2013. For type 2 diabetes the data are less precise because of the difficulty in ascertaining the precise date of diabetes onset. In the UKPDS cohort of newly diagnosed patients, the rate of renal replacement therapy or death from renal failure was 0.6% at 10.4 years.

Screening for nephropathy

There are conflicting views on the utility of routine screening for nephropathy. Current NICE and ADA guidance suggests annual screening using an early morning urine specimen for an albumin:creatinine ratio in all people with diabetes, with a positive moderate test repeated for confirmation. Testing should commence after 5 years for people with type 1 and immediately after diagnosis for people with type 2 diabetes. A simultaneous plasma creatinine with eGFR estimation should also be performed.

Because of the variability of urine albumin and the recognition of so-called normoalbuminuric CKD there has been an intensive search for other biomarkers of early nephropathy, but few have been shown to be superior and none more practical. This is a fast-moving field, however, and newer tests are sure to be validated in the future.

Pathology and pathophysiology

The classic pathological lesions of nodular glomerulosclerosis were first described in 1936. The earliest pathological feature of diabetic nephropathy is thickening of the glomerular capillary basement membrane (GBM) due to an accumulation of matrix material, and this is detectable within 5 years of diabetes onset in patients with type 1 diabetes (Figures 16.4–16.6).

Increasing proteinuria is preceded and accompanied by further accumulations of matrix material (mostly type IV collagen and laminin) in the mesangium (called diffuse glomerulosclerosis), due to both overproduction and reduced breakdown and clearance. Ultimately this process obliterates the capillary and reduces filtration, leading to renal failure.

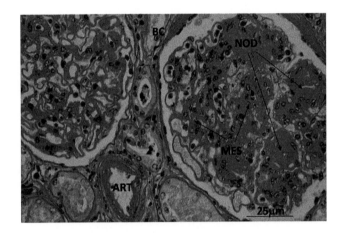

Figure 16.4 Nodular glomerulosclerosis in a patient with type 1 diabetes and severe albuminuria. ART, arteriole with hyalinosis; BC, thickened Bowman's capsule; MES, mesangial expansion; NOD, nodules.

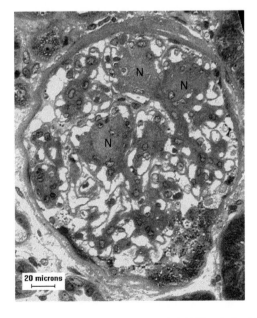

Figure 16.5 Nodular glomerulosclerosis (Kimmelstiel–Wilson lesions) in a patient with diabetic nephropathy. N= nodules.

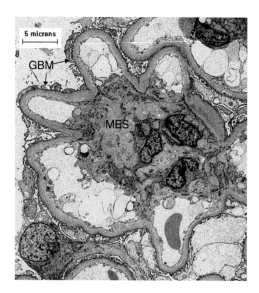

Figure 16.6 Electron micrograph of the glomerulus from a patient with diabetes, showing basement membrane thickening (GBM) and mesangial expansion with extracellular matrix accumulation (MES).

Arteriolar hyalinosis leading to glomerular ischaemia, glomerular epithelial cell (podocyte) loss and tubulointerstitial inflammation and fibrosis are also features of established nephropathy.

The pathophysiology of these changes has been partly covered in Chapter 14. Essentially, metabolic and haemodynamic factors combine to stimulate a cascade of processes that result in the release of profibrogenic cytokines ultimately leading to nephropathy and end stage renal disease (Figure 16.7). In experimental and human diabetes, renal blood flow is increased and there is a relative dilatation of the afferent compared to the efferent glomerular arteriole. This leads to an increase in glomerular capillary pressure which has been closely related to the development of glomerulosclerosis in diabetic animals. Angiotensin II blockade relaxes the efferent arteriole, whereas SGLT2 inhibition restores normal tubulo-glomerular feedback and reduces afferent arteriolar dilatation, both actions effectively lowering intraglomerular capillary pressure (Figure 16.2).

The interaction of these changes on structure and capillary pressure underpin the development of albuminuria (Figure 16.8). The glomerular capillary has an inherent size and molecular charge selectivity. In structural terms the endothelium lining the capillary is fenestrated and has a complex glycocalyx of proteins on its surface. The glomerular basement membrane (GBM) is a meshwork of mainly type IV collagen which is cross-linked in a lattice formation. Finally, the epithelial surface comprises the podocytes which have a series of interdigitating foot processes connected by a filtration membrane. Charge selectivity is located mainly at the endothelial and epithelial surfaces, whereas size selectivity is thought to reside within the GBM structure (Figure 16.8)

The glomerular barrier normally retains most circulating proteins of the size and charge of albumin. Glycation of the glycocalyx proteins, disruption of the GBM lattice by matrix accumulation, and podocyte loss allow filtration of increasing amounts of albumin and larger macromolecules, which characterises progressive nephropathy. There is evidence that the increased presentation of proteins in the filtrate to tubular cells leads to tubulointerstial inflammation and fibrosis, contributing to declining GFR.

Risk factors for nephropathy

Prospective observational studies have shown a consistent association between glycaemia and known duration of diabetes, and development of nephropathy. The role of hypertension has been mentioned earlier; blood pressure rises as nephropathy develops in type 1 and plays a more causative role in type 2 diabetes (Box 16.1).

A meta-analysis of studies of directly measured GFR in type 1 diabetes found a significant link between hyperfiltration and later development of nephropathy but there was marked heterogeneity and the relationship was weakened when glycaemic control was taken into account.

Ethnicity plays an important but ill-understood role. Rates of nephropathy are much higher in Native American, South Asian, some Pacific Islander, non-Ashkenazi Jewish, and Afro-Caribbean diabetic patients compared to their white Europid age- and duration-matched controls. Some of this increased risk relates to increased rates of hypertension (e.g. in Afro-Caribbean patients), and some may be related to the low birthweight (thrifty phenotype) hypothesis (see Chapter 7) which has been linked to higher adult blood pressures and nephropathies generally, as well as to type 2 diabetes *per se*. Studies of Australian aboriginals and other populations suggest that nephron size and number may be lower than in Europid populations resulting in an increased vulnerability to nephropathy in those who go on to develop diabetes.

Sibling studies in multiplex families with type 1 diabetes have shown an increased incidence of nephropathy in siblings of a proband with the condition compared to those of a proband with normal albuminuria. These observations do not completely rule out environmental factors but the heritability of a risk for nephropathy is supported by the observation that a positive family history of hypertension and cardiovascular disease is more likely in the parents of type 1 patients with nephropathy compared to parents of type 1 patients without nephropathy (Figure 16.9). Estimates of the heritability of albuminuria and GFR range from 0.3–0.44 and 0.6–0.75 respectively. Extensive search for candidate genes and genome-wide scanning have so far yielded some positive associations (notably with polymorphisms in the angiotensin converting enzyme gene) but on the whole, these relationships are not very strong and no

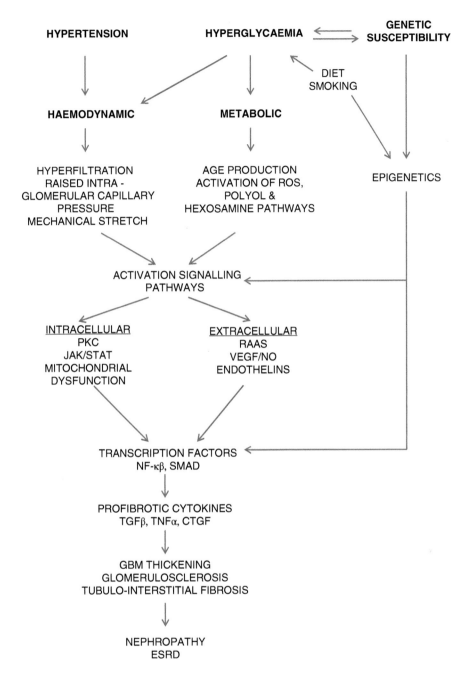

Figure 16.7 Schematic to show how metabolic and haemodynamic factors combine to cause nephropathy in diabetes. AGE = advanced glycation end products. ROS = reactive oxygen species. PKC = Protein Kinase C. JAK/STAT = Janus kinase/signal transducer and activator of transduction. RAAS = renin angiotensin aldosterone system. VEGF/NO = vascular endothelium growth factor/nitric oxide. NF-κβ = nuclear factor-κβ. TGFβ = transforming growth factor β. TNFα = tumour necrosis factor α. CTGF = connective tissue growth factor. ESRD = end stage renal disease.

major gene effect has yet been identified. Part of the problem lies with the difficulty in defining a precise phenotype of nephropathy, albuminuria alone is not sufficient because of its variability, and end stage renal disease is complicated by a survival bias.

There is increasing interest in the role of epigenetics, (defined by some as the study of heritable non coding changes in DNA that impact on gene expression) and its possible role on the 'metabolic memory effect' of a period of improved glycaemic control on subsequent development of complications, perhaps best illustrated by the DCCT (Figure 16.10 and see Chapter 14). In this construct, early good glycaemic control has a positive effect on genes that influence pathways involved in the development of complications, and this benefit continues should blood glucose levels deteriorate at a later time.

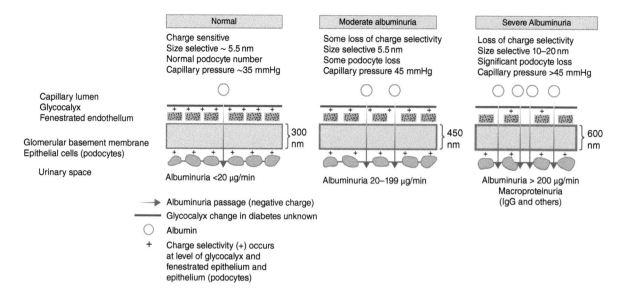

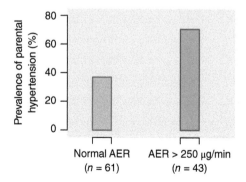

Figure 16.8 Schematic of changes in selectivity of glomerular capillary to albumin in diabetic nephropathy. A rise in capillary pressure and thickening of the glomerular basement membrane (GBM), together with loss of podocytes, result in increasing passage of circulating proteins into the urinary space. Most charge selectivity takes place at the endothelium and epithelium, size selectivity at the GBM. The precise constitution and role of the glycocalyx in diabetes remains unclear. Charge selectivity resides at the endothelial and epithelial (podocyte) barrier. IgG, immunoglobulin G.

Box 16.1 Factors associated with the development of diabetic nephropathy.

- Glycaemia
- Diabetes duration
- Hypertension
- Hyperfiltration
- Ethnicity
- Genetics
- Diet (meat protein intake)

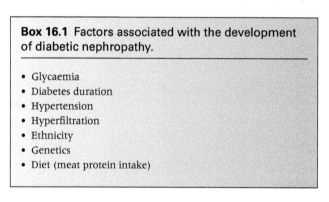

Figure 16.9 Prevalence of parental hypertension in type 1 patients with normoalbuminuria and nephropathy (defined as albuminuria ≥250 μg/min)

Management
Glycaemic control

The DCCT/EDIC Study provides incontrovertible evidence that good glycaemic control can prevent the development of moderate albuminuria, reduce the incidence of hypertension, and reduce the numbers developing renal impairment, and this benefit was apparent for at least 8–10 years after the studies concluded (Figure 16.10). A similar benefit was seen in the UKPDS. There is very little evidence, however, to suggest that it can prevent or delay the clinical progression of nephropathy once it is established. This is probably because after nephropathy has been initiated (by largely glucose-dependent mechanisms), it is continued by pathways that are no longer sensitive to changes in glycaemia. Moreover, the ACCORD study of tight glycaemic control in people with type 2 diabetes and high cardiovascular risk, showed an increased mortality in those in the intensive arm, and this was particularly evident in those with CKD at baseline. This has led to a graded target of HbA1c by the ADA of ≤48 mol/mol (6.5%) for those of a younger age, with a shorter duration of diabetes and with few, if any, complications; and <64 mol/mol (8.0%) for older people with complications and a shorter life expectancy. The latest KDIGO (Kidney Disease Improving Global Outcomes) guidance recommends individual HbA1c targets in people with diabetes and CKD of between 47 mmol/mol (6.5%) and 64 mmol/mol (8.0%) depending upon factors such as age, comorbidities and life expectancy. For those patients on renal replacement therapy (RRT) there are no prospective studies to guide therapy. There are retrospective data showing improved survival on haemodialysis for those patients with an HbA1c <64 mmol/mol (<8.0%). Many of these patients have cardiovascular disease and hypoglycaemic unawareness so the prudent course would be to achieve the best and safest level of glycaemic control as per the ADA guidance.

Intriguingly, in a small group of type 1 pancreas transplant recipients, renal pathology improved in their native kidneys after 10 (but not 5) years of normoglycaemia, implying that

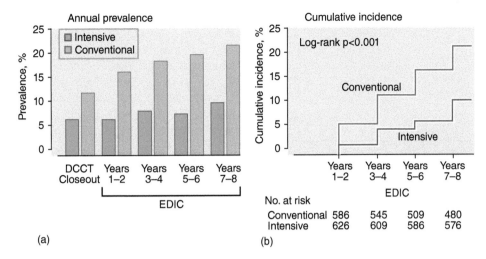

Figure 16.10 (a) Prevalence and (b) cumulative incidence of moderate albuminuria (microalbuminuria) in the DCCT/EDIC study showing continuing benefit of intensive diabetic control for up to 8 years after the main study concluded. Data from DCCT/EDIC Research Group. JAMA 2003; 290:2159–2167.

not only is complete normalisation of blood glucose required to reverse pathological changes, but also the lesions take almost as long to resolve as they do to develop.

The choice of agent is also unclear. Most patients with advanced CKD will either require or be using insulin. Over 50% of exogenously injected insulin is renally excreted so doses should be reduced as GFR declines, with some groups recommending a reduction of 50% for those with CKD stage 5. Practically speaking, doses should be adjusted based not only on overall glycaemic control but also on incidence of hypoglycaemia. There are no data supporting any particular insulin regimen or analogue in CKD patients. Oral agents and GLP-1 injectables have variable renal excretion and product characteristics should be checked before prescribing. There are no hard data supporting the use of any particular class of oral agent in patients with CKD and this was confirmed in a recently published Cochrane review. Metformin is not recommended for those with an eGFR < 30 ml/min/1.73m² because of a potential risk of lactic acidosis. SGLT2 inhibitors are thought to be ineffective at CKD stage 4 or worse but may have a non-glycaemic mediated benefit at earlier stages (see below).

Blood pressure

Target blood pressure for people with diabetes is discussed in more detail in chapter 19. Many guidelines set treatment thresholds of ≤140/90 mmHg with higher levels for the older person. Target levels in some guidelines are 120–139 mmHg systolic and 70–79 mmHg diastolic for those with albuminuria. The ACCORD study of intensive blood pressure control showed no benefit and possible harm in those with a target systolic pressure of ≤120 mmHg in terms of numbers developing an eGFR ≤30 mL/min/1.73 m². Because of this, all guidelines agree that the lower limit for reduction is 120 mmHg systolic and 70 mmHg diastolic. Improved control of blood pressure, however, is probably the main reason why

the median duration of clinical nephropathy prior to ESRD has risen from 7 to 14 years since 1980 (Figure 16.11).

Because of the involvement of angiotensin II in the glomerular haemodynamic changes in diabetes, agents which block the RAS feature as first-line therapy in most guidelines. These drugs also reduce albuminuria which would help ameliorate any tubulointerstitial insult caused by increased protein trafficking across the tubular epithelium. Meta-analysis in normotensive patients with type 1 diabetes and moderate albuminuria confirms that angiotensin-converting enzyme inhibitors (ACEI) can reduce the numbers developing severe albuminuria by around 60%, with those having higher levels of albuminuria at baseline showing the most benefit (Figure 16.12). In people with severe albuminuria and poorly controlled type 1 diabetes, captopril reduced the numbers doubling their baseline serum creatinine, or requiring a kidney transplant, or dialysis, or dying. Similar results were obtained with angiotensin receptor blocking agents in type 2 diabetes.

However, there is little evidence that RAS blockade can prevent primary development of moderate albuminuria in type 1 diabetes, and may only be effective in patients with type 2 diabetes who are already hypertensive or at high cardiovascular risk.

Most patients with nephropathy will require two or more agents to achieve blood pressure targets. For more details about blood pressure management, please see Chapter 19.

Proteinuria

There is evidence from intervention trials that patients who have a greater reduction in proteinuria in response to blood pressure treatment do better in terms of rate of decline in renal function. This observation has led to the proposal that reduction of proteinuria to <1 g/day should be a therapeutic target. This is not widely accepted, and there have been no prospective trials of treatment to target albuminuria. Studies

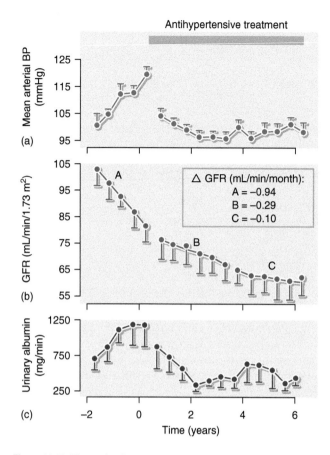

(a)

(b)

(c)

Figure 16.11 Effects of antihypertensive treatment on (a) mean arterial blood pressure, (b) GFR, and (c) urinary albumin excretion in 11 patients with type 1 diabetes and nephropathy. Rates of decline in both GFR and albumin excretion were significantly reduced. From Parving et al. BMJ 1987; 294: 1443–1447.

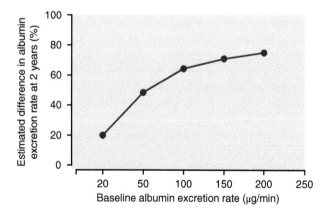

Figure 16.12 Meta-analysis of the effects of angiotensin-converting enzyme (ACE) inhibition on moderate albuminuria (microalbuminuria). Estimated difference in albumin excretion rate between placebo and ACE inhibitor treatment groups at 2 years, according to albuminuric status at baseline. From ACE Inhibitors in Diabetic Nephropathy Trialist Group. Ann Intern Med 2001; 134: 370–379.

of multiple blockade of the RAS using combinations of ACEI, angiotensin type 1 receptor blockers, aldosterone antagonists, and renin inhibitors have shown greater reductions in albuminuria compared to the use of individual agents alone but only at the expense of worse patient outcomes in terms of hyperkalaemia and acute kidney injury. The recently reported FIDELIO study of finerenone (a non-steroidal aldosterone antagonist) in people with type 2 diabetes and moderate or severe albuminuria showed significant reductions in both albuminuria and rate of decline of GFR in combination with other RAS blocking agents. Hyperkalaemia was twice as common in the finerenone group, although rates of acute kidney injury were not increased. The precise role of finerenone remains to be defined but it may prove useful as an adjunct to RAS blockade in those with increasing albuminuria or rapidly declining GFR. Combination RAS blockade is otherwise no longer recommended.

Protein restriction

In experimental diabetes, dietary protein restriction reduces albuminuria and progression to renal failure. Studies in humans have been variable in duration and endpoint. A systematic review has shown a modest reduction in the rate of decline of GFR in type 1 diabetes with a restriction of dietary protein intake to 0.7–1.1 g/kg bodyweight/day. Only one study used mortality and ESRD as endpoints and found a relative risk of 0.23 (95% CI 0.07–0.72). For type 2 diabetes the data were not significant. The latest KDIGO guideline recommends a dietary protein intake of 0.8 g/kg bodyweight/day for CKD stages 1–4.

Anaemia correction

Anaemia secondary to erythropoietin (EPO) deficiency is a feature of CKD generally and some studies suggest that it occurs earlier at a higher GFR in people with diabetes. Hospital clinic-based surveys suggest prevalence rates of WHO-defined anaemia. (<120 g/L women, <130 g/L men) of 15–25%, and many cases were in patients with an eGFR >60 mL/min/1.73 m². Several large trials of anaemia correction using various preparations of EPO have suggested no benefit (and possibly some harm) of achieving a haemoglobin concentration >130 g/L. Below this level, patients feel better, but no conclusive impact on rate of decline in GFR or cardiovascular morbidity/mortality has been demonstrated. Current NICE guidance recommends treatment in all those with CKD who have adequate iron stores and who might clinically benefit, and has set a target of 100–120 g/L.

Other therapies

The SGLT2 inhibitors have both glycaemic and renal haemodynamic effects (Figure 16.2). Results from the EMPA-REG and EMPA-REG RENAL and other studies showed a reduction in both cardiovascular and renal outcomes. In particular, there were lower numbers progressing from moderate to severe albuminuria, and those doubling baseline plasma creatinine or requiring renal replacement therapy (although numbers were small). A recent systematic review and meta-analysis of four large trials showed a consistent reduction in the major outcomes of dialysis, kidney transplantation and/ or renal related death (RR 0.67; 95% CI 0.52-0.86), as well as the development of ESRD (0.65; 0.53–0.81) and acute kidney injury (0.75; 0.66-0.85). These findings have been recently confirmed in CKD patients with and without diabetes in the Dapagliflozin CKD Trial. Although the cardiovascular and albuminuria benfits were seen with most agents (notably not with Ertugliflozin), Canagliflozin had a significantly increased risk of distal amputation in the CREDENCE Trial which remains unexplained. The benefit in terms of reduction of rate of loss of GFR seems to be greater for those with severe albuminuria and only patients with an eGFR >30 ml/min/1.73m² were eligible for most studies (≥25 ml/min/1.73m² for DAPA-CKD; the majority of participants in these trials had an eGFR >60). Intriguingly, the agents do not seem to prevent the new onset of moderate albuminuria (microalbuminuria). Because of these positive data many guidelines are now recommending their use in people with type 2 diabetes and early nephropathy. It is important to remember that all of these trials studied SGLT2 in addition to RAS blockade, and the reported rates of loss of GFR were similar to those reported with ARBs alone.

The effects of SGLT2 inhibitors and GLP1 agonists on numbers of patients developing renal failure (defined as an eGFR <15 ml/min/1.73 m² or need for renal replacement therapy) were compared in a network meta analysis. The benefit of both therapies was confirmed in those at high or very high risk defined as CKD ± severe albuminuria. For SGLT2 inhibitors between 29 and 58 fewer patients developed kidney failure per 1000 patients treated for 5 years; for GLP1 agonists the range was between 19 and 29 per 1000 patients treated for 5 years.

KDIGO also recommend diet and lifestyle changes similar to those for hypertension (Chapter 19)

Other agents that were under investigation include endothelin antagonists (now abandoned), and allopurinol (to reduce hyperuricaemia which is associated with progressive loss of GFR) with no benefit.

Cardiovascular risk factor management

There are no conclusive trial data to support aspirin or lipid-lowering therapy specifically in diabetic nephropathy, but as many patients with diabetes and CKD will have concomitant cardiovascular disease or be classified as being at high risk of developing it, most guidelines support their routine use.

The Steno 2 Study of multifactorial cardiovascular risk intervention in type 2 patients with moderate albuminuria at baseline showed a major impact on mortality, development of severe albuminuria and ESRD, as well as cardiovascular complications including myocardial infarction and amputation

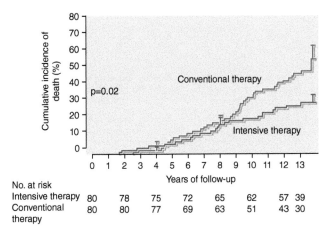

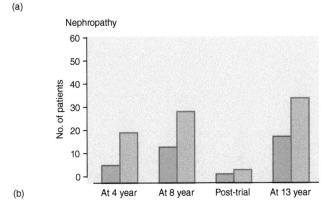

Figure 16.13 (a) Cumulative incidence of death in 160 moderately albuminuric (microalbuminuric) patients with type 2 diabetes randomised to intensive or conventional management of cardiovascular risk factors for 8 years in the Steno 2 trial and for 5 years after the end of the study period. (b) Number of patients developing nephropathy on intensive or conventional treatment during and after the Steno 2 trial. Data from Gaede et al. N Engl J Med 2008; 358: 580–591.

(Figure 16.13). The protocol for the intensive arm was for RAS-blocking drugs in all, lipid-lowering therapy with a target total cholesterol <4.5 mmol/L, intensive glycaemic control with a target HbA1c ≤48 mmol/mol (≤6.5%), low-dose aspirin, antioxidants (vitamins C and E) and lifestyle changes including stopping smoking, weight reduction, and increasing exercise. As with the DCCT/EDIC and UKPDS, these benefits continued beyond the end of the trial, but it was not possible to determine which were the most effective interventions. The latest report from this study has estimated an increase in median life expectancy of 7.9 years in the intensively treated cohort.

Patients with severe albuminuria and CKD Stage 3 or worse are at high risk of foot complications and many undergo amputation both before and after commencing renal replacement therapy. There are data suggesting that regular foot surveillance in people with nephropathy can reduce amputation rates significantly.

Taken together, these studies suggest that the patient with nephropathy should have multifactorial management of all

					Persistent albuminuria categories Description and range		
Guide to Frequency of Monitoring (number of times per year) by GFR and Albuminuria Category					A1	A2	A3
					Normal to mildly increased	Moderately increased	Severely increased
					<30 mg/g <3 mg/mmol	30–300 mg/g 3–30 mg/mmol	>300 mg/g >30 mg/mmol
GFR categories (ml/min/1.73 m²) Description and range	G1	Normal or high	≥90		1 if CKD	1	2
	G2	Mildly decreased	60–89		1 if CKD	1	2
	G3a	Mildly to moderately decreased	45–59		1	2	3
	G3b	Moderately to severely decreased	30–44		2	3	3
	G4	Severely decreased	15–29		3	3	4+
	G5	Kidney failure	<15		4+	4+	4+

Figure 16.14 Frequency of monitoring (number of clinic visits per year) based upon eGFR stage and albuminuria. Reproduced with permission from Kidney Disease Improving Global Outcomes (KDIGO) CKD Work Group. KDIGO 2012 Clinical Practice Guideline for the Evaluation and Management of Chronic Kidney Disease. Kidney Int 2013; Suppl 3: 1–150.

known cardiovascular and diabetic complication risk factors to recommended targets. They also imply that regular follow-up and surveillance for concomitant complications is necessary and a suggested frequency has been proposed by the KDIGO guidelines (Figure 16.14).

Renal replacement therapy (RRT)

The standardised **incidence** rates for commencement of RRT in patients with diabetes was 185 per million population in the USA in 2018, increasing by 3 per million per year from 2009. In the UK, the incidence was 32 per million population in 2018 with an annual increase of 1 per million from 2009. Globally the largest increases have been seen in Mexico and South East Asia. Proportionally, these represent 46.9% and 29.4% respectively of total incident patients starting RRT per year. Incidence rates in the USA have fallen in all ethnic groups over the last few years, but remain two- to threefold higher for Black and Hispanic populations compared to white Europid individuals in those ≥44 years of age.

Overall crude **prevalence** of diabetic ESRD has continued to rise in both the USA and UK at 39 and 17.8% respectively in 2017. The disparity between the two countries is probably a reflection of their different ethnic backgrounds.

Most patients with diabetes on RRT in the UK in 2017 were managed with haemodialysis (58%) compared to 29% with glomerulonephritis and 10% for polycystic kidney disease. Kidney transplantation rates tend to be lower in patients with diabetes compared to patients without diabetes in ESRD, perhaps as a result of greater comorbidities. In

the UK in 2017, the Odds Ratio of being listed for a kidney transplant within two years of commencing RRT was only 0.51. Of patients with diabetes and RRT 35% had a transplant in 2017 compared to 66% of those with glomerulonephritis and 74% with polycystic kidney disease. In the USA 2018, 16.5% of people with diabetes and ESRD < 45 years of age had a transplant, compared to 52.5% of those with glomerulonephritis and 60.9% with cystic kidney disease.

Median overall survival for people with diabetes commencing RRT in the UK is reduced at 3.6 years, compared to 7.3 years for those without diabetes. One-year survival is much lower for people with diabetes aged 18–44 years, but more or less equivalent to those without diabetes in older age groups. At 5 years, survival on all forms of RRT is 72.3 versus 89.5% (18–44-year-olds) and 51.2 versus 68.9% (45–64-year-olds) for those with and without diabetes, respectively. For those aged ≥ 65 years, 5-year survival is broadly equivalent at around 30%. Survival is generally better in kidney transplant recipients, but this is partly explained by selection bias toward fitter patients. There is an increasing trend for live donor related and unrelated transplantation which has increased both availability and improved success rates and short-term survival. The role of pancreas and islet transplantation is discussed in Chapter 34.

As patients approach ESRD, planning for RRT becomes a priority. Patients do much less well if they present in acute on chronic renal failure. All patients with CKD stage 4 (eGFR <30 mL/min/1.73 m²) should be referred for specialist renal assessment. Other indications are shown in Box 16.2.

Is it diabetic nephropathy?

Because type 2 diabetes is a common condition, patients
will also present with non-diabetes related kidney disease.
However, it is likely that <10% with type 2 diabetes and albuminuria have a non-diabetic cause and few of these will have a
specifically treatable disease. Interestingly, those with atypical
or non-diabetic pathologies tend to have a slower rate of decline
in GFR compared to patients with typical glomerulosclerosis.

In the presence of retinopathy and albuminuria >300 mg/
day, it is highly likely that patients have diabetic kidney disease; in the absence of retinopathy and in the presence of
moderate albuminuria then non-diabetic kidney disease

becomes more likely. If patients have signs of systemic disease,
rapidly increasing proteinuria or deteriorating renal function,
or urinalysis suggesting microscopic haematuria, then they
should be referred for specialist review and a non-diabetic
cause of their nephropathy should be considered. NICE guidance for consideration of non-diabetic renal disease in people
with type 1 diabetes is summarised in Box 16.3.

CASE HISTORY

A 32-year-old man with type 1 diabetes, moderate renal impairment (serum creatinine 212 µmol/L, eGFR 34 mL/min/1.73 m²)
and severe albuminuria had a BP of 170/110 mmHg when he first
presented in 1994. His diabetic control was poor and he would
only take insulin once a day in an unusual mixture of lente and
ultralente preparations. He was started on enalapril 10 mg bd with
an immediate response; his BP fell to 120/80 mmHg. Although
there was an initial increase in his serum creatinine, this stabilised
and 15 years later he was still independent of dialysis. His inverse
creatinine chart is shown in Figure 16.15.

During this time his BP was always <140/90 mmHg and usually much less than that. He was working until 2005 as a scaf-
folder but had to stop because of postural dizziness due to
autonomic neuropathy. His HbA1c varied between 64 and
97 mmol/mol (8.0% and 11.0%) over this time. He was the
recipient of a combined kidney pancreas transplant in 2012
after 12 months haemodialysis and is currently insulin independent with good renal function.

Comment: The renal response to therapy in this man is
striking and was achieved despite poor glycaemic control. This
underscores the primacy of BP in driving progression of diabetic
nephropathy once it is established. The initial increase in serum
creatinine is significant but still within a change that is acceptable when commencing RAS-blocking drugs. His blood pressure
response was dramatic which supports the role of angiotensin II
in nephropathy-related hypertension.

Although eGFR is a useful marker of kidney function, a
reciprocal serum creatinine chart like this is also helpful in
monitoring progression and the impact of any interventions,
especially once the level is >150 µmol/L.

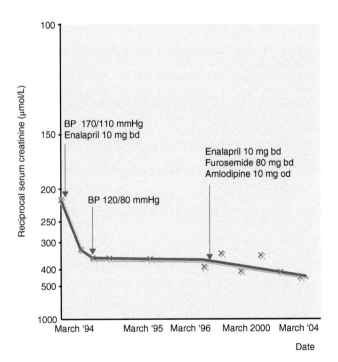

Figure 16.15 Reciprocal serum creatinine plotted against date for the case history.

LANDMARK CLINICAL TRIAL

Mogensen CE. Long-term antihypertensive treatment inhibiting progression of diabetic nephropathy. BMJ 1982; 285: 685–688.

This small observational study in six type 1 diabetic men with clinical nephropathy (severe albuminuria) was published 8 months before the much more widely known study of Parving (shown in Figure 16.11). GFR was measured directly using isotopic clearance methods three or four times in the 20–31 months before commencing antihypertensive therapy, and 12–18 times over the subsequent 28–86 months.

Blood pressure treatment was first line β blockade plus hydralazine in 4 and furosemide in 3. Mean BP readings fell from 162/103 to 144/95 mmHg (range 138–160 mmHg systolic). Rate of fall of GFR was 1.24 mL/min/1.73 m^2/month before antihypertensive therapy and 0.49 mL/min/1.73 m^2/month during treatment. A statistically significant positive relationship was found between achieved BP and rate of decline in GFR. Baseline proteinuria was 3.9 (range 0.5–8.8) g/day and stabilised during treatment. Prior to this there was an average annual increase of 107%.

At the time of this study, there were still concerns that lowering blood pressure in patients with CKD would reduce kidney perfusion and exacerbate renal impairment. This observational study and others that followed showed that BP lowering actually preserved renal function and slowed the otherwise rapid and relentless decline to ESRD. The principle of BP control in CKD is now firmly established, but 35 years ago this was far from the case.

KEY WEBSITES

- GFR calculator https://www.kidney.org/professionals/kdoqi/gfr_calculator
- Diabetes Atlas: www.diabetesatlas.org
- NICE guidance: www.nice.org.uk (CG 182 Chronic kidney disease in adults: assessment and management; NG 8 Chronic kidney disease: managing anaemia; NG 17 Type 1 diabetes in adults: diagnosis and management; NG 28 Type 2 diabetes in adults: management)
- UK Renal Registry: www.renal.org/audit-research/annual-report
- USRDS: www.USRDS.org
- UK Renal Association: www.renal.org
- SIGN Guidelines: www.SIGN.ac.uk

FURTHER READING

Alicic RZ, Rooney MT, Tuttle KR. Diabetic kidney disease: challenges, progress, and possibilities. Clin Am J Soc Nephrol 2017; 13: doi.org/10.2215/CJN.11491116

American Diabetes Association. Standards of medical care in diabetes – 2020. Diabetes Care 2020; 43(Suppl 1): S135–151.

Bilous R. Microvascular disease: what does the UKPDS tell us about diabetic nephropathy? Diabetic Med 2008; 25(Suppl 2): 25–29.

Bilous R, Chaturvedi N, Sjolie AK, et al. Effect of candesartan on microalbuminuria and albumin excretion rate in diabetes: 3 randomised trials. Ann Intern Med 2009; 151: 11–20.

de Boer I on behalf of the DCCT/EDIC Research Group. Kidney disease and related findings in the Diabetes Control and Complications Trial/Epidemiology of Diabetes Interventions and Complications Study. Diabetes Care 2014; 37: 24–30 doi: 10.2337/dc13-2113

de Boer IH, Caramori ML, Chan JCN et al. Executive summary of the 2020 KDIGO Diabetes Management in CKD Guideline: evidence-based advances in monitoring and treatment. Kid Int 2020; 98: 839–48.

Gaede P, Oellgaard J, Cartensen B et al Years of life gained by multifactorial intervention in patients with type 2 diabetes mellitus and microalbuminuria: 21 years follow-up on the Steno-2 randomised trial. Diabetologia 2016; 59: 2298–2307 doi: 10.1007/s00125-016-4065-6

Lo C, Toyama T, Wang Y et al. Insulin and glucose-lowering agents for treating people with diabetes and chronic kidney disease. Cochrane database of Systematic Reviews 2018, Issue 9. Art.No.:CD011798. doi: 10.1002/14651858.CD011798.pub2

Ma RC, Cooper ME. Genetics of diabetic kidney disease- from the worst of nightmares to the light of dawn? J Am Soc Nephrol 2017; 28: 389–93 doi: 10.1681/ASN.2016091028

Neven Bl, Young T, Heerspink HJL et al. SGLT2 inhibitors for the prevention of kidney failure in patients with type 2 diabetes: a systematic review and meta-analysis. Lancet Diabetes Endocrinol 2019; 7: 845–54.

Palmer SC, Tendal B, Mustafa RA et al. Sodium-glucose co-ransporter protein-2 (SGLT2) inhibitors and glucagon-like peptide-1 (GLP-1) receptor agonists for type 2 diabetes: systematic review and network meta-analysis of randomised controlled trials. *BMJ 2021; 372 doi: https://doi.org/10.1136/bmj.m4573*

Prigent A. Monitoring renal function and limitation of renal function tests. Semin Nucl Med 2008; 38: 32–46.

Robertson LM, Waugh N, Robertson A. Protein restriction for diabetic renal disease. Cochrane Database Syst Rev 2007; 2: CD002181. doi: 10.1002/14651858.CD002181.pub2

Russell NDF, Cooper ME. 50 years forward: mechanisms of hyperglycaemia-driven diabetic complications. Diabetologia 2015; 58: 1708–14 doi: 10.1007/s00125-015-3600-1

Stevens LA, Coresh J, Greene T, Levey AS. Assessing kidney function-measured and estimated glomerular filtration rate. New Engl J Med 2006; 354: 2473–83.

UK Renal Registry (2020) UK Renal Registry 22nd Annual Report – data to 31/12/2018, Bristol, UK

United States Renal Data System. 2020 *USRDS Annual Data Report: Epidemiology of kidney disease in the United States.* National Institutes of Health, National Institute of Diabetes and Digestive and Kidney Diseases, Bethesda, MD, 2020

Diabetic neuropathy

Diabetes is one of the most common causes of peripheral neuropathy, a term that encompasses a heterogeneous group of disorders (Figure 17.1). In population-based surveys, diabetic neuropathies are the most prevalent chronic complications of diabetes. Diabetic neuropathy should not be diagnosed solely on the basis of one symptom, physical sign or test; it is recommended that a minimum of two abnormalities be detected (either symptoms, signs or test abnormalities – either nerve conduction, quantitative sensory testing, or quantitative autonomic testing) (Figure 17.2).

Healthy nerves consist of myelinated and unmyelinated nerve fibres or axons. The pathophysiology of diabetic neuropathy is complex, but microvascular disease affecting small vessels (the vasa vasorum) that supply oxygen and nutrients to peripheral nerves results in ischaemic and metabolic neuronal injury via activation of several biochemical pathways, in particular the Polyol pathway, non-enzymatic glycation and formation of advanced glycation endproducts (AGEs), activation of diacylglycerol-protein kinase C-β, transcription factors (e.g. NF-κB) and mitogen-activated protein kinase (MAPK), and the accumulation of reactive oxygen species (ROS) (Figure 17.3).

Chronic sensorimotor neuropathy

Chronic sensorimotor neuropathy is the commonest form of diabetic neuropathy. This results from the distal dying back of axons that begins in the longest nerves; thus, the feet are affected first in a stocking distribution, and later there may be progressive involvement of the upper limbs. Sensory loss is most evident; autonomic involvement is usual, although it is mostly symptomless. Positive painful symptoms tend to be worse at night. Neurological examination shows a symmetrical sensory loss to all modalities, reduced or absent ankle or knee reflexes, and small muscle wasting of the feet and hands (Figure 17.4). The foot at high risk of neuropathic ulceration might have a high arch (pes cavus deformity) and clawing of the toes.

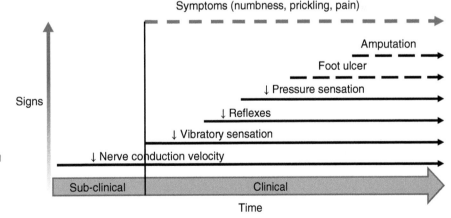

Figure 17.1 Diabetic neuropathy is common and associated with a complex mix of symptoms and signs. With increasing duration of diabetes and associated microangiopathy, diabetic neuropathy may lead to foot ulceration, deformity and/or amputation.

A. Diffuse neuropathy
Diffuse Symmetrical PolyNeuropathy

c Primarily small-fiber neuropathy
c Primarily large-fiber neuropathy
c Mixed small-and large-fiber neuropathy (most common)

Autonomic
Cardiovascular
c Reduced HRV
c Resting tachycardia
c Orthostatic hypotension
c Sudden death (malignant arrhythmia)
  Gastrointestinal
c Diabetic gastroparesis (gastropathy)
c Diabetic enteropathy (diarrhea)
c Colonic hypomotility (constipation)
  Urogenital
c Diabetic cystopathy (neurogenic bladder)
c Erectile dysfunction
c Female sexual dysfunction
  Sudomotor dysfunction
c Distal hypohydrosis/anhidrosis,
c Gustatory sweating
  Hypoglycemia unawareness
  Abnormal pupillary function

B. Mononeuropathy (mononeuritis multiplex) (atypical forms)

Isolated cranial or peripheral nerve (e.g., CN III, ulnar, median, femoral, peroneal)
Mononeuritis multiplex (if confluent may resemble polyneuropathy)

C. Radiculopathy or polyradiculopathy (atypical forms)
Radiculoplexus neuropathy (a.k.a. lumbosacral polyradiculopathy, proximal motor amyotrophy)
Thoracic radiculopathy

D. Nondiabetic neuropathies common in diabetes
Pressure palsies
Chronic inflammatory demyelinating polyneuropathy(CIDP)
Radiculoplexus neuropathy
Acute painful small-fiber neuropathies (treatment-induced)

Figure 17.2 Classification of diabetic neuropathy.

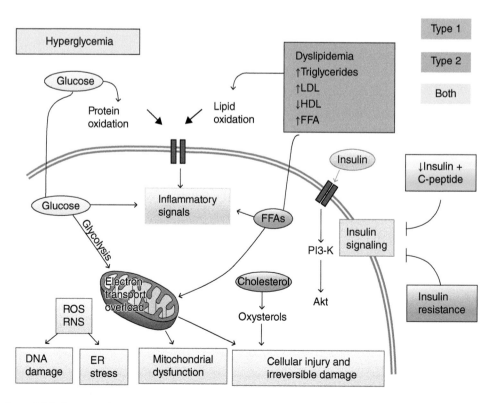

Figure 17.3 Mechanisms of diabetic neuropathy.

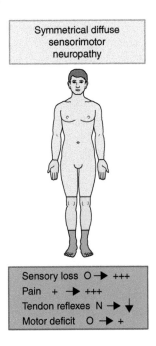

Figure 17.4 Clinical pattern of distal symmetrical neuropathies.

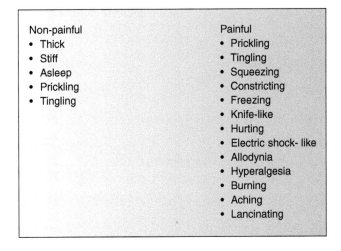

Figure 17.6 Positive sensory symptoms; painful neuropathy.

A simple staging system has been developed for diabetic neuropathy (Figure 17.5).

Positive sensory symptoms can arise spontaneously or as a response to stimulation, and they are often classified into painful and non-painful descriptors (Figure 17.6). Numbness and prickling are the most common symptoms, and they usually occur earlier. Allodynia is the perception of pain from a non-noxious stimulus. The prevalence of painful symptoms varies from 3–20%. The natural history of painful neuropathy is unclear, but there is some suggestion

Stage 0:	No signs or symptoms
Stage 1:	Asymptomatic neuropathy
1a:	No symptoms or signs but nerve conduction velocity abnormalities or autonomic test abnormalities
1b:	N1a criteria + neurological examination abnormality. Vibration detection threshold abnormality
Stage 2:	Symptomatic neuropathy
2a:	Symptoms, signs and tests abnormality*
2b:	N2a criteria + signifi cant weakness of ankle dorsiflexion
Stage 3:	Disabling polyneuropathy

* Tests include nerve conduction, quantitative sensory testing and quantitative autonomic testing

Figure 17.5 Staging the severity of diabetic neuropathy.

that the intensity of symptoms may subside with worsening quantitative measures of nerve function. Similarly, risk factors for painful neuropathy are ill-defined. Hypoaesthetic neuropathy is associated with minimal or negative sensory symptoms, and therefore is best detected by quantitative sensory testing

In identifying feet at risk of ulceration, the 10 g monofilament has a sensitivity of 86-100%. These are patients who are unable to feel the monofilament when applied with sufficient pressure at the handle to buckle the filament (Figure 17.7). The monofilament should be applied to the sole of each foot in four places (over the hallux and metatarsal heads 1, 3, 5). More sophisticated instruments for measuring vibration detection threshold (VDT) and quantitative sensory testing (three modalities - vibration, thermal and pain thresholds) are also useful for predicting patients with neuropathy who are at high risk of ulceration and amputation.

Positive symptoms of neuropathy are distressing, often at night, disabling, and difficult to treat. Patients with painful peripheral neuropathy often have warm, dry feet because of autonomic involvement, which results in dilated arteriovenous shunts and absent sweating. The most important complications are:
• Foot ulceration
• Neuropathic oedema, caused by increased blood flow in the foot, which has reduced sympathetic innervation
• Charcot arthropathy, with chronic destruction, deformity and inflammation of the joints and bones of the mid-foot. There is reduced bone density, possibly because of increased blood flow (Figure 17.8) (see Chapter 21).

Various topical and systemic therapies have been tried for painful diabetic peripheral neuropathy, but few have been subjected to well-designed randomised controlled trials

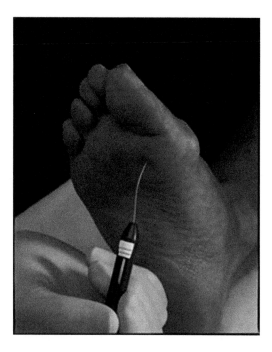

Figure 17.7 A 10g monofilament is simple, easy to use in the clinic and is much better than clinical assessment for identifying patients at risk of foot ulceration.

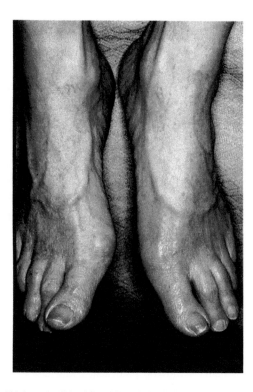

Figure 17.8 Increased blood flow (distended veins) on the dorsum of the foot of a diabetic patient with painful peripheral neuropathy.

(RCTs). The U.S Food and Drug Administration (FDA) have received regulatory approval for the treatment of neuropathic pain in the U.S, Europe and Canada. Combination therapy, including combinations with opioids, may provide effective treatment for diabetic neuropathic pain at lower doses. In addition to those listed in the Figure, acupuncture may be helpful and the antioxidant, alpha-lipoic acid, is used in some countries (Table 17.1).

Pressure palsies comprise focal lesions of peripheral nerves that occur at sites of entrapment or compression (Figure 17.9). Diabetic nerves are thought to be more susceptible to mechanical injury. The most common is the carpal tunnel syndrome (median nerve compression), in which paraesthesiae and sometimes numbness occur in the fingers and hands. Discomfort can radiate into the forearm. Examination can show wasting and weakness of the thenar muscles, with loss of sensation over the lateral three-and-a-half fingers. The diagnosis can be confirmed by nerve conduction studies. Most patients respond to surgical decompression.

Ulnar nerve compression at the elbow causes numbness and weakness of the fourth and fifth fingers and wasting of the interossei muscles (Figure 17.10). Lateral popliteal nerve compression can cause foot drop.

In mononeuropathies, single nerves or their roots are affected and, in contrast to distal symmetrical neuropathy, these conditions are of rapid onset and reversible, which suggests an acute, possibly vasculitic or inflammatory origin rather than chronic metabolic disturbance. The most well-known is femoral neuropathy or diabetic amyotrophy (Figures 17.11 and 17.12). There is multifocal involvement of the lumbosacral roots, plexus and femoral nerve. Typically, the patient is over 50 years of age with continuous thigh pain, wasting and weakness of the quadriceps, and sometimes weight loss. The knee jerk reflex is lost.

Other mononeuropathies include cranial nerve palsies of the third or sixth nerves (causing sudden-onset diplopia). The cause is thought to be a localized infarct that involves brainstem nuclei or nerve roots. Older people are affected mainly.

In patients with long-standing diabetes, numerous abnormalities can be demonstrated in organs that receive an autonomic innervation (Figure 17.13). Often, autonomic abnormalities are found in those with distal sensory neuropathies. Symptoms are unusual, occurring mostly in those with poorly controlled type 1 diabetes. Common manifestations are gustatory sweating over the face, induced by eating cheese or other foods, postural hypotension (systolic blood pressure fall >30 mmHg on standing), blunting of physiological heart-rate variations, diarrhoea, and erectile dysfunction. The efficacy of the topical antimuscarinic agent glycopyrrolate in the treatment of gustatory sweating was confirmed in a randomized controlled trial, and daily application attenuates this complication in most patients for at least

Table 17.1 Treatments for symptomatic diabetic polyneuropathy pain-dosing and side effects.

Drug Class	Drug	Dose	Side Effects
Tricyclics	Amitryptyline	50-150 QDS	Somnolence, dizziness, dry mouth, tachycardia
	Nortriptyline	50-150 QDS	constipation, urinary retention, blurred vision
	Imipramine	25-150 QDS	Confusion
	Desipramine	25-150 QDS	
SSRIs	Paroxetine	40 OD	Somnolence, dizziness, sweating, nausea, anorexia
	Citalopram	40 OD	diarrhea, impotence, tremor
SNRIs	Duloxetine	60 OD	Nausea, somnolence, dizziness, anorexia
Anticonvulsants	Gabapentin	300-1200 TID	Somnolence, dizziness, Confusion, ataxia
	Pregabalin	50-150 TID	Somnolence, confusion, edema, weight gain
	Carbamazepine/ Oxcarbezepine	Up to 200 QDS	Dizziness, somnolence, Nausea, leukopenia
	Topiramate	Up to 400 OD	Somnolence, dizziness, ataxia, Tremor
Opioids	Tramadol	50-100 BID	Nausea, constipation, HA Somnolence
	Oxycodone CRTapentadol ER	10-30 BID Up to 500 QD	Somnolence, nausea, constipation, HA Constipation, nausea, somnolence, dizziness
Topical	Capsaicin	0.075% QDS	Local irritation
	Lidocaine	0.04% OD	Local irritation
Injection	Botulinum toxin		None

Aaron Vinik, Endotext; www.endotext.org, 2018.

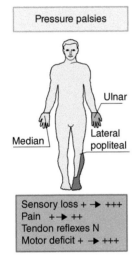

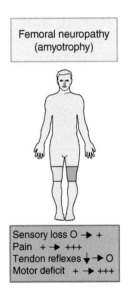

Figure 17.9 Clinical pattern of pressure palsies in patients with diabetes.

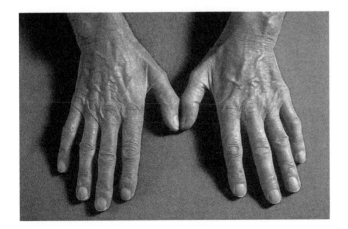

Figure 17.10 Generalised wasting of the interossei (and hypothenar eminence) caused by bilateral ulnar nerve palsies in a diabetic patient.

Figure 17.11 Diabetic amyotrophy, showing marked quadriceps wasting, and clinical pattern (inset).

24 hours. Midodrine, a peripheral, selective, direct a1-adrenoreceptor agonist, is an FDA-approved drug for the treatment of postural hypotension. Low-dose fludrocortisone may also be beneficial in supplementing volume repletion in some patients with postural hypotension, but there is risk of risk of supine hypertension, leg odema and hypokalaemia. Gastroparesis (delayed gastric emptying and vomiting) and bladder dysfunction are rare but are potentially debilitating complications of diabetes. The evaluation of patients suspected of gastroparesis should include withdrawal of potential offending drugs such as Opiods, GLP-1 agonist, Leva-dopa, Anti-cholinergics, octretotide; exclusion of function causes and, in some cases, nutritional and psychological

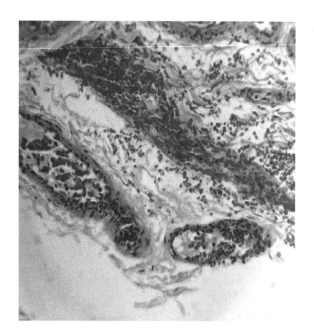

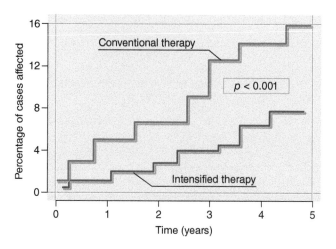

Figure 17.14 Effects of intensified insulin therapy and strict glycaemic control on the incidence of neuropathy in type 1 diabetic patients (DCCT). From Diabetes Control and Complications Trial Research Group. Ann Intern Med 1995; 122: 566–568.

Figure 17.12 Histological changes associated with diabetic amyotrophy. In particular, an inflammatory cell infiltrate, occlusion of epineurial blood vessels and features of necrotising vasculitis. This H&E section shows inflammatory infiltrate affecting arterioles and venules. Courtesy of Dr R. Malik.

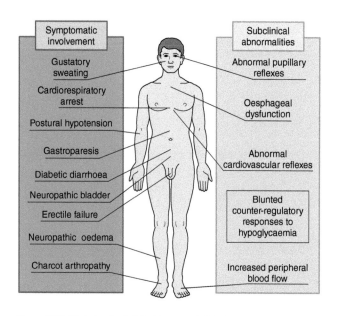

Figure 17.13 Clinical and subclinical features of diabetic autonomic neuropathy.

evaluation. Diagnosis is made by gastric emptying study. Only metoclopramide, a prokinetic agent, is approved by the FDA for the treatment of gastroparesis, but in view of potential long-term adverse effects, treatment is not recommended beyond 5 days. The mainstay of treatment for all types of autonomic neuropathy is a multifactorial approach targeting glycemia and other risk factors for cardiovascular disease in people with diabetes. In some cases, patients may require feeding through a jejunostomy until the stomach recovers or with gastric pacing.

Management of diabetic neuropathy begins with explanation and empathy, the exclusion of other causes of neuropathy (e.g. alcoholism, vitamin B12 deficiency and uraemia), and then the institution of tight glycaemic control. Both the DCCT and UKPDS trials show that strict glycaemic control can decrease the risk of developing neuropathy, as judged by objective measures such as nerve conduction velocity. However, the main complaint of patients with neuropathy is pain, and there is as yet little evidence that improving diabetic control influences the intensity of neuropathic pain (Figure 17.14).

CASE HISTORY

A 55-year-old man with 6-year history of type 2 diabetes presents to his family doctor with unpleasant symptoms of prickling discomfort, numbness, and tingling over both lower limbs and feet. These symptoms often disturb his sleep, and he has noticed excessive discomfort when putting his feet into a warm bath. There are no symptoms in his hands, he is a non-smoker and drinks 6 units of alcohol per week. There are no symptoms to suggest autonomic dysfunction. He has background diabetic retinopathy, and his diabetes is managed with metformin 1g bid and gliclazide MR 120mg daily (HbA1c 8.5%). Clinical examination shows some distal muscle wasting in the feet, but no ulceration. He is unable to feel the 10g monofilament placed over the metatarsal heads. Pedal pulses are present. His height is 6' 1", BMI 29.

Comment: This patient presents with typical symptoms and signs of diabetic peripheral neuropathy, including allodynia when he puts his feet into warm water. Risk factors include age, duration of diabetes, and HbA1c, and peripheral neuropathy is more common in tall people (longer nerves are more susceptible to damage). Alcohol consumption may aggravate his symptoms. He also has evidence of microvascular complications in the eye. Improving HbA1c is important, and his feet are at high risk of ulceration. Appropriate foot care education is needed. This man may also need symptomatic treatment, e.g. pregabalin, gabapentin, or amitriptyline would be reasonable choices.

LANDMARK CLINICAL TRIALS

Dyck PJ, et al. Risk factors for severity of diabetic polyneuropathy: intensive longitudinal assessment of the Rochester Diabetic Neuropathy Study cohort. Diabetes Care 1999; 22: 1479–1486.

EURODIAB IDDM Study Group. Prevalence of diabetic peripheral neuropathy and its relation to glycaemic control and potential risk factors: the EURODIAB IDDM complication study. Diabetologia 1996; 39: 1377–1386.

Ismail-Beigi F et al.; ACCORD trial group. Effect of intensive treatment of hyperglycaemia on microvascular outcomes in type 2 diabetes: an analysis of the ACCORD randomised trial. Lancet 2010; 376: 419–430

DCCT Research Group. The effect of intensive diabetes therapy on the development and progression of neuropathy. Ann. Intern. Med. 1995; 122: 561–568.

Backonja m et al. Gabapentin for the symptomatic treatment of painful neuropathy in patients with diabetes mellitus: a randomized controlled trial. JAMA 1998; 280: 1831–1836

Low PA et al. Midodrine Study Group. Efficacy of midodrine vs placebo in neurogenic orthostatic hypotension. A randomized, doubleblind multicenter study. JAMA 1997; 277: 1046–1051

KEY WEBSITES

- https://www.niddk.nih.gov/health-information/health-communication-programs/ndep/health-care-professionals/practice-transformation/specific-outcomes/neuropathy/Pages/default.aspx
- http://www.ninds.nih.gov/disorders/diabetic/diabetic.htm
- https://www.nice.org.uk/guidance/cg173/evidence/neuropathic-pain-pharmacological-management-full-guideline-191621341
- http://www.sign.ac.uk/guidelines/fulltext/55/section7.html

FURTHER READING

Veves A, et al. Painful diabetic neuropathy: epidemiology, natural history, early diagnosis and treatment options. Pain Med. 2008; 9: 660–674.

Dyck PJ et al. Toronto Expert Panel on Diabetic Neuropathy. Diabetic polyneuropathies: update on research definition, diagnostic criteria and estimation of severity. Diabetes Metab Res Rev 2011; 27: 620–628

Callaghan BC et al. Diabetic neuropathy: clinical manifestations and current treatments. Lancet Neurol 2012; 11: 521–534

Tesfaye S et al; Toronto Diabetic Neuropathy Expert Group. Diabetic neuropathies: update on definitions, diagnostic criteria, estimation of severity, and treatments. Diabetes Care 2010; 33: 2285–2293

Diabetic Neuropathy. Position statement by the American Diabetes Association Diabetes Care 2017; 40: 136–154 | DOI: 10.2337/dc16-2042

Finnerup NB et al. Pharmacotherapy for neuropathic pain in adults: a systematic review and meta-analysis. Lancet Neurol 2015; 14: 162–173

Callaghan BC, et al. Role of neurologists and diagnostic tests on the management of distal symmetric polyneuropathy. JAMA Neurol 2014; 71: 1143–1149

Blood lipid abnormalities

Abnormalities of blood lipids are common in patients with type 2 diabetes, even when there is reasonable glycaemic control. The characteristic dyslipidaemia of type 2 diabetes consists of elevated total and VLDL (very low-density lipoprotein) triglyceride (TG) levels, reduced HDL (high-density lipoprotein), and minimal change in total and LDL (low-density lipoprotein) cholesterol concentrations. Overproduction of TG-rich VLDL by the liver and impaired TG clearance by endothelial lipoprotein lipase are contributory factors. Although total and LDL-cholesterol levels in patients with type 2 diabetes are no different to those in non-diabetic subjects, the profile of LDL subfractions in patients with type 2 diabetes is more atherogenic due to a greater proportion of small, dense LDL particles (known as the 'type B' pattern) which are more susceptible to oxidation; oxidised LDL plays a major role in atherogenesis. Improved glycaemic control results in less VLDL-triglyceride synthesis in the liver, but these lipid abnormalities are not completely resolved by HbA1c-lowering (Figure 18.1).

The dyslipidaemia of type 2 diabetes is frequently accompanied by other metabolic and biochemical abnormalities indicative of insulin resistance, chronic low-grade inflammation (e.g. increased high-sensitivity C-reactive protein (hsCRP) and elevated cytokines such as interleukin-6 and tumour necrosis factor-α) and a prothrombotic state (increased levels of fibrinogen and plasminogen activator inhibitor-1, PAI-1). Collectively, these abnormalities interact to substantially increase the risk of cardiovascular disease (Figure 18.2).

In non-obese, well-controlled patients with type 1 diabetes, serum lipid, and lipoprotein concentrations are similar to those in non-diabetic people. In poorly controlled type 1 diabetes, hypertriglyceridaemia can occur because insulin deficiency causes increased lipolysis, overproduction of nonesterified fatty acids and VLDL, and decreased activity

Figure 18.1 Features of Diabetic dyslipidaemia. In the German PROCAM study, 39% of diabetic patients had fasting serum TG concentrations >2.3 mmol/L (vs 21% in non-diabetics) and 27% had HDL-cholesterol levels <0.9 mmol/L (vs 16% in non-diabetics).

of endothelial lipoprotein lipase, which reduces clearance of triglyceride-containing VLDL and chylomicrons. Very high triglyceride levels (>20 mmol/L) can occur in poorly controlled or newly presenting patients with type 1 diabetes, often in association with ketoacidosis. Complications include eruptive xanthomas in the skin (Figure 18.3), acute pancreatitis and lipaemia retinalis (a milky appearance of the retinal vessels seen on ophthalmoscopy). The main determinants of hyperlipidaemia in type 1 diabetes are age, obesity, poor glycaemic control, and nephropathy.

The relationship between total cholesterol levels and coronary heart disease (CHD) mortality was first identified in the screening database of male subjects for the Multiple Risk Factor Intervention Trial (MRFIT) (Figure 18.4). Over 360,000 healthy men were screened, and for both diabetic and non-diabetic subjects there was a continuous relationship between cholesterol and CHD death rates over the subsequent 10-year period. This observational epidemiology

Handbook of Diabetes, Fifth Edition. Rudy Bilous, Richard Donnelly, and Iskandar Idris.
© 2021 John Wiley & Sons Ltd. Published 2021 by John Wiley & Sons Ltd.

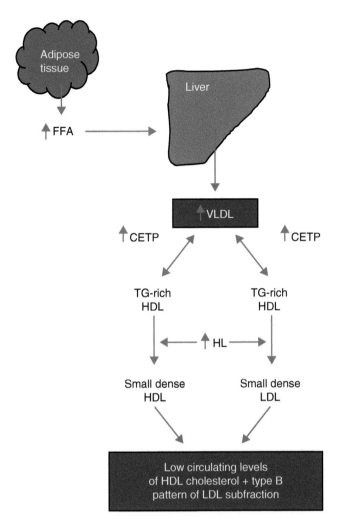

Figure 18.2 The pathogenesis of diabetic dyslipidaemia involves increased release of free fatty acids (FFAs) from expanded adipose tissue depots (obesity), which in turn fuels the hepatic synthesis of TG-rich very-low-density-lipoprotein (VLDL) particles. The increase in circulating VLDL is a reflection of increased synthesis and secretion of VLDL from the liver, and decreased lipoprotein lipase-mediated clearance in peripheral tissues. Cholesterol ester transfer protein (CETP, which is increased in diabetes) transfers TG from VLDL to HDL and LDL in exchange for cholesterol, thus generating TG-rich HDL and LDL particles. These particles are a substrate for hepatic lipase (HL), which cleaves TG leaving small dense HDL and LDL.

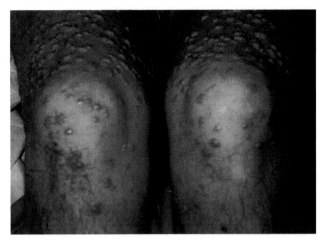

Figure 18.3 Eruptive xanthomata. This young patient with type 1 diabetes presented with ketoacidosis, severe hypertriglyceridaemia and eruptive xanthomata. (Photograph courtesy of Pictures in Lipidology, MedNet, www. mednet.gr/pim/lipid.htm).

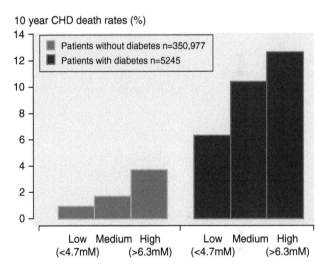

Figure 18.4 The MRFIT screening study enrolled >360,000 men in the 1960s-70s, and showed the relationship between serum total cholesterol (classified as low, medium or high) and 10-year CHD mortality for diabetic and non-diabetic subjects. For any given level of cholesterol, CHD mortality is much higher in diabetic men.

provided strong evidence for cholesterol as a risk factor, and suggested that, among diabetic patients, for any given level of cholesterol the CHD mortality was three to four-fold higher. Subsequently, high quality evidence has shown that LDL-cholesterol is a reliable and surrogate marker in the relationship between statins and CHD risk. Whether this applies to non-statin therapy remains unclear but recent negative trials with non-statin lipid-lowering therapies such as niacin and the CETP inhibitor, torcetrapib suggest that non all LDL-C lowering strategies are equal in their ability to reduce the risk of CHD. Nevertheless, a systematic review

and meta-analysis have reported that statin and non-statin therapy that act by up-regulating the LDL receptor have similar effects on LDL-C lowering and the risk of CHD events (Figure 18.5).

Statins (HMG-CoA reductase inhibitors) are the drugs of first choice for lowering cholesterol levels and CHD risk, especially in patients with diabetes (Figure 18.6). Examples include simvastatin, rosuvastatin, and atorvastatin. They work by inhibiting an early step in cholesterol synthesis, reducing hepatic cholesterol production by up to 50%, which secondarily upregulates LDL receptor synthesis and

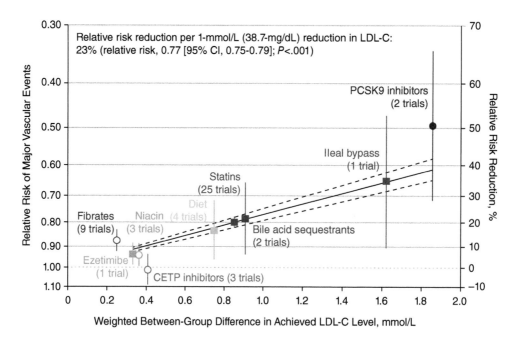

Figure 18.5 The importance of LDL cholesterol lowering to reduce major vascular events has been confirmed using combined data from several large statins and non-statin trials. Each type of intervention is plotted based on the between-group difference in achieved LDL-C level (weighted across all the trials in the class) and the relative risk (with vertical lines depicting the 95% CIs) derived from meta-analysis of all trials in that class. The square data markers indicate the established interventions that lower LDL-C predominantly through upregulation of LDL receptor expression. The meta-regression slope (predicted RR for degree of LDL-C reduction) is represented by the solid black line and the 95% CIs by the dashed lines, both of which are derived from a trial-level analysis of all established interventions. CETP indicates cholesteryl ester transfer protein; PCSK9, proprotein convertase subtilisin/kexin type 9). Adapted from Silverman et al. *JAMA.* 2016;316(12):1289–1297.

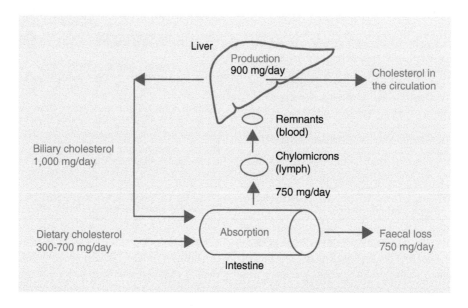

Figure 18.6 Circulating cholesterol is derived from two sources: de novo synthesis in the liver (statins block the rate-limiting enzyme in cholesterol synthesis, HMG CoA reductase), and intestinal absorption of dietary cholesterol and cholesterol contained in bile. Intestinal (re)absorption of cholesterol is blocked by ezetimibe, which can be used in combination with a statin to maximise cholesterol reduction. Other cholesterol-lowering drugs include nicotinic acid, which blocks lipolysis in adipose tissue thereby lowering free fatty acid levels and hepatic VLDL-TG synthesis.

thus promotes the removal of LDL cholesterol and VLDL remnant particles from the blood. LDL-cholesterol levels fall by up to 50% and triglycerides by about 20%. Second and third generation statins are more effective at lowering triglyceride levels. The drugs are generally safe and well tolerated, but generalised muscle aches and pains are more common than previously thought. Myositis however is a rare adverse effect, but is more common when statins are used with fibrates, nicotinic acid, or cyclosporin.

The initial placebo-controlled trials of statins for primary and secondary cardiovascular prevention included only a small proportion of patients with diabetes. Subsequently, the CARDS trial (atorvastatin versus placebo) was undertaken solely in patients with type 2 diabetes, and the larger Heart Protection Study (HPS) included approximately 25% of patients with diabetes. These trials have demonstrated that statins have a powerful effect on lowering cardiovascular mortality and morbidity among patients with diabetes, even at relatively low baseline levels of cholesterol, and the relative risk reductions in major CV events are at least as high in diabetics compared with non-diabetics. Most clinical guidelines now recommend statin therapy for all patients with diabetes; target levels of lipids should be a total cholesterol <4 mmol/L and LDL-cholesterol <2 mmol/L. Given that most patients have baseline untreated levels of total cholesterol >6 mmol/L, these targets are often difficult to achieve using standard doses of first-generation statins such as simvastatin 40mg (Figure 18.7).

Fibric acid derivatives (bezafibrate, fenofibrate, gemfibrozil) are useful for the treatment of hypertriglyceridaemia and mixed hyperlipidaemia, lowering serum triglyceride and increasing HDL cholesterol concentrations. Their mechanism of action involves binding to the nuclear receptor, peroxisome proliferator activated receptor (PPAR-α). This forms a complex with another nuclear receptor, retinoid X receptor (RXR), and interacts with the response elements of several genes that control lipoprotein metabolism (e.g. increasing the expression of the lipoprotein lipase gene and thus increasing triglyceride breakdown). Several trials show

that fibrates reduce CHD events in diabetes, and they appear particularly beneficial in patients with low HDL-cholesterol, central obesity and other features of the metabolic syndrome.

Ezetimibe, an inhibitor of cholesterol intestinal absorption, is another LDL-cholesterol lowering agent. Ezetimibe in combination with a statin is effective in decreasing LDL-cholesterol, lowering triglyceride and raising high density lipoprotein cholesterol levels. Ezetimibe plus statin achieve LDL-C targets in a greater proportion of patients than statin monotherapy. The Results from the Improved Reduction of Outcomes: Vytorin Efficacy International Trial (IMPROVE-IT) suggest that, in high-risk (post–myocardial infarction) patients, lowering LDL-cholesterol with the combination of moderate-intensity statin therapy and ezetimibe provides a modest and predictable clinical benefit. However in a sub-analysis of the study, the non-diabetics surprisingly showed little benefit with ezetimibe. In contrast, the 4933 people with diabetes in the study showed a significant 24% reduction in myocardial infarction and a 39% reduction in ischaemic stroke.

The proprotein convertase subtilisin kexin 9 (PCSK9) inhibitors is a new class of cholesterol lowering drug which have gained interest. It inhibit PCSK9 and decrease intrahepatic degradation of internalised LDL receptors, producing elevated hepatic expression of LDL receptors and a reduced level of circulating LDL-C. A meta-analysis of phase 3 trials in people with diabetes have shown a mean LDL-cholesterol reduction by 55%. The findings were similar across diabetes subgroups based on glycaemia, insulin use, renal function, and cardiovascular status. Alirocumab and evolocumab are examples of this drug class. Both drugs have been evaluated in patients with diabetes and have been proven to be safe and efficient for decreasing LDL-C concentrations in monotherapy or when given in combination with statins, with or without ezetimibe. They have also been authorised as additional therapy for patients with ASCVD or familial hypercholesterolaemia who are taking the maximally tolerated dose of statins but who require a further reduction in their levels of LDL-C. FOURIER and ODYSSEY OUTCOMES showed a reduced number of cardiovascular events after treatment with evolocumab and alirocumab, respectively, related to the degree of further LDL-C lowering. Unlike statins, which have shown a dose-dependent relationship with risk of new-onset diabetes, clinical trials with PCSK9 inhibitors have not shown a higher incidence of diabetes or metabolic worsening in diabetic patients.

For patients who are unable to tolerate statins due to muscle symptoms and therefore have high cholesterol levels, a new class of drug – Bempedoic acid, a pro-drug that inhibits ATP-citrate lyase, an enzyme upstream of β-hydroxy β-methylglutaryl-coenzyme A reductase in the cholesterol biosynthesis pathway has been shown to significantly reduced low-density lipoprotein cholesterol, non–high-density lipoprotein cholesterol, total cholesterol, apolipoprotein B and high-sensitivity C-reactive protein and well tolerated (Figure 18.8).

Relative risk reduction per 1 mmol/L reduction in LDL-cholesterol	
• All-cause mortality	9%
• Major fatal or non-fatal CV events	21%
• MI or coronary death	22%
• Coronary revascularisation	25%
• Stroke	21%

Figure 18.7 A meta-analysis of cholesterol-lowering therapy in 18 686 patients with diabetes has quantified the risk reductions per 1 mmol/L reduction in LDL-cholesterol (Lancet 2008; 371: 117–125). In individual patients, statin therapy will typically reduce LDL-cholesterol by 1-2 mmol/L.

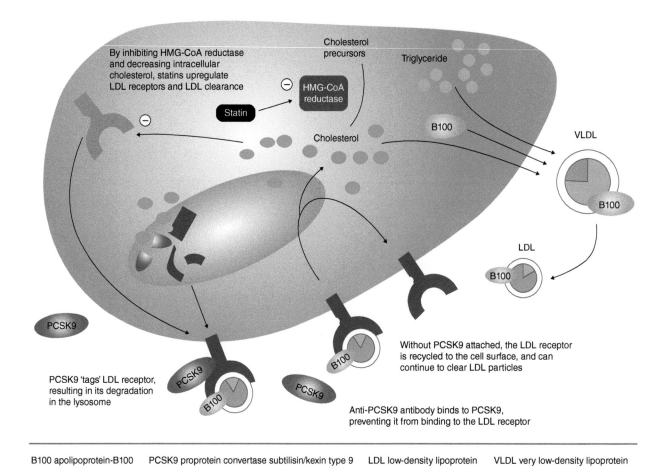

| B100 apolipoprotein-B100 | PCSK9 proprotein convertase subtilisin/kexin type 9 | LDL low-density lipoprotein | VLDL very-low-density lipoprotein |

Figure 18.8 The mechanism of action of statins and PCSK9 monoclonal antibodies. Adapted from Page et al. Australian Prescrib. V39; 2016 Oct.

VLDL is secreted by the liver and converted to LDL, which delivers cholesterol to peripheral tissues and is atherogenic. LDL particles are taken up via LDL receptors, primarily on hepatocytes, and degraded. The production of LDL receptors is decreased by intracellular cholesterol, so lowering intracellular cholesterol with statins results in increased LDL receptors and LDL uptake. LDL-receptor degradation is enhanced by PCSK9, so inhibiting PCSK9 with antibodies increases LDL-receptor recycling and LDL uptake.

CASE HISTORY

A 62-year-old woman with obesity and type 2 diabetes presents for annual review. She is taking NPH insulin twice daily and metformin 1g bid, with a past history of angina, gall stones and type 2 diabetes for 8 years. Her fasting blood tests show total cholesterol 4.8mmol/L, HDL-cholesterol 0.65mmol/L, LDL-cholesterol 3.5mmol/L and triglycerides 3.8mmol/L. HbA1c 8.8%. She is already taking simvastatin 40mg o.d, aspirin 75mg, bendroflumethiazide 2.5mg, ramipril 10mg, and atenolol 100mg. BP 166/92mmHg. Examination shows no signs of hypothyroidism. Renal and liver function are normal; she takes no alcohol. Her dietary compliance is eratic.

Comment: This lady has the typical pattern of dyslipidaemia associated with obesity, insulin resistance, and type 2 diabetes, in particular the low HDL and high fasting triglycerides. Improving her HbA1c will help improve these lipid abnormalities, and both thiazide diuretics and beta blockers can adversely affect HDL / TG levels. She has established angina, and therefore her CV risk is very high. Despite simvastatin 40mg, her total and LDL-cholesterol levels are above target. Dietetic input would be helpful, but she is likely to require further changes to her lipid lowering treatment: (1) either add-on treatment with ezetimibe 10mg od to block cholesterol absorption; or (2) a switch to atrovastatin or rosuvastatin, which are more potent statins that also lower TG levels; or (3) it may be worth trying a higher dose of simvastatin, e.g. 80mg od.

LANDMARK CLINICAL TRIALS

Cannon CP et al. Ezetemibe added to statin therapy after acute coronary syndromes. NEJM 2015; 372: 2387–2397

Silverman MG et al. Association between lowering LDL-C and cardiovascular risk reduction among different therapeutic interventions: a systematic review and meta-analysis. JAMA. 2016; 316(12): 1289–1297

Cholesterol treatment trialists collaboration. Efficacy of cholesterol-lowering therapy in 18,686 people with diabetes in 14 randomised trials of statins: a meta-analysis. Lancet 2008; 371: 117–125.

Colhoun HM, et al. Primary prevention of cardiovascular disease with atorvastatin in type 2 diabetes in the Collaborative Atorvastatin Diabetes Study (CARDS): multicentre, randomised placebo-controlled trial. Lancet 2004; 364: 685–696.

Stamler J, et al. Multiple Risk Factor Intervention Trial Research Group: Diabetes, other risk factors and 12 year cardiovascular mortality for men screened in the multiple risk factor intervention trial (MRFIT). Diabetes Care 1993; 16: 434–444.

Heart Protection Study Collaborative Group: MRC/BHF Heart Protection study of cholesterol-lowering with simvastatin in 5,963 people with diabetes: a randomised placebo-controlled trial. Lancet 2003; 361: 2005–2016.

Knopp RH, et al. Efficacy and safety of atorvastatin in the prevention of cardiovascular endpoints in subjects with type 2 diabetes: the Atrovastatin Study for Prevention of Coronary Heart Disease Endpoints in non-insulin-dependent diabetes (ASPEN). Diabetes Care 2006; 29: 1478–1485.

Sabatine MS et al.; FOURIER Steering Committee and Investigators. Evolocumab and clinical outcomes in patients with cardiovascular disease. N Engl J Med. 2017; 376(18): 1713–22.

Schwartz GG et al. Alirocumab and Cardiovascular Outcomes after Acute Coronary Syndrome N Engl J Med. 2018; 379: 2097–2107.

KEY WEBSITES

- www.diabetes.org/diabetescare
- http://www.dtu.ox.ac.uk/index.php?maindoc=/LDS/index.php
- https://www.nice.org.uk/guidance/cg67
- http://heart.bmj.com/content/91/suppl_5/v1

FURTHER READING

Clinical Practice Recommendations American Diabetes Association Diabetes Care 2015 Jan; 38(Supplement 1): S49–S57. https://doi.org/10.2337/dc15-S011

Lloyd-Jones DM etal. Writing Committee. 2016 ACC expert consensus decision pathway on the role of non-statin therapies for LDL-cholesterol lowering in the management of atherosclerotic cardiovascular disease risk: a report of the American College of Cardiology Task Force on Clinical Expert Consensus Documents. J Am Coll Cardiol. 2016;68(1):92–125.

Sattar N. et al. Lipid lowering efficacy of the PCSK9 inhibitor evolocumnab (AMG 145) in patients with type 2 diabetes: a meta-analysis of individual patient data. The Lancet Diabetes & Endocirnology 2016; V4:403–410.

Heart Protection Study Collaborative Group. Lifetime cost-effectiveness of simvastatin in a range of risk groups and age groups derived from a randomised trial of 20,536 people. Br. Med. J. 2006; 333: 1145–1148.

Keech AC, et al. Effect of fenofibrate on the need for laser treatment for diabetic retinopathy (FIELD study): a randomised controlled trial. Lancet 2007; 370: 1687–1697.

The FIELD study investigators. Effects of longterm fenofibrate therapy on cardiovascular events in 9795 people with type 2 diabetes mellitus (the FIELD study): randomised controlled trial. Lancet 2005; 366: 1849–1861.

Betteridge DJ. Treating dyslipidaemia in the patient with type 2 diabetes. Eur. Heart J. 2004; 6 (Suppl. C): C28–C33.

Handelsman Y et al. PCSK9 Inhibitors in Lipid Management of Patients With Diabetes Mellitus and High Cardiovascular Risk: A Review J Am Heart Assoc. 2018; 7(13): e008953.

Chapter
19

Hypertension in diabetes

KEY POINTS

- Hypertension is more common in people with diabetes; both conditions are components of the so-called metabolic syndrome.
- Hypertension increases the cardiovascular risk in diabetic patients by 2–3-fold.
- Insulin resistance and oxidative stress provide two common potential causative mechanisms for hypertension and diabetes.
- The accepted definition of hypertension in people with diabetes in the UK is a BP ≥140/90 mmHg and in the US ≥130/80 mmHg.

- The target should be 120–129/70–79 if < 65 years of age and 130–139/70–79 mmHg if aged >65 yrs.
- Diet and lifestyle interventions can have a significant impact on blood pressure and should be recommended first-line therapy for all.
- Most patients will require three or more drugs to achieve target blood pressure; agents which block the renin angiotensin system, calcium channel blockers or diuretics are first line.

Diabetes and hypertension have been termed the 'bad companions' for cardiovascular disease risk. Diabetes alone increases this risk two–four-fold; in the presence of hypertension, the risk for coronary heart disease is further trebled, and for stroke, doubled. There is also a close relationship with microvascular disease; in the UKPDS, for every 10 mmHg increase in systolic pressure, there was a 13% increase in the combined microvascular endpoints involving the retina and kidney. Moreover, in the UKPDS, up to 50% of people with type 2 diabetes were hypertensive or on antihypertensive therapy at diagnosis. In cross-sectional studies, up to 75% of adults with diabetes are hypertensive, increasing to 80% if they have moderate albuminuria (microalbuminuria) and over 90% if they have severe albuminuria (clinical nephropathy). For people with type 1 diabetes, 30–43% of adults have hypertension, but this is almost always in the presence of nephropathy.

Causative links

Type 2 diabetes and hypertension are constituents of the so-called metabolic syndrome which is underpinned by

insulin resistance. There are several plausible reasons why this might lead to hypertension as well as glucose intolerance (Box 19.1). However, not all epidemiological studies have demonstrated a positive link between fasting plasma insulin levels and blood pressure (or cardiovascular risk); moreover, patients with insulinomas, who have high circulating plasma insulin levels, do not consistently have high blood pressure. There are also ethnic differences in estimates of insulin resistance and blood pressure levels.

The common role of oxidative stress for both hypertension and diabetes has been proposed (Box 19.2). Again, there are plausible mechanisms linking the two. However, oxidative stress is hard to measure in humans, there are few data on the benefit or otherwise of antioxidant therapies, and the observed reduction in some measures of oxidative stress in response to antihypertensive therapy does not prove causality.

As can be seen from Box 19.2 and Figure 19.1, there is some overlap of potential causative mechanisms for hypertension and it is possible that both insulin resistance and oxidative stress play a role, with a different predominance in individual patients. There is also a strong influence of ethnicity, for

Handbook of Diabetes, Fifth Edition. Rudy Bilous, Richard Donnelly, and Iskandar Idris.
© 2021 John Wiley & Sons Ltd. Published 2021 by John Wiley & Sons Ltd.

Box 19.1 Potential causative links between insulin resistance, hyperinsulinaemia and hypertension.

- Sodium retention secondary to stimulated renal tubular reabsorption.
- Raised intracellular sodium secondary to increased Na^+/K^+ ATPase.
- Hypertrophy of vascular smooth muscle cells by direct trophic action.
- Increased intracellular calcium leading to increased contractility of vascular smooth muscle cells.
- Increased sympathetic nervous system stimulation.
- Decreased vascular endothelial nitric oxide generation.

Box 19.2 Potential causative links between oxidative stress and hypertension.

- Quenching of nitric oxide.
- Generation of vasoconstrictor lipid peroxidation products (e.g. F_2 isoprostanes).
- Depletion of tetrahydrobiopterin (BH_4), a nitric oxide synthase co-factor.
- Direct endothelial cell damage leading to increased permeability.
- Direct vascular smooth muscle cell damage.
- Increased intraceullar calcium leading to increased contractility of vascular smooth muscle cells.
- Stimulation of inflammation and growth factors.

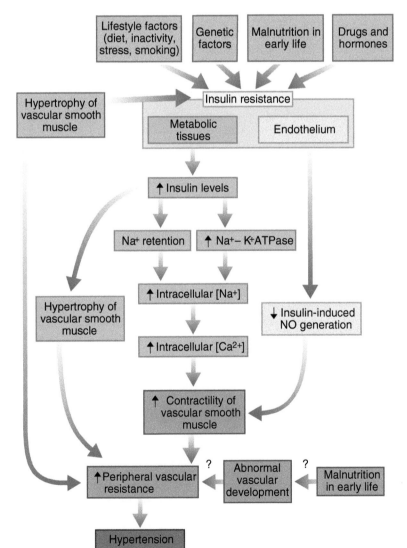

Figure 19.1 Suggested mechanisms linking insulin resistance to the development of systemic hypertension. NO = nitric oxide.

example Afro-Caribbean and Chinese populations have high prevalences of both hypertension and diabetes.

For type 1 diabetes, hypertension is almost invariably a consequence of nephropathy and the processes that lead to it. Many of these will share the potential causative mechanisms of insulin resistance and oxidative stress. Interestingly, the DCCT/EDIC 8-year follow-up showed a significantly lower number of patients with hypertension in the original intensively treated arm (29.9% versus 40.3%), almost certainly as a consequence of fewer cases of nephropathy in this cohort.

Definition of hypertension and targets

With the increasing numbers of antihypertensive agents and large trials, the close relationship between level of blood pressure and cardiovascular disease risk has resulted in the definition of hypertension being revised downwards, from 160/95 mmHg in the 1980s to 140/90 mmHg today.

For every 20/10 mmHg increase in blood pressure above 115/75, the risk for cardiovascular disease in the population doubles. For people with type 2 diabetes, for every 10 mmHg increase in blood pressure, there is an 18% increase in risk of myocardial infarction, and 29% for stroke. Intervention trials have not shown the magnitude of benefit on cardiovascular disease that might have been predicted from the epidemiological studies (Figure 19.2). This has led to a revision of blood pressure targets in many published guidelines with

a broad, but by no means uniform, consensus (Table 19.1) There have been a plethora of meta-analyses and systematic reviews which have either supported the consensus or argued for lower diagnostic thresholds and treatment targets. A recent meta-analysis explored the impact of baseline and achieved blood pressure on cardiovascular outcomes in people with diabetes who had taken part in randomised controlled clinical trials (RCTs) of anti-hypertensive therapies. In 49 trials with 73,738 people with diabetes they found a definite benefit for all cause and cardiovascular mortality in those with an entry systolic blood pressure > 140 mmHg and who achieved levels of 130–140 mmHg during the trial. Below these thresholds, there was no evidence of benefit and evidence of possible harm. Based on these and other data, it seems appropriate to use a diagnostic threshold of 140/90 mmHg (in those <65 years of age) and a target of 130–140/80–90 mmHg. Patients who have achieved lower blood pressures and who are otherwise well with no adverse side effects should not have their therapy relaxed. There is general agreement that blood pressure should not be lowered below 120 mmHg systolic and/or 70 mmHg diastolic. The latest available National Diabetes Audit data for primary care in England and Wales for 2017/18 show that 91% of people with type 1 and 96% with type 2 diabetes had their blood pressure measured and 75% and 74% respectively had a reading of ≤140/80 mmHg. The World Health Organisation (WHO) has published cardiovascular risk tables to guide therapeutic targets and to help inform patients (Figure 19.3).

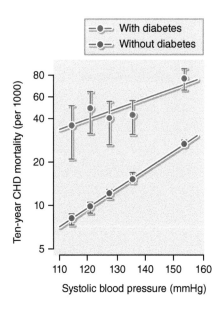

Figure 19.2 Additive effects of diabetes and hypertension on deaths from coronary heart disease (CHD). Data from 342,815 subjects without diabetes and 5163 subjects with diabetes aged 35–57 years, free from myocardial infarction at entry. From Pickup & Williams. *Textbook of Diabetes*, 2nd edition. Blackwell Publishing Ltd, 1997.

Diagnosis of hypertension

The latest NICE guidelines suggest that hypertension should be diagnosed in those with a clinic reading >140/90 mmHg and after an average ambulatory and/or home blood pressure recording of ≥135/85 mmHg. The latest US Guidance defines hypertension as ≥130/80 mmHg. Automated blood pressure recording devices are recommended, mercury sphygmomanometers should no longer be used (Box 19.3). Aneroid devices should be calibrated six-monthly. Current NICE guidance suggests offering ambulatory blood pressure monitoring (ABPM) to confirm the diagnosis. At least 14 measurements during waking hours should be available and the threshold for diagnosis is 135/85 mmHg. Home blood pressure measurement (HBPM) is an alternative if patients cannot tolerate ABPM or it is not available. Home readings should be checked at least twice, one minute apart, on at least two occasions during the day for 4–7 days.

All people diagnosed with hypertension should undergo a full assessment looking for any evidence of end organ damage (Box 19.4). Secondary causes of hypertension such as Cushing's syndrome, acromegaly, phaeochromocytoma,

Table 19.1 Comparison of guidelines for diagnostic thresholds and treatment targets for hypertension in people with diabetes.

GUIDELINE	NICE	ASH/ACC	JNC 8	ADA	ESH/ESC	ISH
Publication	2019	2017	2014	2020	2018	2020
Diagnostic threshold (mmHg)	140/90 (clinic) 135/85 (ABPM/HBPM)	130/80	140/90 30-59y 150/90 ≥60y	140/90	140/90	140/90 (clinic) 130/80 (ABPM) 135/85 (HBPM)
Treatment target (mmHg)	<140/90 <80y (clinic) <138/85 (ABPM/HBPM) <150/90 >80y (clinic) <145/85 (ABPM/HBPM)	<130/80 if tolerated	<140/90 30-59y <150/90 ≥60y	<140/90 <130/80 if at high CV risk and safe/tolerated	<130/80 <65y <140/80 ≥65y	<130/80 <65 y <140/80 ≥65y
First line therapy	ACEI/ARB (ARB in Afro Caribbean)	ACEI/ARB CCB or Thiazide	Thiazide or CCB or ACEI/ARB ACEI/ARB if CKD	ACEI/ARB CCB or Thiazide if no albuminuria ACEI/ARB if albuminuria	ACEI/ARB + CCB or Thiazide	ACEI/ARB + CCB or Thiazide

NB All guidelines suggest lower limit for treatment of 120 mmHg systolic and 70 mmHg diastolic.
NICE: National Institute for Clinical and Healthcare Excellence. ASH: American Society of Hypertension. ACC: American College of Cardiology ISH: International Society of Hypertension. JNC 8: Eighth Joint National Committee. ADA: American Diabetes Association.
ESC: European Society of Cardiology. ESH: European Society of Hypertension.
ABPM: Ambulatory Blood Pressure Monitoring. HBPM: Home Blood Pressure Monitoring.
ACEI: angiotensin converting enzyme inhibitor. ARB: angiotensin receptor blocker. CCB: dihydropyridine calcium channel blocker. CKD: chronic kidney disease
For references, see end of chapter.

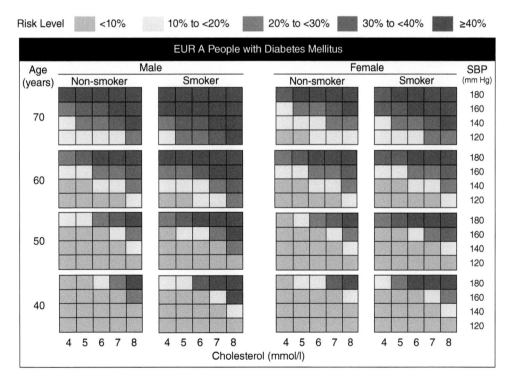

Figure 19.3 World Health Organisation/International Society for Hypertension risk prediction chart for cardiovascular disease in people with diabetes based upon age, gender, smoking status, systolic blood pressure, and total blood cholesterol concentrations. Reproduced with permission from: Prevention of cardiovascular disease pocket guidelines for the assessment and management of cardiovascular risk. WHO Geneva 2007.

Box 19.3 Recommended practice for measuring blood pressure adapted from International Society of Hypertension.

- Use a calibrated and validated instrument.
- Quiet room.
  - No smoking, exercise or caffeine for 30 mins.
  - Measure after 5 minutes in a seated position, feet on floor.
- Arm should be free of tight clothing and at heart level.
- Cuff bladder should cover >80% of arm circumference.
- Take 3 measurements, 1 min apart and average last 2.
- Check both arms (always use the arm with higher reading).
- Check standing blood pressure to detect autonomic neuropathy and/or drug-induced postural hypotension.

Adapted from International Society of Hypertension.

Box 19.4 Assessment and investigation of the patient with hypertension.

- Measurement of height and weight (for BMI); or waist circumference.
- Examination of the:
  - heart for evidence of left ventricular hypertrophy
  - lungs for heart failure
  - abdomen for pulsatile masses, renal enlargement or bruits
  - fundi for signs of retinopathy
- Auscultation for carotid and femoral arterial bruits.
- Examination of peripheral pulses (to exclude co-arctation or peripheral vascular disease).
- Investigations to include ECG, urinalysis (including for microalbuminuria), serum electrolytes, urea and creatinine (and calculation of eGFR), HbA1c, fasting blood lipid profile, chest X-ray or echocardiogram to confirm left ventricular hypertrophy if suspected from ECG. Consider referral for specialist opinion in those with signs or symptoms to exclude secondary causes of hypertension.

Adapted from NICE NG136 Hypertension in adults: diagnosis and management.

Table 19.2 Stages of hypertension.

Stage 1 hypertension
Clinic blood pressure ranging from 140/90 mmHg to 159/99 mmHg and subsequent ABPM daytime average or HBPM average blood pressure ranging from 135/85 mmHg to 149/94 mmHg.
Stage 2 hypertension
Clinic blood pressure of 160/100 mmHg or higher but less than 180/120 mmHg and subsequent ABPM daytime average or HBPM average blood pressure of 150/95 mmHg or higher.
Stage 3 or severe hypertension
Clinic systolic blood pressure of 180 mmHg or higher or clinic diastolic blood pressure of 120 mmHg or higher.

From NICE NG136 Hypertension in Adults: Diagnosis and Management 2019.

guidance on hypertension stresses the importance of dietary salt reduction. Average daily salt intake is 9–12g which is more than twice the WHO recommendation of 5g/d (equivalent to 2000 mg of sodium). Many staple foods and snacks have a significant sodium content: 250 mg/100g bread, 1500 mg/100g popcorn or pretzels, 20,000 mg/100g stock cubes or bouillon for example. WHO also recommends increasing dietary potassium to 3510 mg/d (90 mmol) by consuming more peas, beans, green vegetables, nuts, and fruits such as bananas, but care should be taken if the patient has chronic kidney disease or is taking medication (such as ACE inhibitors) that cause potassium retention.

Regular alcohol consumption is associated with high blood pressure and alcohol associated hypertension is often resistant to medical therapies. A careful alcohol history should be taken in all cases of therapy resistant hypertension. Table 19.3 lists lifestyle factors known to have an impact on blood pressure. It should be remembered that most of these data have come from populations without diabetes or from mixed populations of people with and without type 1 and type 2 diabetes.

Table 19.3 Lifestyle changes and the magnitude of reported reduction in blood pressure.

Modification	Systolic/diastolic blood pressure effect (mmHg)
Weight loss	2.0/1.0 per kg
Dietary Approaches to Stop Hypertension (DASH) diet	8.0/6.0
Potassium intake >3.5 g/d	1.8./1.1
Sodium intake <2.4 g (6 g sodium chloride)/day and normal diet	5.0/2.7
Alcohol ≤30 mL ethanol (3 units)/day men ≤15 mL ethanol (1.5 units)/day women	3.3/2.0
Exercise 30–60 minutes moderate × 4–7/week	4.0/2.0
Dietary fibre supplement (11.5 g/day)	1.1/1.3
Multiple modifications (DASH diet, weight loss, low sodium intake, physical activity) – 9-week trial	12.1/6.6

renal artery stenosis, or co-arctation of the aorta, although rare, should be considered if the history or examination are suggestive. A low or low normal serum potassium (especially if the serum bicarbonate is raised) should prompt consideration of primary hyperaldosteronism (Conn's syndrome).

Management

Initial management depends upon the stage and severity. NICE has classified hypertension as Stage 1, Stage 2, and Stage 3 (severe) (Table 19.2).

Lifestyle changes can be remarkably effective and should be adopted by all. The World Health Organisation (WHO)

Box 19.5 Drugs and behaviours that increase blood pressure.

Drugs
- Corticosteroids
- Cyclo-oxygenase (COX-2) inhibitors
- Non-steroidal anti-inflammatory drugs
- Erythropoietin
- Oral contraceptive pill
- Serotonin reuptake inhibitors
- Monoamine oxidase inhibitors

Behaviours
- Alcohol excess
- Tobacco (smoking/snuff)
- Liquorice

Some medicines and behaviours are known to increase blood pressure (Box 19.5) and treatments may need to be adjusted and lifestyle modified.

Drug treatment

Lifestyle changes should be adopted by all, but current NICE Guidance suggests offering drug treatment immediately after diagnosis to patients with hypertension who have concomitant diabetes. Those with stage 2 hypertension should be offered treatment with two agents initially and those with Stage 3 (severe hypertension) should be referred for urgent specialist assessment.

Drugs which block the renin angiotensin system (RAS)

The RAS has been closely linked to the development of micro and macrovascular complications. Activation both locally at the tissue level and systemically has been described in people with diabetes. The pathway generating aldosterone is complex and involves many steps which can now be blocked or modified by medications (Figure 19.4). Angiotensin II (AII) is a potent vasoconstrictor and has profibrogenic properties in both the kidney and myocardium. Aldosterone causes salt and water retention and is also profibrogenic. Moreover, several of the breakdown products of angiotensin I (AI) and II have vasoactive properties. The rate-limiting step for AII production in the RAS is renin activation. Although renin is an enzyme, together with its precursor prorenin it now appears to have its own receptor

Angiotensin-converting enzyme (ACE) is responsible for most AII production from AI, but other enzymes such as

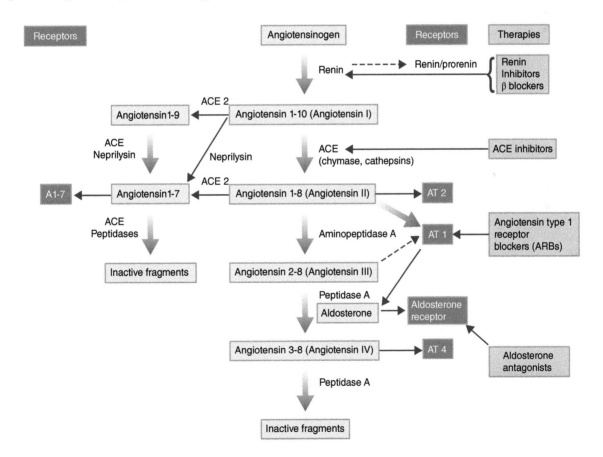

Figure 19.4 Schematic diagram of the renin-angiotensin system. Dotted lines refer to possible or minor actions. Angiotensin 1–7 acts via a separate receptor system and antagonises AT1 actions. AT1 activation results in vasoconstriction, aldosterone release, cell growth, matrix accumulation, inflammation and sympathetic nervous system activation. AT2 activation antagonises some AT1 actions, promotes apoptosis, and possibly promotes inflammation. AT4 activation results in vasodilatation, decreased renal tubular sodium transport, and possibly inflammation. Renin/prorenin receptor activation promotes fibrosis and AII production (not yet confirmed in humans). ACE, angiotensin converting enzyme; AT, angiotensin II type receptor. Prevention of cardiovascular disease: pocket guidelines for the assessment and management of cardiovascular risk. WHO Geneva 2007. © 2007, WHO.

chymases may also operate and be upregulated in the presence of ACEI drugs. ACE2 is a newly described enzyme not inhibited by ACEI and responsible for production of angiotensin 1–7.

By blocking AII action at the type 1 receptor, angiotensin receptor blocking agents (ARB) may up-regulate the type 2 receptor but also increase angiotensin 1–7 production via ACE2.

Finally, both spironolactone and eplerenone block aldosterone action by direct antagonism at its receptor and nonsteroidal aldosterone antagonists such as finerenone are now available and shown benefit in people with type 2 diabetic nephropathy.

With the development of a direct renin inhibitor (aliskiren), blockade of the RAS is possible at almost all levels although its use has not been shown to add benefit compared to ACE inhibitors or ARBs alone. Neprilysin inhibitors in combination with ARBs have recently been licensed for use in heart failure and are undergoing trials in hypertension.

Theoretically, the choice of agent should be determined by where in the RAS it is active and the likely consequences of blockade in terms of physiological outcome. In practice, however, because the agents were developed historically, there is much more information available on ACEI and ARBs (Table 19.4).

In experimental animals, ACEI and ARBs reduce glomerular intracapillary pressure and subsequent glomerulosclerosis. Based on these and other data, many studies of RAS blockade in people with diabetes have focussed on renal outcomes and have consequently been performed in those with varying severity of nephropathy at baseline. The results confirm a positive effect in terms of reducing albuminuria, and

also slowing the progressive loss of GFR towards end stage renal failure in those with more advanced nephropathy at baseline. ACE inhibitors and ARBs appear to be broadly equivalent in terms of efficacy. The impact on all cause and CV mortality has been less clear cut. Results from meta analyses of RCTs that have recruited people with diabetes with and without nephropathy suggest that RAS blocking agents are not more effective than other antihypertensive therapies in terms of effects on CV outcomes such as myocardial infarction and stroke. However, because of their potential for benefit in terms of microvascular complications, ACE inhibitors or ARBs are usually recommended as first line therapy for hypertension in people with diabetes. Combination therapy with two or more RAS blocking agents are no longer recommended because of the risks of acute kidney injury and hyperkalaemia. The exception is that of spironolactone at step 4 in NICE guidance, and perhaps finerenone, but regular monitoring of serum electrolytes and renal function is mandatory in this instance (Figure 19.5). The role of aliskiren is uncertain following the neutral results of the ALTITUDE trial.

Side effects

All RAS-blocking agents can cause hyperkalaemia and regular serum potassium monitoring is required when initiating or adjusting therapy. An acute reduction in GFR can occur as part of the lowering of glomerular pressure.

An acute increase in serum creatinine of up to 30% of baseline (equivalent to a GFR fall of 25%) is acceptable, but above this either a reduction in concomitant diuretic dose or investigation for possible renal artery stenosis should be considered. Although many type 2 patients at postmortem

Table 19.4 RAS-blocking agents.

Class	Indications	Contraindications	Precautions/side effects
ACEI	Nephropathy (type 1 diabetes) Heart failure Younger patients <55 years Post myocardial infarction	Renal artery stenosis Hyporeninaemic hypoaldosteronism Aortic stenosis Pregnancy (or risk of)	First dose hypotension Acute deterioration in renal function Hyperkalaemia Angio-oedema (especially Afro-Caribbean) Cough (10–15%)
ARB	Nephropathy (type 2 diabetes) Intolerance of ACEI (cough, angio-oedema) Heart failure	Renal artery stenosis Hyporeninaemic hypoaldosteronism Aortic stenosis Pregnancy (or risk of)	Acute deterioration in renal function Hyperkalaemia
Renin inhibitors	Not established	Renal artery stenosis Hyporeninaemic hypoaldosteronism Aortic stenosis Pregnancy (or risk of)	GI side effects Hyperkalaemia
Aldosterone antagonists	Resistant hypertension Heart failure	Renal impairment (relative)	Hyperkalaemia GI side effects Gynaecomastia (spironolactone)

Offer lifestyle advice and continue to do so periodically
Use clinical judgement for those with frailty or multiple co-morbidities

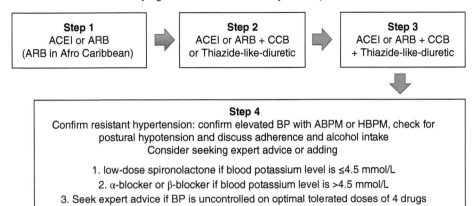

Step 1
ACEI or ARB
(ARB in Afro Caribbean)

Step 2
ACEI or ARB + CCB
or Thiazide-like-diuretic

Step 3
ACEI or ARB + CCB
+ Thiazide-like-diuretic

Step 4
Confirm resistant hypertension: confirm elevated BP with ABPM or HBPM, check for
postural hypotension and discuss adherence and alcohol intake
Consider seeking expert advice or adding

1. low-dose spironolactone if blood potassium level is ≤4.5 mmol/L
2. α-blocker or β-blocker if blood potassium level is >4.5 mmol/L
3. Seek expert advice if BP is uncontrolled on optimal tolerated doses of 4 drugs

For women who are pregnant or considering pregnancy or breastfeeding see guideline Hypertension in Pregnancy
For people with CKD see guideline Chronic Kidney Disease
For people with heart failure see guideline Chronic Heart Failure

Figure 19.5 Summary of antihypertensive drug management in people with diabetes based upon NICE NG136 Hypertension in Adults: diagnosis and management 2019. Optimise dosage at each step before proceeding to the next. If spironolactone is added at Step 4 then regular monitoring of serum potassium and renal function is advised.

have evidence of renal artery atheroma and stenosis, this is functional in only a minority of individuals. If there is a suspicion of stenosis from a rapid deterioration in renal function after RAS blockade, renal arterial Doppler ultrasound or renal angiography should be undertaken. Trials in patients with renal artery stenosis have shown no consistent benefit of angioplasty or stenting on rate of decline of GFR. Some patients may experience hypotension with the first dose of an RAS-blocking drug. Because of this the first dose should be given at night.

Hyporeninaemic hypoaldosteronism (also known as type IV renal tubular acidosis) is more common in people with diabetes with developing nephropathy and is probably a result of tubulointerstitial disease. It often only becomes apparent when patients are challenged with RAS-blocking agents and they become markedly hyperkalaemic. Patients suspected to have this problem should be referred for specialist advice and their RAS blockade discontinued. Fludrocortisone may be helpful to control serum potassium levels.

Calcium channel blockers

There are two groups: dihydropyridine and non-dihydropyridine; both are vasodilators and useful in systolic hypertension (Table 19.5). However, they can increase albuminuria in nephropathy and are less effective than ARB in preserving renal function in patients with type 2 diabetes and clinical nephropathy.

The non-dihydropyridines also slow heart rate and for this reason they should not be used with β-blockers. They can worsen heart failure. Verapamil has been shown to be less effective in reducing albuminuria than the ACEI trandolapril.

Diuretics

These also fall into two main groups: thiazides and loop diuretics (Table 19.6). Thiazides are very effective first-line agents in uncomplicated essential hypertension, as shown in the ALLHAT trial. However, they do have side effects, including glucose intolerance, and have been linked to the development of hyperosmolar hyperglycaemic state (HHS; see Chapter 12). In patients with an eGFR <60 mL/min/1.73 m²

Table 19.5 Calcium channel-blocking agents.

Class	Indications	Contraindications	Precautions/side effects
Dihydropyridines	Systolic hypertension Afro-Caribbean	Heart failure Aortic stenosis	Peripheral oedema Flushing
Non-dihydropyridines	Angina	Heart block β-Blocker use	Constipation Bradycardia Postural hypotension

Table 19.6 Diuretics.

Class	Indications	Contraindications	Precautions/side effects
Thiazides	Heart failure Addition to RAS blockers Elderly	Gout	Hypokalaemia/hyponatraemia Hyperuricaemia Postural hypotension Erectile dysfunction
Loop diuretics	Heart failure eGFR <60 Addition to RAS blockers	Hypovolaemia Gout	Constipation Bradycardia Hypokalaemia/hyponatraemia Postural hypotension Hyperuricaemia

Table 19.7 β-Blockers.

Class	Indications	Contraindications	Precautions/side effects
Cardioselective	Post MI Heart failure Angina	Heart block Asthma (relative) Severe peripheral vascular disease Less effective in elderly Hypoglyaemic unawareness (relative)	Bronchospasm Cold hands/feet Altered hypoglycaemic symptoms (rare) Fatigue

they are rarely effective in producing a diuresis and more potent loop diuretics are required. Diuretics act in synergy with RAS-blocking agents.

β-Blockers

These drugs reduce cardiac output, slow heart rate and reduce renin release in the kidney (Table 19.7). They are of proven benefit in angina, post-MI and in heart failure. Non-cardioselective β-blockers can worsen bronchospasm and are contraindicated in people with asthma. They can also blunt some symptoms of hypoglycaemia and exacerbate symptomatic peripheral vascular disease. For these reasons only cardioselective β-blockers should be used in diabetes. β-Blockers are associated with the development of glucose intolerance and type 2 diabetes and are no longer first-line therapy in the latest guidelines. However, they are indicated post myocardial infarction or for control of angina, and in those patients with symptomatic heart failure.

Other agents

α-Blocking drugs were associated with more heart failure in the ALLHAT study and should not be used as monotherapy. They may be helpful in men with prostatic symptoms by improving urine flow. Labetolol (a combined α- and β-blocking agent) is recommended in pregnancy and can be used parenterally in hypertensive emergencies.

Neprilysin inhibitors in combination with RAS blocking agents have been shown to be effective in short term studies in patients with essential hypertension and in patients with heart failure. They are not currently licensed for use in

hypertension and there are no active studies in diabetes or diabetic nephropathy.

Centrally acting drugs are limited to patients who cannot tolerate first-line agents. However, they have problems with drowsiness, postural hypotension and depression. Methyldopa is completely safe in pregnancy and is useful as an alternative to contraindicated agents such as RAS blockers.

Combination therapy

The UKPDS showed that most patients require three or more agents to achieve a modest target of 144/82 mmHg. Data from the 2015/16 National Diabetes Audit in the UK showed that 89.1% type 1 and 95.7% type 2 diabetic patients had their blood pressure recorded and 74.2% and 73.6% had readings <140/80 mmHg. In the USA, the NHANES survey revealed that 53% of people with diabetes had a recorded blood pressure <130/80 in 2009–12.

Current NICE recommendations are for either an RAS or calcium channel-blocking agent or thiazide as first line, with the addition of another class if target is not reached (Figure 19.5). Few guidelines suggest a β-blocker as first line but suggest that they have a place in those with concomitant ischaemic heart disease or heart failure. Most suggest titration of dose of each class to the maximum effective tolerated level before adding another agent, although this does run the risk of more side effects. The latest ISH guidelines suggest combinations of half maximal doses may improve adherence. In order to reduce the numbers of tablets, combination medications have been developed (such as RAS blockers and diuretics, β-blockers and diuretics) in an attempt to improve compliance.

A 59-year-old man with type 2 diabetes of 9 years' duration was referred to our clinic because of difficult-to-control hypertension. He was overweight (BMI 31 kg/m²) and despite being prescribed ramipril 10 mg, bendroflumethiazide 5 mg, and amlodipine 5 mg, his blood pressure was 164/102 mmHg. His glycaemic control was also outside target, his HbA1c was 68 mmol/mol (8.4%) on gliclazide 80 mg bd. His ECG suggested left ventricular hypertrophy confirmed on chest X-ray. Fundoscopy showed some AV nipping and a few microaneurysms. Examination was otherwise normal apart from his obesity. Investigations showed normal biochemistry, eGFR was 84 mL/min/1.73 m², albumin:creatinine ratio was 9 mg/mmol.

A careful history revealed that he had developed a persistent cough since starting ramipril; he had read the patient information which warned him of this side effect and had discontinued the tablets. He had some prostatic symptoms and consequently only took his diuretic intermittently. Because he was a shift worker, he ate mainly convenience foods and his estimated sodium intake was around 8 g/d (20 g sodium chloride). He had never had a formal dietary review or diabetes education.

He was highly motivated because he did not want to go onto insulin and his mother had recently suffered a disabling stroke.

His BP was confirmed at 164/102 mmHg which is well over the threshold (20/10 mmHg above target) for immediately commencing medication. He was started on an ARB and his amlodipine was changed to an α-blocker (he was found to have benign prostatic hypertrophy). His diuretic was maintained, and he was ultimately switched to an ARB/diuretic combination when doses were stabilised. Formal dietary review led to a significant reduction in his sodium intake and he was able to lose 4 kg in weight over 6 months. His BP came down to 140/86 mmHg.

Comment: There are several points here. Many people with type 2 diabetes are on multiple therapies and find it hard to comply, hence our use of a combination tablet. Many patients do not take their medication as prescribed, often because of side effects. A really careful drug history is essential in these situations. Cough is much less common (but still occurs) on ARBs and this patient required a RAS-blocking agent because of his microalbuminuria. Although α-blockers are not recommended as monotherapy, they are effective for minor prostatic symptoms and enabled this man to continue his diuretics. This is important because they have a synergy with RAS blockers, but neither is effective if dietary sodium intake is high. It is possible to use potassium chloride instead (Lo-salt), but careful monitoring of serum potassium would be required because of the propensity for retention on RAS blockers. Education and awareness of the role of sodium in hypertension and its treatment are crucial. This man was well motivated and the information, support and follow-up he received helped him to significantly reduce his cardiovascular risk (30% for MI, 45% for stroke).

UK Prospective Diabetes Study Group. Tight blood pressure control and risk of macrovascular and microvascular complications in type 2 diabetes: UKPDS 38. BMJ 1998; 317: 703–713.

The UKPDS has been referred to many times in this handbook, but this report was the first to demonstrate not only the link between hypertension and micro- and macrovascular complications, but also that blood pressure lowering *per se* could benefit both types of tissue damage, notably retinopathy.

A total of 1148 patients who were hypertensive (>160/94 mmHg) or on antihypertensive therapy at the time of diagnosis of their type 2 diabetes were randomised to less tight (*n* = 390, target <180/105 mmHg) or tight (*n* = 758, <150/85 mmHg) blood pressure management. In the event, achieved mean BP was 154/87 and 144/82 mmHg for the less tight and tight cohorts, respectively. There was a 21% (95% CI 41, −7%; p NS) relative risk reduction (RRR) in MI and 44% (65,11%; p = 0.013) for stroke; for the combined microvascular endpoint (renal failure, death from renal disease, vitreous haemorrhage or retinal photocoagulation) the reduction was 37% (56,11%; p = 0.0092). The RRR for moderate albuminuria (microalbuminuria) and severe albuminuria (clinical nephropathy) after 6 years was 29% and 39% respectively.

Subsequent analysis and papers revealed a 13% decrease in the microvascular endpoint, 12% for MI, and 19% for stroke for every 10 mmHg decrease in systolic BP. Recently, the 10-year post original study follow-up showed that this benefit of tight control did not persist once the less tight cohort were managed to the same BP target (i.e. no 'memory' effect, unlike for glycaemia).

It is hard to overemphasise the impact the UKPDS has had on the management of type 2 diabetes.

FURTHER READING

Adler AI, Stratton IM, Neal HAW, et al. Association of systolic blood pressure with macrovascular and microvascular complications of type 2 diabetes (UKPDS 36) A prospective observational study. BMJ 2000; 321: 412–419.

American Diabetes Association. Standards of medical care in diabetes – 2020. Diabetes Care 2020; 43(Suppl 1): S111–S134.

Arguedas JA, Leiva V, Wright JM. Blood pressure targets for hypertension in people with diabetes mellitus. Cochrane Database of Systematic Reviews 2013, Issue 10. art. No.:CD008277 doi: 10.1002/14651858.CD008277.pub2.

Brunstrom M & Carlsberg B. Effect of antihypertensive treatment at different blood pressure levels in patients with diabetes mellitus: systematic review and meta-analyses. BMJ 2016;352:i717 http://dx.doi.org/10.1136/bmj.i717

Grossman A & Grossman E. Blood pressure control in type 2 diabetic patients. Cardiovascular Diabetes 2017; 16.3 doi: 10.1186/s12933-016-0485-3

James PA, Oparil S, Carter BL et al 2014 Evidence-based guideline for the management of high blood pressure in adults. Report from the panel members appointed to the Eighth Joint National Committee (JNC8). JAMA 2014; 311: 507–20 doe:10.1001/jama.2013.284427

NICE NG136. Hypertension in adults: diagnosis and management. Published 2019. www.nice.org.uk/guidance/ng136. Accessed 5th June 2020

Sharma G, Ram CVS, Yang E. Comparison of the ACC/AHA and ESC/ESH hypertension guidelines. https://www.acc.org/latest-in-cardiology/articles/2019/11/25/08/57/comparison-of-the-acc-aha-and-esc-esh-hypertension-guidelines

Unger T, Borghi C, Charchar F et al. International Society of Hypertension global hypertension practice guidelines. J Hypertens 2020; 38: 982–1004 doi:10.1097/HJH.0000000000002453

UK Prospective Diabetes Study Group. Tight blood pressure control and risk of macrovascular and microvascular complications in type 2 diabetes: UKPDS 38. BMJ 1998; 317: 703–713.

Weber MA, Schiffrin EL, White WB et al. Clinical practice guidelines for the management of hypertension in the community. A statement by the American Society of Hypertension and the International Society of Hypertension. J Clin Hypertension 2014; 16: 14 -26 doi: 10.1111/jch.12237

Williams B, Mancia G, Spiering W et al. 2018 ESC/ESH guidelines for the management of arterial hypertension. Eur Heart J 2018; 39: 3021–3104. https://doi.org/10.1093/eurheart/ehy339

Macrovascular disease in diabetes

Atherosclerosis

For any given age, level of cholesterol or BP, the risk of atherosclerotic cardiovascular disease (CVD) is three to fivefold higher among patients with diabetes compared with non-diabetic subjects. Macrovascular complications include fatal and non-fatal coronary heart disease (CHD) events, stroke, and peripheral arterial disease (PAD). CVD accounts for most (>75%) of the premature mortality and shortened life expectancy among patients with diabetes. It affects both genders equally, and in particular the protective effect of premenopausal status is lost in women with diabetes. Within the diabetic population, hypertension and especially proteinuria (nephropathy) have a multiplying effect on CVD risk and there is a strong inverse relationship between urinary albumin excretion rate and survival (Figures 20.1 and 20.2). Some ethnic groups are particularly susceptible to CVD complicating diabetes (e.g. South Asians in the UK and blacks in the USA), while others are relatively protected (e.g native Americans, such as the Pima Indians, and Hispanic whites in the USA).

Histologically, atherosclerotic disease in patients with diabetes is similar to that in non-diabetics, but plaques tend to be more diffuse in nature and involve more distal, smaller arteries, which often makes revascularisation (angioplasty/stenting or bypass) less feasible. In patients with diabetes, atherosclerotic disease occurs at a younger age, progresses more rapidly, and plaque rupture leading to superimposed thrombus and major vessel occlusion is more common (Figure 20.3). Outcomes from acute myocardial infarction (AMI) and stroke are all consistently worse in patients with diabetes compared with non-diabetics, e.g. rates of coronary reperfusion and re-occlusion, left ventricular function, and sudden death. There is also an inflammatory component to atherosclerotic disease progression and plaque rupture, and several studies have shown a relationship between the risk of CVD events and circulating inflammatory biomarkers such as high-sensitivity C-reactive protein (hsCRP)

PAD in patients with diabetes typically involves multiple vessels with diffuse, distal narrowing, and there is a fortyfold increased risk of lower limb amputation. The smaller arteries and arterioles are damaged further by microvascular disease affecting the vasa vasorum (the tiny nutrient vessels which supply oxygen to the arterial wall itself), which makes the medial layer of arteries prone to calcification – known as 'Mönckeberg's medial sclerosis', which is often seen in the digital arteries of diabetic patients with nephropathy and/or neuropathy (Figure 20.4).

Glycaemic vascular injury

Observational epidemiological studies have shown a continuous linear relationship between HbA1c and CVD mortality which extends into the non-diabetic range of glucose levels, but the excess macrovascular risk in diabetes reflects multiple components of the diabetes syndrome as well as hyperglycaemia (e.g. BP, lipids, proteinuria, and inflammatory markers) (Figures 20.5). In addition, there is some concern that HbA1c may underestimate the link between glycaemia and macrovascular outcomes; postprandial glucose levels may be a better indicator of CVD risk.

There are four principal mechanisms by which hyperglycaemia causes the structural and functional vascular abnormalities associated with diabetes: (i) non-enzymatic glycation of tissue proteins and formation of Advanced Glycosylation Endproducts (AGEs), which bind to specific receptors for AGEs (RAGEs) especially on endothelial cells and smooth muscle cells, (ii) metabolism of glucose via the aldose reductase pathway, (iii) excess formation of reactive oxygen species (ROS) leading to oxidative stress and formation of highly atherogenic end products such as oxidised-LDL, and (iv) increased *de novo* synthesis of diacylglycerol

Handbook of Diabetes, Fifth Edition. Rudy Bilous, Richard Donnelly, and Iskandar Idris.
© 2021 John Wiley & Sons Ltd. Published 2021 by John Wiley & Sons Ltd.

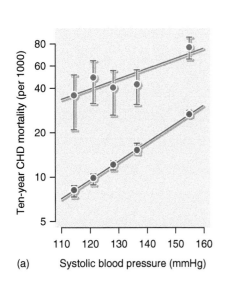
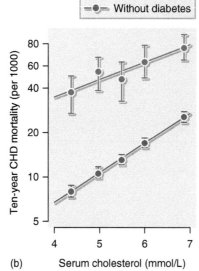

(a) Systolic blood pressure (mmHg)

(b) Serum cholesterol (mmol/L)

Figure 20.1 Relationships between systolic BP (a) and serum cholesterol (b) and CHD mortality for diabetic and non-diabetic subjects in the Multiple Risk Factor Intervention Trial (MRFIT) screening programme. For any given level of BP or lipids, the risk of death from CHD is three to fivefold higher among patients with diabetes. This excess risk is evident from the time of diagnosis of diabetes.

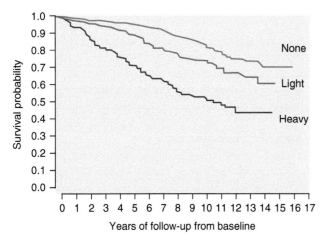

Figure 20.2 Among patients with diabetes, those who develop nephropathy and micro- or macro-proteinuria have an even higher risk of fatal or non-fatal CVD events. From the WHO Multinational Study of Vascular Disease in diabetes, urinary albumin excretion rate is a powerful prognostic indicator of CVD risk. Leakage of protein at the glomerulus probably reflects widespread endothelial barrier dysfunction and atherosclerotic disease activity.

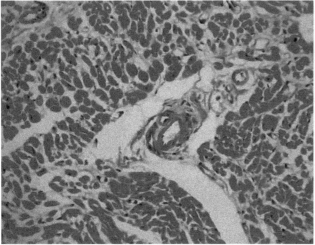
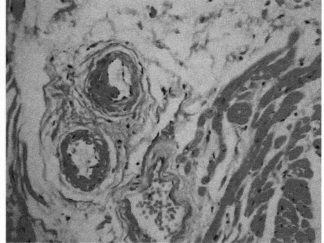

Figure 20.3 Arteriolar changes in diabetes in the myocardium of a woman who died from macrovascular disease associated with diabetic nephropathy. Basement membrane thickening, vascular smooth muscle hypertropathy and intravascular thrombus reflect widespread atherosclerosis accelerated by diabetes, hypertension and proteinuria.

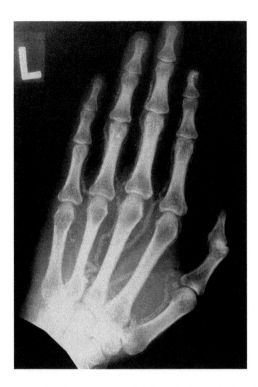

Figure 20.4 Medial calcification of the digital arteries in a diabetic patient with widespread arterial disease and nephropathy.

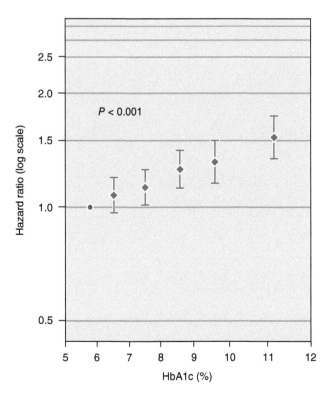

Figure 20.5 New Zealand cohort study showing the relationship between CVD mortality and HbA1c among 48,000 patients with type 2 diabetes. Adapted from Elley et al. *Diabet. Med.* 2008; 25: 1295–1301.

(DAG) from intermediate steps in glycolysis, which in turn leads to activation of protein kinase C, especially PKC-β. These pathways are not mutually exclusive, and indeed all four probably contribute and interact to influence the development, progression, and complications from macrovascular disease (Figures 20.6 and 20.7).

Evidence for glucose lowering in CVD prevention

There is considerable interest in the effects of glucose-lowering therapy on macrovascular disease outcomes. In the original UKPDS population, intensive versus conventional glycaemic control strategies (average HbA1c 7.0% vs 7.9%) had no significant effect on diabetes-related deaths (principally due to CVD). More recent and much larger randomised controlled trials (ACCORD, ADVANCE, VADT and PROACTIVE) have now provided a total study population of >33,000 patients from which to assess the benefits versus harms of intensive glucose lowering. Overall, the meta-analysis showed that intensive glycaemic control (on average HbA1c was 0.9% lower in intensively treated patients) resulted in a 17% reduction in non-fatal myocardial infarction, but no significant effect on stroke or all-cause mortality. Of note however, one of these studies, the ACCORD study, was stopped prematurely. This was because, the group that was allocated tight glucose control experienced excess premature mortality compared with less tight control. The reason for this is unclear and crucially, this observation was not seen in the other studies. The discordance on the results is likely explained by differences in the study population, i.e. studies which have shown no benefit with tight glucose control tended to be studies where the study cohort had longer duration of diabetes with majority of them on insulin therapy at recruitment, whereas studies which reported potential benefits were performed in patients at earlier diagnosis of diabetes and not on insulin therapy. A sub-analysis of these studies has indirectly implicated hypoglycaemia as an independent predictor of adverse outcomes irrespective of which treatment allocations patients received. However, hypoglycaemia as a mediator of adverse outcomes in these studies remains speculative. Nonetheless, the optimal HbA1c target should be individualised – tight glucose control in early diabetes and not on insulin therapy (HbA1c ~6.5%), and less tight control with increased disease duration and/ or receiving insulin therapy (Hba1c ~7.5%) (Figure 20.8).

The cardiovascular benefits of tight glycaemic control in the first few years after diagnosis of type 1 and type 2 diabetes may not be evident until 10+ years later. This has been well illustrated by the DCCT-EDIC trial in type 1 diabetes and the UKPDS in type 2 diabetes. In both trials, long after study closeout, and despite near-identical post-trial HbA1c levels in the two groups, those patients who were previously assigned to intensive glycaemic control obtained lasting benefits on survival. The 10 years follow-up of the original

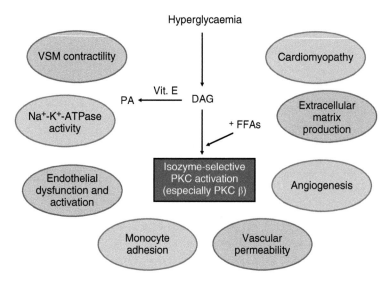

Figure 20.6 DAG-mediated activation of protein Kinase C-β results in phosphorylation and altered function of numerous proteins, enzymes and/or receptors involved in endothelial and vascular smooth muscle function, cardiac hypertrophy, contractility and fibrosis. Inhibitors of PKC-β (e.g ruboxistaurin) have undergone clinical trials to block hyperglycaemia-induced vascular disease in patients with diabetes. Free fatty acids (FFA) enhance DAG-PKC activation, and vitamin E can help reduce DAG via conversion to phosphatidic acid (PA).

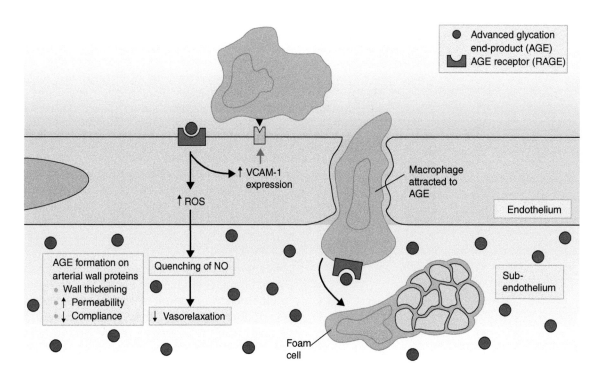

Figure 20.7 Advanced glycation end products (AGEs) have a number of unwanted effects on vascular structure and function. In particular, AGEs bind to specific receptors (RAGEs) and, via decreased nitric oxide bioavailability, increase arterial stiffness and reactive oxygen species (ROS) formation. AGEs also attract macrophages and promote foam cell formation. Foam cells contribute to atherosclerotic disease progression.

UKPDS trial showed a significant 15% relative risk reduction of developing myocardial infarction (P=0.014) and a 13% relative risk reduction of all-cause mortality (P=0.006). These observation of long-term benefits of optimal glucose control has been described as a 'legacy effect of hyperglycaemia' in type 2 diabetes and 'glycaemic memory in type 1 diabetes. They reinforce the importance of tight glycaemic control in the early stages of type 1 and type 2 diabetes.

More recently, several landmark trials have reported significant cardiovascular and mortality reduction with glucose lowering therapies. The first of the study is the EMPA-REG study, which reported significant reduction in composite of death from cardiovascular causes, nonfatal myocardial infarction, or nonfatal stroke, as well as hospitalization for hearth failure, with the sodium glucose transported (SGLT)-2 inhibitor, Empagliflozin. This was followed

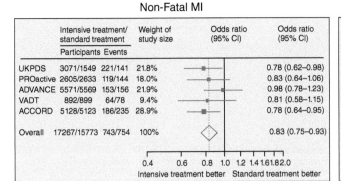

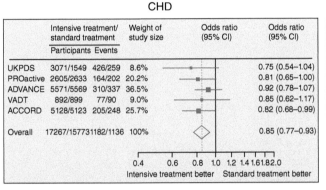

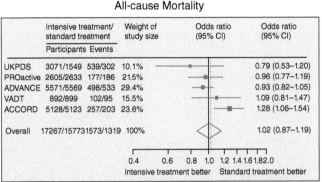

Figure 20.8 A meta-analysis of five prospective randomised controlled trials of intensive glucose lowering in a total of 33,040 patients with type 2 diabetes. On average, HbA1c was 0.9% lower in intensively treated patients, which resulted in modest significant benefits in terms of preventing CHD and non-fatal AMI, but all-cause mortality and stroke events were not significantly different between intensive and conventional glycaemic control. These effects contrast with BP-lowering and cholesterol-lowering interventions which have a more powerful effect on macrovascular outcomes in patients with diabetes. Adapted from Ray et al, Lancet 2009; 373: 1765–72.

by the LEADER study, which reported that the rate of the first occurrence of death from cardiovascular causes, nonfatal myocardial infarction, or nonfatal stroke among patients with type 2 diabetes mellitus was lower with the Glucagon like peptide (GLP)-1 analogue, Liraglutide compared with placebo. More recently, the CANVAS study also reported significant reduction in the composite major outcome of cardiovascular death, non-fatal myocardial infarction or non-fatal stroke with the SGLT2 inhibitor, Canagliflozin compared with placebo. However, this finding was slight tainted by the unexplained observation of an increased risk of lower limb amputation with Canagliflozin. Another SGLT2 inhibitor, Dapagliflozin also reported benefits in reducing cardiovascular event in the DECLARE study. With regards to GLP-1 analogues, three other drugs have shown benefits in reducing cardiovascular events, namely, Semaglutide, Albiglutide, and Dulaglutide, all of which are once weekly GLP-1 formulations. While most of these studies were performed in patients with active cardiovascular diseases, the studies with Dulaglutide (REWIND) and Dapagliflozin (DECLARE)

included the majority of patients without overt cardiovascular diseases (Figures 20.9 and 20.10).

Macrovascular disease remains the leading cause of death among patients with diabetes. The presentation of ischaemic heart disease in diabetes includes angina, acute myocardial infarction (AMI) and heart failure, as it does in the non-diabetic population. However, angina and AMI may be relatively painless ('silent') in patients with diabetes, especially in older people (perhaps because of neuropathic damage to the autonomic nerves that serve the myocardium); symptoms such as malaise, sweating, nausea, dyspnoea, and syncope may be ignored or confused with hypoglycaemia. Both immediate and long-term mortality from myocardial infarction are increased in diabetes, largely through the increased risk of heart failure in diabetes (because of diabetic cardiomyopathy, superimposed hypertension, and loss of functioning myocardium after coronary occlusion). Nevertheless, considerable progress has been made over the last 10–20 years in improving outcomes from macrovascular events in patients with diabetes.

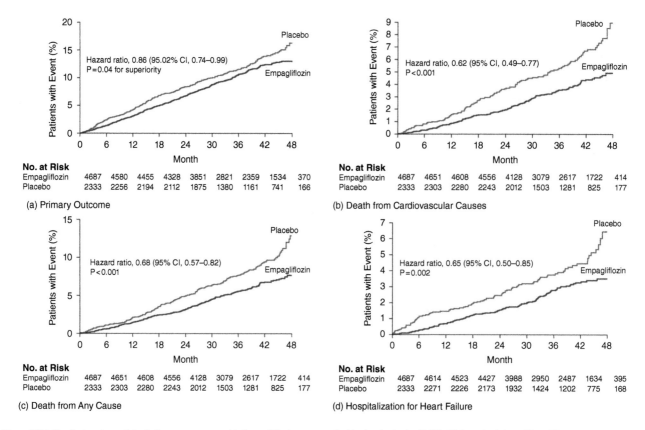

Figure 20.9 Cardiovascular and death from any course with Empagliflozin compared with placebo in the EMPA-REG study. Adapted from Zinman et al. N Engl J Med 2015; 373: 2117–2128. DOI: 10.1056/NEJMoa1504720.

Multiple risk factor intervention

Despite recent evidence on the efficacy of glucose lowering therapies in preventing cardiovascular events, evidence pertaining to the benefits of tight control of BP and lipids is more established than tight glycaemic control in preventing deaths from macrovascular disease. In practice however, a multi-factorial intervention strategy, aggressively lowering all three risk factors, is the mainstay of best practice for cardiovascular protection (Figure 20.11). Thus, international guidelines set tough targets for treated diabetic patients that include BP<130/80mmHg, LDL-cholesterol <2.0mmol/L (total-cholesterol <4.0mmol/L) and HbA1c <6.5–7%. In those with established nephropathy, optimum BP targets are even lower.

Transient ischaemic attacks and stroke are also common in diabetes, and mortality and disability after a stroke are greater in diabetes compared to non-diabetic people. This might be because of the high blood glucose levels that follow a stroke.

The role of low-dose aspirin in the (primary) prevention of macrovascular events among asymptomatic patients with diabetes is still unclear and the major international guidelines offer differing advice. In those patients who have symptoms (e.g. angina, or claudication or previous TIA),

there is no doubt that aspirin confers significant benefits for secondary prevention, but primary prevention is more doubtful, bearing in mind that low-dose aspirin is not without side effects. The ASCEND trial investigated the efficacy and safety of enteric-coated aspirin at a dose of 100 mg daily, as compared with placebo, in persons who had diabetes without manifest cardiovascular disease at trial entry. The study showed that while Aspirin use prevented serious vascular events in persons who had diabetes and no evident cardiovascular disease, it also caused major bleeding events. Overall, the absolute benefits were largely counterbalanced by the bleeding hazard.

Individual analysis of glucose lowering trials and cardiovascular outcomes have shown that SGLT2 inhibitor did not reduce stroke in people with diabetes. However, some evidence of benefits in reducing stroke events have been reported in studies with the GLP-1 analogue Liraglutide (LEADER study) and the PPAR-γ receptor agonist, Pioglitazone (IRIS – Insulin resistance After Ischaemic Stroke, trial) (Figures 20.12 and 20.13).

Peripheral arterial disease (PAD) in the legs typically presents with intermittent claudication (i.e. calf pain on walking) (Figure 20.14). Buttock pain may occur if the iliac vessels are affected and may be associated with erectile

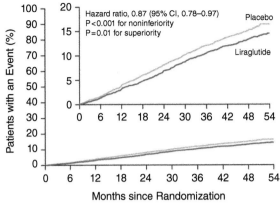

(a)

No. at Risk

Liraglutide	4668	4593	4496	4400	4280	4172	4072	3982	1562	424
Placebo	4672	4588	4473	4352	4237	4123	4010	3914	1543	407

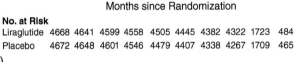

(b)

No. at Risk

Liraglutide	4668	4641	4599	4558	4505	4445	4382	4322	1723	484
Placebo	4672	4648	4601	4546	4479	4407	4338	4267	1709	465

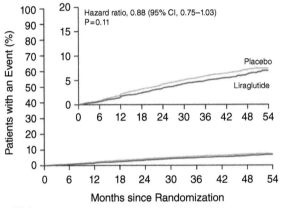

(c)

No. at Risk

Liraglutide	4668	4609	4531	4454	4359	4263	4181	4102	1619	440
Placebo	4672	4613	4513	4407	4301	4202	4103	4020	1594	424

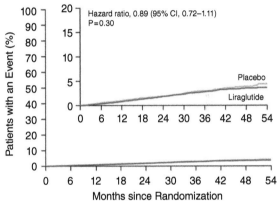

(d)

No. at Risk

Liraglutide	4668	4624	4564	4504	4426	4351	4269	4194	1662	465
Placebo	4672	4222	4558	4484	4405	4314	4228	4141	1648	445

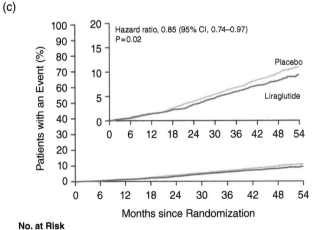

(e)

No. at Risk

Liraglutide	4668	4641	4599	4558	4505	4445	4382	4322	1723	484
Placebo	4672	4648	4601	4546	4479	4407	4338	4268	1709	465

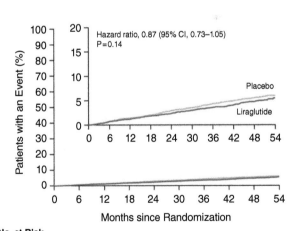

(f)

No. at Risk

Liraglutide	4668	4612	4550	4483	4414	4337	4258	4185	1662	467
Placebo	4672	4612	4540	4464	4372	4288	4187	4107	1647	442

Figure 20.10 Primary and exploratory outcomes with Liraglutide vs Placebo in the LEADER study. Marso et al. N Engl J Med 2016; 375: 311–322. DOI: 10.1056/NEJMoa1603827.

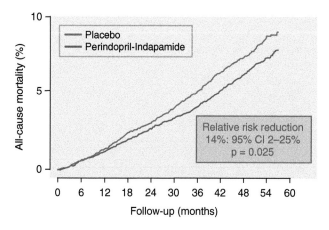

Figure 20.11 The ADVANCE study randomised approximately 20,000 high-risk patients with type 2 diabetes to usual care + add-on angiotensin converting enzyme (ACE) inhibitor/diuretic combination (perindopril + indapamide) or add-on placebo, on top of usual BP-lowering therapies. Baseline BP for the study population was quite good (average BP 140/77mmHg), and the active therapy resulted in a modest further BP reduction, 6/2mmHg on average over 5 yrs. This effect translated into a 14% risk reduction in all-cause mortality, due largely to a reduction in macrovascular events. The treatment effect may have been at least partly BP-independent, but the trial emphasises that small differences in BP matter. Adapted from Patel et al. Lancet 2007; 370: 829.

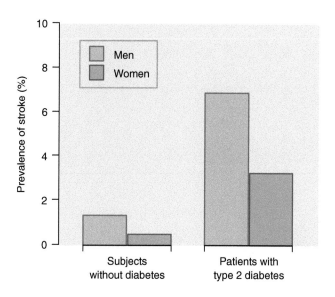

Figure 20.12 Age-adjusted prevalence of previous stroke among type 2 diabetes patients compared with non-diabetic subjects (45–64 yrs of age). Small vessel cerebral ischaemia, as well as internal carotid artery stenosis, are more common among patients with diabetes. Data from Pyörälä et al. Diabet Metab Rev 1987; 3: 463–524.

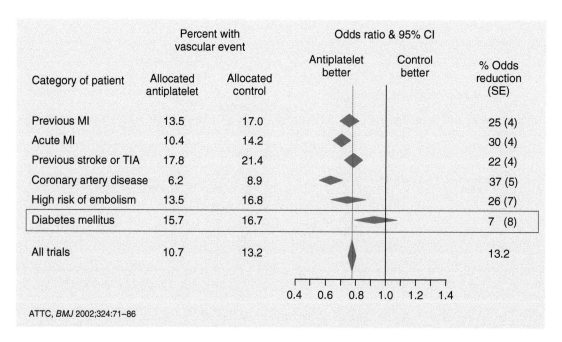

Category of patient	Percent with vascular event		Odds ratio & 95% CI		% Odds reduction (SE)
	Allocated antiplatelet	Allocated control	Antiplatelet better	Control better	
Previous MI	13.5	17.0			25 (4)
Acute MI	10.4	14.2			30 (4)
Previous stroke or TIA	17.8	21.4			22 (4)
Coronary artery disease	6.2	8.9			37 (5)
High risk of embolism	13.5	16.8			26 (7)
Diabetes mellitus	15.7	16.7			7 (8)
All trials	10.7	13.2			13.2

ATTC, *BMJ* 2002;324:71–86

Figure 20.13 From the Antithrombotic Trialists Collaboration, there is no clear evidence for the routine use of low-dose aspirin for primary prevention of macrovascular disease in patients with diabetes, but international guidelines do not all agree. In contrast, low-dose aspirin is highly effective in those patients with previous AMI, stroke or symptomatic angina. Adapted from ATTC, Br. Med. J. 2002; 324: 71–86.

dysfunction (Leriche's syndrome). Decreasing claudication distance or rest pain may indicate critical ischaemia. PAD in diabetics tends to be more diffuse and distal in nature, therefore less amenable to percutaneous intervention (i.e.

angioplasty or stenting). People with diabetes have an approximately sixteenfold higher risk of lower limb amputation than non-diabetic people. About 20% of those with PAD die within two years of the onset of symptoms, mostly

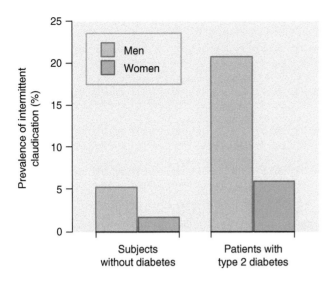

Figure 20.14 Age-adjusted prevalence of intermittent claudication in patients with type 2 diabetes (45–64 yrs of age). Data from Pyörälä et al. Diabet Metab Rev 1987; 3: 463–524.

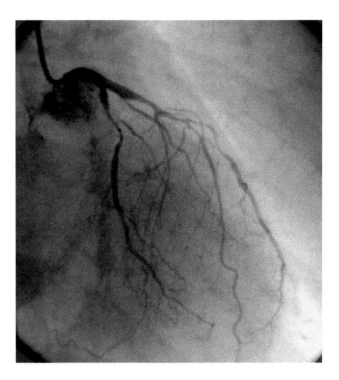

Figure 20.15 Diffuse coronary artery disease in a 49-year-old woman with type 1 diabetes. There is widespread narrowing of the mid-portions of the left anterior descending coronary artery and circumflex artery.

from myocardial infarction. Because of increased calcification and stiffness, measurements of ankle-brachial pressure index (ABPI; ankle systolic BP divided by branchial systolic BP) may be artificially raised and therefore underestimate the severity of PAD in patients with diabetes. Fibrate therapy has been shown to reduce amputation rates in diabetics with PAD.

Coronary heart disease and diabetes

In patients admitted with acute myocardial infarction, blood glucose should be controlled tightly using IV insulin infusion (Figure 20.15). The Diabetes Mellitus Insulin Glucose Infusion in Acute Myocardial Infarction (DIGAMI) study showed a 30% reduction in mortality in diabetic patients treated with insulin soon after infarction, compared with conventional management. This involves an insulin–glucose solution infused intravenously to maintain blood glucose levels of 7–11 mmol/L for at least 24–48 hours. However, uncertainty exists with regards to the mechanism of any potential benefit. For example, the design of the study was such that the decrease in mortality could potentially be attributed to either the insulin-glucose infusion, the 4/ day subcutaneous insulin alone, or due to the cessation of sulfonylurea therapy. Unfortunately, subsequent studies to address this have continued to yield conflicting findings.

Until recently, the optimum management of patients with diabetes and stable ischaemic heart disease was uncertain. In particular, there has been uncertainty about the extent to which asymptomatic patients with diabetes

should be screened for coronary artery disease; and there has been uncertainty about the role of revascularisation, on prognostic grounds, in patients with stable and/or minimal angina symptoms. The BARI-2D study (a Randomised trial of therapies for type 2 diabetes and coronary artery disease) randomised patients with established macrovascular disease who were eligible for either percutaneous coronary intervention (PCI) or coronary artery bypass grafting (CABG). In a 2x2 factorial design, patients were assigned to undergo either prompt revascularization or medical therapy, and separately randomised to either insulin-sensitization treatment or insulin-provision treatment to achieve HbA1c <7%. Overall, there was no significant difference in the rates of death and major cardiovascular events between patients who had prompt revascularization versus those managed by medical therapy, and nor was there a difference in CV outcomes between the two strategies of HbA1c-lowering. Thus, revascularisation is likely to be used mainly for those patients with an acute coronary syndrome and those with unstable or troublesome symptoms despite medical treatment. In the DIAD study, screening of asymptomatic patients with diabetes for coronary disease using myocardial perfusion imaging was of no clinical benefit (the DIAD study).

CASE STUDY

A 57-year-old man with obesity and longstanding type 2 diabetes (15+ years) presents with macrovascular complications. He is known to have hypertension, diabetic nephropathy, and dyslipidaemia, but on his annual review he presents with symptoms of intermittent claudication and cold feet. Clinical examination shows loss of pedal pulses and some early ischaemic ulceration at the tips of his toes on the left foot. Measurement of ankle-brachial pressure index (ABPI) is 0.56 in the left leg and 0.65 in the right leg, but Duplex scanning shows diffuse distal disease and arterial calcification in both legs, especially the left, with evidence of critical ischaemia. In addition, there is a proximal 75% stenosis of the left superficial femoral artery that is amenable to percutaneous intervention and stenting. Two days following this procedure, perfusion to the left foot is improved but he develops atypical chest pain and ECG shows a non-ST-elevation myocardial infarction (serum troponin-I 0.18). He is treated in hospital with aspirin, clopidogrel, and enoxaparin (7 days).

Comment: This man has features of the metabolic syndrome, and proteinuria as well as hypertension increase his macrovascular risk. ABPI can be unreliable in patients with diabetes. Although his ABPI measurements confirm PAD, 0.56, and 0.65 probably underestimate the severity of his disease. Stenting of a proximal lesion in the left leg is aimed at preserving tissue viability, healing the ischaemic ulceration and preventing sepsis and amputation. His symptoms of acute myocardial infarction were not typical – which is often the case in diabetes – but biomarkers and ECG confirmed non-ST elevation infarction. This is treated with combination antiplatelet therapy and short-term low molecular weight heparin. Optimum secondary prevention requires a statin, tight BP control, ideally with an ACE inhibitor, and antiplatelet therapy. A low-dose beta blocker for cardio-protection will probably have minimal adverse effect on his PAD.

LANDMARK CLINICAL TRIALS

Ray KK, et al. Effect of intensive control of glucose on cardiovascular outcomes and death in patients with diabetes mellitus: a meta-analysis of randomised controlled trials. Lancet 2009; 373: 1765–1772.

Rajamani K, et al. Effect of fenofibrate on amputation events in people with type 2 diabetes mellitus (FIELD study): a prespecified analysis of a randomised controlled trial. Lancet 2009; 373: 1780–1788.

The BARI-2D Study group. A randomised trial of therapies for type 2 diabetes and coronary artery disease. N. Engl. J. Med. 2009; 360: 2503–2515.

Antithrombotic Treatment Trialists Collaboration (ATTC). Aspirin in the primary and secondary prevention of vascular disease: collaborative meta-analysis of individual participant data from randomised trials. Lancet 2009; 373: 1849–1860.

The DCCT/EDIC Study Research Group. Intensive diabetes treatment and cardiovascular disease in patients with type 1 diabetes. N. Engl. J. Med. 2005; 353: 2643–2653.

Young LH, et al. The DIAD study. Cardiac outcomes after screening for asymptomatic coronary artery disease in patients with type 2 diabetes. JAMA 2009; 301: 1547–1555.

The ACCORD study Group. Effects of intensive glucose lowering in type 2 diabetes. N. Engl. J. Med. 2008; 358: 2545–2559.

Selvin E, et al. Cardiovascular outcomes in trials of oral diabetes medications. Arch. Intern. Med. 2008; 168: 2070–2080.

Gaede P, et al. Effect of a multifactorial intervention on mortality in type 2 diabetes. N. Engl. J. Med. 2008; 358: 580–591.

The ADVANCE Collaborative Group. Intensive blood glucose control and vascular outcomes in patients with type 2 diabetes. N. Engl. J. Med. 2008; 358: 2560–2572.

KEY WEBSITES

- http://diabetes.niddk.nih.gov/dm/pubs/stroke/
- http://www.americanheart.org/presenter.jhtml?identifier=3044762
- http://www.diabetes.org/diabetes-heart-disease-stroke.jsp

FURTHER READING

Elley CR et al, Glycated haemoglobin and cardiovascular outcomes in people with type 2 diabetes: a large prospective cohort study. Diabet. Med. 2008; 25: 1295–1301.

Antithrombotic treatment trialists collaboration. Br. Med. J. 2002; 324: 71–86.

Patel A, et al. Effects of a fixed combination of perindopril and indapamide on macrovascular and microvascular outcomes in patients with type 2 diabetes mellitus (the ADVANCE study): a randomised controlled trial. Lancet 2007; 370: 829–840.

Cubbon RM, et al. Temporal trends in mortality of patients with diabetes mellitus suffering acute myocardial infarction: a comparison of over 3000 patients between 1995 and 2003. Eur Heart J. 2007; 28: 540–545.

Cubbon RM, et al. Aspirin and mortality in patients with diabetes sustaining acute coronary syndrome. Diabetes Care 2008; 31: 363–365.

Selvin E, et al. Meta-analysis: glycosylated haemoglobin and cardiovascular disease in diabetes mellitus. Ann. Intern. Med. 2004; 141: 421–431.

Law MR, et al. Use of blood pressure lowering drugs in the prevention of cardiovascular disease: meta-analysis of 147 randomised trials in the context of expectations from prospective epidemiological studies. Br. Med. J. 2009; 338 (doi:10.1136/bmj.b1665).

Do Lee C, et al. Cardiovascular events in diabetic and nondiabetic adults with or without history of myocardial infarction. Circulation 2004; 109: 855–860.

Belch J, et al. The prevention of progression of arterial disease and diabetes (POPADAD) trial: factorial randomised placebo-controlled trial of aspirin and antioxidants in patients with diabetes and asymptomatic peripheral arterial disease. Br. Med. J. 2008; 337: 1030–1038.

The ASCEND study Collaborative group. Effects of Aspirin for primary prevention in persons with diabetes mellitus. NEJM 2018; 379:1529–1539.

Chapter 21

Foot problems in diabetes

The lifetime risk of a person with diabetes developing foot ulceration is around 25%. Recent studies suggest that the population-based incidence of diabetic foot ulcers is 1–4% with a prevalence of 4–10%. The risk of amputation is ten to thirtyfold higher in people with diabetes compared with the general population, and global estimates suggest that one million people with diabetes every year undergo some sort of lower limb amputation. The majority of limb amputations (85%) are preceded by foot ulceration, and the mortality rate following an amputation is reported to be in the region of 15–40% at 1 year and 39–80% at 5 years. The risk of foot ulceration may be lower in South Asians compared with Europeans living in the UK. There is increased evidence that providing an integrated foot care pathway, with trained staff in foot protection services in the community and speedy access to multidisciplinary specialist teams, considerably lowers risk of amputation (Figure 21.1).

Diabetic foot ulcers are caused mainly by neuropathy (motor, sensory and autonomic) and/or ischaemia, and frequently complicated by infection. Loss of pain sensation can damage the foot directly (e.g. from ill-fitting shoes) and motor neuropathy leads to a characteristic foot posture – raised arch, clawed toes and pressure concentrated on the metatarsal heads and heel. Skin thickening (callus) is stimulated at these pressure points and the haemorrhage or necrosis, which is common within callus, can break through to form an ulcer. Callus is therefore an important predictor of ulcers (Figure 21.2).

Diabetic neuropathy is present in at least half of patients over 60 years of age, and increases the risk of foot ulceration sevenfold. Since peripheral nerve damage is often insidious and asymptomatic, regular inspection of the foot by patients themselves and healthcare professionals is essential to identify early signs of impending ulceration. Sensory neuropathy often renders the diabetic foot 'deaf and blind'. Therefore, effective and simple education about footwear, and strategies to minimise ulcer risk, are important aspects of diabetes care, especially in high-risk individuals with a history of previous ulceration and/or several risk factors (Figures 21.3).

The 'diabetic foot' refers to a mix of pathologies

- Diabetic neuropathy
- Peripheral arterial disease
- Charcot's neuroarthropathy
- Foot ulceration
- Osteomyelitis
- Limb amputation

Figure 21.1 The 'diabetic foot' refers to a mix of pathologies.

Motor neuropathy leads to muscle atrophy, foot deformity, altered biomechanics, and a redistribution of foot pressures. This in turn leads to ulceration. Sensory neuropathy affects pain and discomfort, which predisposes the foot to repetitive trauma. Autonomic nerve damage leads to reduced sweating, which leads to dry and cracked skin and fissures, and so allows the entry and spread of infection. Damage to the sympathetic innervation of the foot leads to arteriovenous shunting and distended veins. This bypasses the capillary bed in affected areas and may compromise nutrition and oxygen supply. Microvascular disease may also interfere with nutritive blood supply to the foot tissues (Figure 21.4).

Classification of diabetic foot ulcers

Diabetic foot ulcers can be neuropathic, ischaemic, or neuro-ischaemic (Figures 21.5–21.7). Neuropathic foot ulcers frequently occur on the plantar surface of the foot

Handbook of Diabetes, Fifth Edition. Rudy Bilous, Richard Donnelly, and Iskandar Idris.

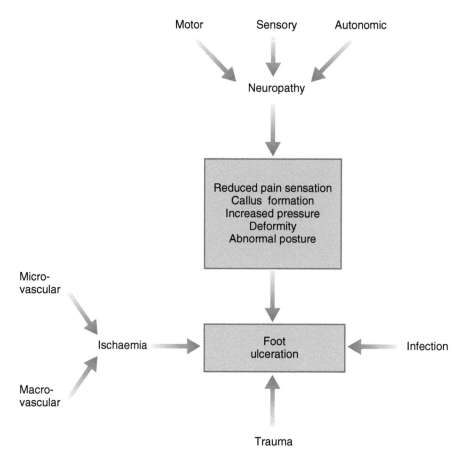

Figure 21.2 Major components in the aetiology of foot ulceration.

Risk factors for diabetic foot
complications

- Neuropathy
- Peripheral arterial disease
- Trauma
- Infection
- Poor glycaemic control
- Ill-fitting footwear
- Older age, smoking, low socio-economic status

Figure 21.3 Risk factors for diabetic foot complications.

in high-pressure areas, e.g. overlying the metatarsal heads, or in other areas overlying a bony deformity. They account for >50% of diabetic foot ulcers, and are often painless with a 'punched out' appearance. Ischaemic or neuro-ischaemic ulcers are more common on the tips of the toes or the lateral border of the foot. Neuropathic ulcers with overlying callus and necrosis should be regularly debrided, and infection

should be treated promptly with antibiotics. In addition to the underlying aetiology, the description of an ulcer should also include characteristics of the ulcer, including size, depth, appearance, and location. This would aid management and follow up. There are many classification systems used to depict ulcers that can aid in developing a standardized method of description. These classification systems are based on a variety of physical findings.

One classification is the Wagner Ulcer Classification System, which is based on wound depth and the extent of tissue necrosis but the disadvantage of this system is that it only accounts for wound depth and appearance and does not consider the presence of ischemia or infection. The University of Texas system is another classification system that addresses ulcer depth and includes the presence of infection and ischemia. Wounds of increasing grade and stage are less likely to heal without vascular repair or amputation.

Progressive arterial disease (PAD) in the lower limb is often diffuse and distal, involving the tibio-peroneal trunk and crural arteries, and vascular insufficiency may be overlooked until signs of critical ischaemia develop. Cutaneous trophic changes such as corns, calluses, ulcers, or frank

HOW TO DO AN ANNUAL FOOT CHECK:

- ✓ Remove shoes and socks/stockings.
- ✓ Test foot sensations using 10g monofilament or vibration with a tuning fork or recognised device.
- ✓ Palpate foot pulses.
- ✓ Inspect for any deformity or discolouration.
- ✓ Inspect for significant callus.
- ✓ Check for signs of ulceration.
- ✓ Ask about any previous ulceration.
- ✓ Inspect footwear.
- ✓ Ask about any pain.
- ✓ Tell patient how to look after their feet and provide written information.
- ✓ Tell patient their risk status and what it means. Explain what to look out for and provide emergency contact numbers.

ADVICE THE PATIENT TO:

- ➢ Check their feet every day.
- ➢ Be aware of loss of sensation.
- ➢ Look for changes in the shape of their foot.
- ➢ Not use corn removing plasters or blades.
- ➢ Know how to look after their toenails.
- ➢ Wear shoes that fit properly.
- ➢ Maintain good blood glucose control.
- ➢ Attend their annual foot review.
- ➢ Look for discolouration.

Figure 21.4 Annual foot review for everyone with diabetes above 12 years old.

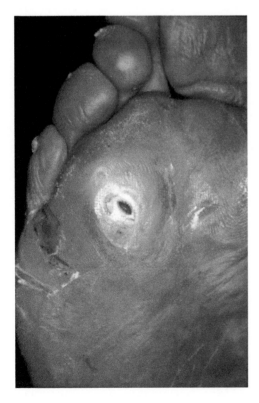

Figure 21.5 Typical neuropathic ulcer with surrounding callus.

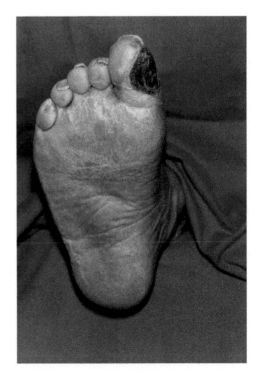

Figure 21.6 *Neuroischaemic damage caused by tightly fitting shoes.*

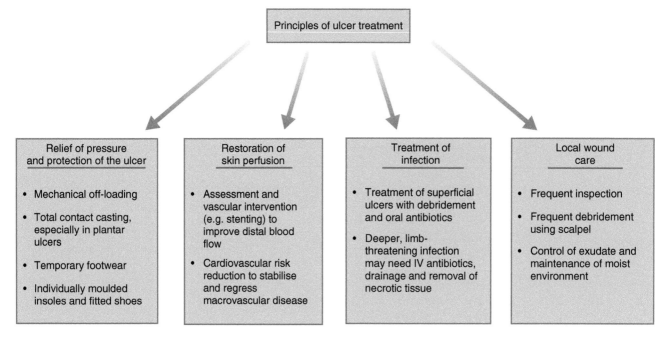

Figure 21.7 Principles of ulcer treatment, in addition to providing education and good metabolic control.

digital gangrene occur (Figure 21.8). Ulceration is typically painful and at the distal extremities of the toes. Ankle-brachial pressure index (ABPI) is easily measured and useful (ABPI<0.9 indicates PAD; critical ischaemia is often reflected by ABPI<0.5), but it can be falsely elevated and underestimate the degree of arterial disease in diabetic patients with calcified vessels. Measurements of toe pressure and transcutaneous oxygen pressure (TcPo2) are also helpful. The probability of an ulcer healing is determined by perfusion, as indicated by measurements of ABPI, toe pressure and TcPo2.

Charcot's arthropathy is a rare complication of severe neuropathy in long-standing diabetes (Figure 21.9). The initiating event may be an injury (perhaps unnoticed) that causes bone fracture in the mid-foot. Repeated minor trauma in pain-insensitive feet and possibly enhanced blood flow caused by sympathetic denervation result in decreased bone density and bony destruction. Excessive osteoclast activity leads to bone resorption, coalescence, and remodelling, which leads to the characteristic deformity and instability. Over months, the patient may notice the foot changing shape or the sensation of the bones crunching on walking. In the later stages a large effusion may surround disrupted joints and bone fragments – often giving the 'bag of bones' appearance on plain X-ray (Figure 21.10). The length of time it takes for charcot foot to heal varies but generally goes through three phases:

1. Active phase (0–3 months). Total contact casting is the most effective treatment, until the hyperaemia and swelling have settled. No weight bearing at all. Bisphosphonate therapy have also been advocated for the acute treatment of charcots with some studies reporting reduced bone

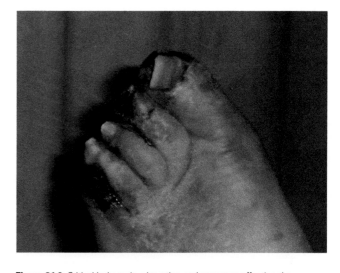

Figure 21.8 Critical ischaemia, ulceration and gangrene affecting the extremities.

turnover markers and skin temperature. However, bisphosphonates did not reduce immobilisation time and its long-term efficacy, specifically that regarding the occurrence of deformities and ulcerations, remains to be demonstrated as no follow-up studies have been published.

2. Healing phase (4–8 months): Gradual weight bearing but foot should remain in plaster cast or walking brace.

3. Rehabilitation (After 8 months): Increase weight bearing, protect foot with special insoles and support shoes. If there is a large change in shape, surgery maybe necessary, including the possibility of amputation.

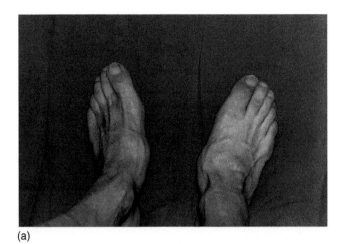

(a)

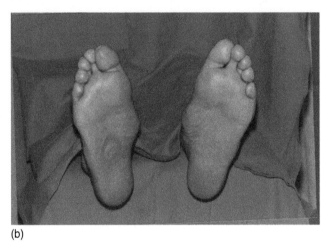

(b)

Figure 21.9 Bilateral Charcot neuroarthropathy in the cuneiform-metatarsal area has resulted in the characteristic deformity of the mid-foot: (a) dorsal and (b) plantar views.

Table 21.1 NICE has recommended this risk stratification system with appropriate frequency of foot assessments.

Risk category	Clinical Features	Frequency of foot assessment
Low risk	Normal sensation Palpable pulses	Annually
Moderate risk	Evidence of deformity, Neuropathy and/or absence pulses	3–6 monthly
High risk	Previous ulceration, previous Amputation, renal replacement Therapy, neuropathy and non-critical limb ischaemia, neuropathy, signs of deformity, or skin changes	1–2 monthly
Very high risk	Active foot ulceration	1–2 weekly

Modified from NICE clinical guideline NG19, 2015.

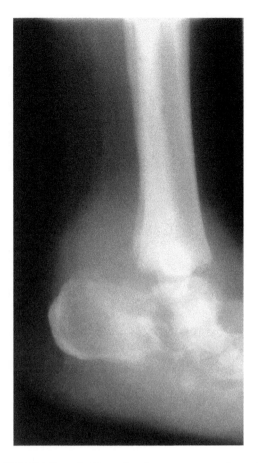

Figure 21.10 Plain X-ray of a Charcot foot demonstrates gross destruction, deformity and instability of the ankle joint + effusion. The 'bag of bones' appearance.

The UK National Institute for Clinical Excellence (NICE) has suggested a risk stratification system for diabetic foot ulceration and appropriate follow-up. Educating patients about foot care, footwear, and self-inspection, is essential. Early intervention at the first sign of ulceration is important, and those patients with a history of previous ulcers are at the highest risk for recurrent ulcer formation (Table 21.1).

Off-loading refers to interventions that relieve pressure from the wound area and redistribute pressure to healthy areas of skin. The simplest method of offloading is through strict bed rest, but this is impractical, difficult to enforce, and associated with other complications (e.g. deep venous thrombosis). Non-removable casting such as Total contact casting (TCC) is the most effective and evidence-based method for offloading (Figure 21.11). This should be offered to offload plantar neuropathic, non-ischaemic, uninfected forefoot and midfoot diabetic foot ulcers. TCC facilitates mobility, but needs changing regularly, limits patients (e.g. in terms of bathing) and does not easily allow regular inspection of the ulcer. An alternative device for offloading the acute active stage of CN is a prefabricated removable walking

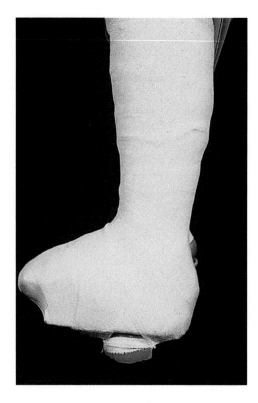

Figure 21.11 Total contact plaster cast for 'offloading' a neuropathic ulcer. Also used in Charcot arthropathy.

cast or 'instant TCC' technique, which transforms a removable cast walker to one that is less easily removed.

Management of infected foot ulcers includes cleaning the wound, and regular debridement of necrotic, unhealthy, and infected material. Weekly debridement using a scalpel is associated with quicker ulcer healing. All hospital, primary care, and community setting should have antibiotic guidelines covering the care pathway for managing diabetic foot infections that take into account local patterns of resistance. If diabetic foot infection is suspected and a wound is present, send a deep tissue aspirate or bone sample from the based on the debrided for microbiological examination and start antibiotic as soon as possible. Do not rely on 'superficial would swab.' Thereafter, decide the targeted antibiotic regimen for diabetic foot infections based on the clinical response to antibiotics and the results of the microbiological examination. Generally, for mild diabetic foot infections, initially offer oral antibiotics with activity

against gram-positive organisms and for mild to severe infection, initially offer antibiotics with activity against gram-positive and gram-negative organisms, including anaerobic bacteria. If necessary, start treatment with intravenous therapy. Offer prolonged antibiotic treatment (usually 6 weeks) to people with diabetes and osteomyelitis, according to local protocols (Figure 21.12).

- Mild diabetic foot infection: Flucloxacillin or if penicillin allergy, Clarithromycin, Erythromycin or Doxycycline

- Moderate or severe diabetic foot in fection: Flucloxacillin with or without Gentamicin and/or Metronidazole; Co-amoxyclav with or without Gentamicin; Co-trimoxazole (in penicllllin allergy) with or without Gentamicin and/or Metronidazole; Ceftriaxone with Metronidazole

- Additional antibiotic of Pseudomonas aeruginosa is suspected guided by microbiological result: Piperacillin with Tazobactam; Clindamycin with Ciprofloxacin and/or Gentamicin

- IF MRSA is suspected (due to lack of response) or confirmed: Vancomycin; Teicoplanin; Linezolid

---

Figure 21.12 The following clinical scenario and anti-microbial agents that have demonstrated clinical effectiveness, alone or in combination, in published prospective studies that include patients with diabetic foot infections. Antibiotic choice however should follow local antimicrobial guidance.

Table 21.2 Wagner Ulcer Classification System.

Grade	Lesion
1	Superficial diabetic ulcer
2	Ulcer extension involving ligament, tendon, joint capsule, or fascia with no abscess or osteomyelitis
3	Deep ulcer with abscess or osteomyelitis
4	Gangrene to potion of forefoot
5	Extensive gangrene of foot

Table 21.3 University of Texas Wound Classification System.

Stages	Description
Stage A	No infection or ischemia
Stage B	Infection present
Stage C	Ischemia present
Stage D	Infection and ischemia present
Grading	**Description**
Grade 0	Epitheliazed wound
Grade 1	Superficial wound
Grade 2	Wound penetratres to trendon or capsule
Grade 3	Wound penetrates to bone or joint

CASE HISTORY

A 56-year-old man with type 2 diabetes presents for annual review. He has required laser photocoagulation to the left eye, but has no history of macrovascular disease. Body mass index is 28.1, HbA1c is 8.5%, BP 142/90mmHg, and LDL-cholesterol 2.7mmol/L. He is on metformin and sitagliptin therapy. On questioning him, he denies any foot symptoms but described features of intermittent claudication in his right calf. On examination using a 10g monofilament and tuning fork he has markedly reduced sensation. Inspection reveals a 1cm 'punched out' ulcer with surrounding callus on the plantar surface of the right foot.

Comment: It is not uncommon for patients with severe neuropathy to report no symptoms in the feet (they have very little sensation), so it is important to remove the socks and shoes and inspect the feet. While this is typical of a neuropathic foot ulcer (punched-out appearance, painless, surrounding callus), the symptoms of intermittent claudication merits further vascular investigation. The ulcer requires cleaning, debridement of callus using a scalpel, oral antibiotics, and offloading. Given his elevated HbA1c levels and obesity, consideration of additional glucose lowering therapy may also be required. A sodium glucose transporter (SGLT)-2 inhibitor may be an option due to its favourable effect on glucose, weight, and blood pressure lowering.

KEY WEBSITES

- http://www.diabetes.nhs.uk/downloads/NDST_Diabetic_Foot_Guide.pdf
- http://guidance.nice.org.uk/CG10
- www.diabetes.org.uk/putting-feet-first
- https://www.diabetes.org.uk/Professionals/Resources/Feet/
- https://www.diabetes.org.uk/Professionals/Resources/shared-practice/Footcare/
- http://www.iwgdf.org/files/2015/website_infection.pdf

For more information about the minimum skills framework: *Putting Feet First: National minimum skills framework*, Diabetes UK and NHS Diabetes, 2011 http://www.diabetes.org.uk/About_us/What-we-say/Improving-services-standards/

LANDMARK CLINICAL TRIALS

Lincoln NB, et al. Education for secondary prevention of foot ulcers in people with diabetes: a randomised controlled trial. Diabetologia 2008; 51: 1954–1961.

Neal B et al. Canagliflozin and cardiovascular and renal events in type 2 diabetes. New England J of Medicine June 12, 2017 / DOI:10.1056/NEJMoa1611925

Hinchliffe RJ, et al. A systematic review of the effectiveness of interventions to enhance the healing of chronic ulcers of the foot in diabetes. Diabetes Metab. Res. Rev. 2008; 24 (Suppl. 1): S119–144.

Rubio JA, Aragon-Sanchez J, Jimenez S, et al. Reducing major lower extremity amputations after the introduction of a multi-disciplinary team for the diabetic foot. Int J Low Extrem Wounds 2014; 13: 22–26.

Ince P, et al. Use of the SINBAD classification system and score in comparing outcome of foot ulcer management on three continents. Diabetes Care 2008; 31: 964–967.

Treece KA, et al. Validation of a system of foot ulcer classification in diabetes mellitus. Diabet. Med. 2004; 21: 987–991.

Ince P, et al. Rate of healing of neuropathic ulcers of the foot in diabetes and its relationship to ulcer duration and ulcer area. Diabetes Care 2007; 30: 660–663.

FURTHER READING

Boulton AJ, et al. Clinical practice: Neuropathic diabetic foot ulcers. N. Engl. J. Med. 2004; 351: 48–55.

Boulton AJ, et al. The global burden of diabetic foot disease. Lancet 2005; 366: 1719–1724.

Cavanagh PR, et al. Treatment for diabetic foot ulcers. Lancet 2005; 366: 1725–1735.

Falanga V. Wound healing and its impairment in the diabetic foot. Lancet 2005; 366: 1736–1743.

Butalia S, et al. Does this patient with diabetes have osteomyelitis of the lower extremity? JAMA 2008; 299: 806–813.

Kerr, M, 2012, Footcare for people with diabetes: The economic case for change, NHS Diabetes and Kidney Care

Holman N, Young RJ, Jeffcoate WJ. "Variation in the recorded incidence of amputation of the lower limb in England", Diabetologia 2012.

Schaper NC, Van Netten JJ, Apelqvist J, Lipsky BA, Bakker K. Prevention and management of foot problems in diabetes: a summary guidance for daily practice based on the 2015 IWGDF guidance documents.

Boulton AJ. The diabetic foot: grand overview, epidemiology and pathogenesis. Diab. Metab. Res. Rev. 2008; 24 (Suppl. 1): S3–S6.

Sexual problems in diabetes

Symptoms of sexual dysfunction affect both men and women with diabetes. The commonest problem among men is erectile dysfunction (ED), which is defined as 'the inability to achieve or maintain an erection sufficient for sexual intercourse'. ED occurs 10–15 years earlier in people with diabetes compared with men without diabetes, has a greater impact on quality of life and is less responsive to oral treatment. The prevalence of ED among men with diabetes varies from 35–90%, and the age-adjusted incidence is twofold higher in men with diabetes compared with those without diabetes. Advancing age and longer duration of diabetes are major risk factors for ED, but ED occurs more often in those men with macro- and/or microvascular and neuropathic complications. It is also associated with obesity, hypertension, and antihypertensive therapies. In women, however, female sexual dysfunction (FSD) is related more closely to psychosocial factors than metabolic variables, and the presence of depression is a key predictor of sFSD (Figure 22.1).

ED is the most common sexual problem that affects men with diabetes. The age-related decline in erectile function is enhanced in diabetes, particularly in men with cardiovascular, microvascular, or neuropathic complications. Depression is a common underlying problem that may predispose to, or exacerbate, ED, and multiple drug therapies, especially antihypertensive drugs, often accentuate or unmask ED. One-third of diabetic men with ED still experience morning erections, which suggests that there may also be a significant psychological component to their ED. The International Index of Erectile Function (IIEF), and its short form (IIEF-5), also known as the Sexual Health Inventory for Men (SHIM) (see Figure 22.2), are validated assessment tools for establishing the presence and severity of ED (Rosen et al. Urology 1997; 49: 822–30, and Int. J. Impot Res. 1999; 11: 319–326). In the erectile function domain of IIEF, men scoring <25 are classified as having ED and those >25 are considered not to have ED.

The principal neural mediator of the erectile response is nitric oxide (NO), which is released by vascular endothelial cells in response to cholinergic and non-cholinergic, non-adrenergic nerve fibre stimulation. NO-mediated relaxation of vascular smooth muscle in the corpus cavernosum of the penis leads to engorgement of the cavernosal space and compression of venous outflow. The post-receptor pathway that mediates NO-induced smooth muscle relaxation involves activation of the intracellular enzyme guanylate cyclase and formation of the second messenger cyclic GMP (cGMP). cGMP is broken down by phosphodiesterase-5, which converts cGMP to guanosine monophosphate (GMP) (Figure 22.3).

In men with diabetes, multiple factors can contribute to ED (Figure 22.4). Macrovascular disease, hypertension, and other CV risk factors (e.g. smoking) impair blood flow to the penis and cause endothelial dysfunction (in which the bioavailability of NO and/or the smooth muscle responsiveness to NO may be reduced). Microangiopathy in diabetes affects both somatic and autonomic nerve function leading to neuropathy. Autonomic neuropathy is strongly associated with ED. Hypogonadism is often associated with type 2 diabetes (up to 35% of diabetic men with ED may have serum total testosterone levels <8nmol/L). Although normal testosterone levels are needed for libido, the role of testosterone in erectile function is unclear. In addition, local and psychosocial factors can be important contributors.

A detailed history should be taken in men who complain of impotence, particularly to exclude related problems, such as premature ejaculation and loss of libido, which the patient may confuse with ED, and to identify associated drugs and risk factors such as smoking. Specifically asking about sexual dysfunction, especially ED in men, should be a routine part of the annual complications' assessment. Patients often suffer in silence and hope that the healthcare

Handbook of Diabetes, Fifth Edition. Rudy Bilous, Richard Donnelly, and Iskandar Idris.
© 2021 John Wiley & Sons Ltd. Published 2021 by John Wiley & Sons Ltd.

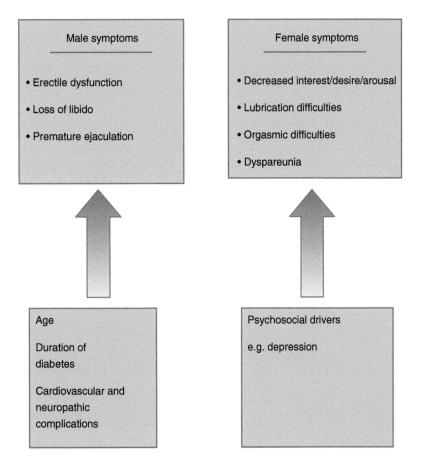

Figure 22.1 The most common symptoms of sexual dysfunction in men and women with diabetes.

professional will ask about sexual function and/or provide an opportunity for them to indicate a possible problem. It is often helpful to have the partner present when discussing symptoms and possible treatment options. A full drug history should be taken.

Patients reporting ED should be examined. General physical examination may give clues to the aetiology (e.g. hypogonadism), or indicate associated conditions such as balanitis, phimosis, or Peyronie's disease. The integrity of the lower limb circulation and any features of peripheral or autonomic neuropathy should be noted. Obesity and features of the metabolic syndrome, independent of diabetes, are associated with ED.

Investigations include serum testosterone and gonadotropin hormones when there is reduced libido or suspected hypogonadism. Testosterone has been shown to enhance the efficacy of PDE5 inhibitors (below) in hypogonadal men. In addition, some studies have shown that testosterone replacement in hypogonadol men can improve ED even without PDE5 inhibitors. Therefore, for managing ED in hypogonadol men, testosterone levels needs to be optimal prior to initiation of PDE5 inhibitors. An assessment of cardiovascular, peripheral arterial, renal and lipid status, and a review of glycaemic control is also important investigation for patients with ED.

In terms of the management of ED, lifestyle modifications are considered to be first-line therapy. Regular exercise, weight loss, reduction in alcohol intake and smoking improve endothelial function, self-confidence, and raise the overall sense of well-being. Any drugs likely to worsen ED, e.g. beta blockers, may be changed or discontinued to minimise the adverse effects on erectile function. There is generally no need for a psycho-sexual counsellor, except when there is a failing relationship, severe anxiety (including performance anxiety), and fear of intimacy. Several treatment options are available. Each has advantages, disadvantages, and limitations (Figure 22.5).

Phosphodiesterase-5 (PDE5) is the primary second line treatment for ED. PDE5 inhibitors work best if taken on an empty stomach, prior to sexual stimulation. Sildenafil (Viagra) and Vardenafi (Levitra) have a shorter duration of action (4–6h) than Tadalafil (Cialis) (36–48h). All of them have shown their efficacy in patients with diabetes, although it has been reported that diabetic men with ED are less responsive to PDE5 inhibitors when compared with nondiabetic men with ED due to diminished NO generation in the penile nerves and/or endothelium, as well as the low testosterone levels of patients with diabetes. A randomized,

SEXUAL HEALTH INVENTORY FOR MEN (SHIM)

PATIENT NAME: _____   TODAY'S DATE: _____

PATIENT INSTRUCTIONS

Sexual health is an important part of an individual's overall physical and emotional well-being. Erectile dysfunction, also known as impotence, is one type of very common medical condition affecting sexual health. Fortunately, there are many different treatment options for erectile dysfunction. This questionnaire is designed to help you and your doctor identify if you may be experiencing erectile dysfunction. If you are, you may choose to discuss treatment options with your doctor.

Each question has several possible responses. Circle the number of the response that **best describes** your own situation. Please be sure that you select one and only response for **each question**.

OVER THE PAST 6 MONTHS:

1. How do you rate your confidence that you could get and keep an erection?		VERY LOW	LOW	MODERATE	HIGH	VERY HIGH
		1	2	3	4	5
2. When you had erections with sexual stimulation how often were your erections hard enough for penetration (entering your partner)?	NO SEXUAL ACTIVITY	ALMOST NEVER OR NEVER	A FEW TIMES (MUCH LESS THAN HALF THE TIME)	SOMETIMES (ABOUT HALF THE TIME)	MOST TIMES (MUCH MORE THAN, HALF THE TIME)	ALMOST ALWAYS OR ALWAYS
	0	1	2	3	4	5
3. During sexual intercourse, how often were you able to maintain your erection after you had penetrated (entered) your partner?	DID NOT ATTEMPT INTERCOURSE	ALMOST NEVER OR NEVER	A FEW TIMES (MUCH LESS THAN HALF THE TIME)	SOMETIMES (ABOUT HALF THE TIME)	MOST TIMES (MUCH MORE THAN, HALF THE TIME)	ALMOST ALWAYS OR ALWAYS
	0	1	2	3	4	5
4. During sexual intercourse, how difficult was it to maintain your erection to completion of intercourse?	DID NOT ATTEMPT INTERCOURSE	EXTREMELY DIFFICULT	VERY DIFFICULT	DIFFICULT	SLIGHTLY DIFFICULT	NOT DIFFICULT
	0	1	2	3	4	5
5. When you attempted sexual intercourse, how often was it satisfactory for you?	DID NOT ATTEMPT INTERCOURSE	ALMOST NEVER OR NEVER	A FEW TIMES (MUCH LESS THAN HALF THE TIME)	SOMETIMES (ABOUT HALF THE TIME)	MOST TIMES (MUCH MORE THAN, HALF THE TIME)	ALMOST ALWAYS OR ALWAYS
	0	1	2	3	4	5

Add the numbers corresponding to questions 1–5   TOTAL: _____

The Sexual Health Inventory for Men further classifies ED severity with the following breakpoints:

1–7 Severe ED   8–11 Moderate ED   12–16 Mild to moderate ED   17–21 Mild ED

Figure 22.2 Sexual Health Inventory for Men (SHIM).

placebo-controlled trial, involving 268 diabetic men with ED, reported improved erections in 56% of patients taking sildenafil in a dose-dependent manner, compared with 10% of those in the control group. In two other multicentre, placebo-controlled studies, treatment with vardenafil (10 mg and 20 mg), or tadalafil (10 mg and 20 mg), improved erections in 57% and 72%, and 56% and 64% of patients, respectively, as compared with improvements in 13% and 25% among those in the placebo arms. In individuals who have persistent resistance to PDE5, findings from both experimental and

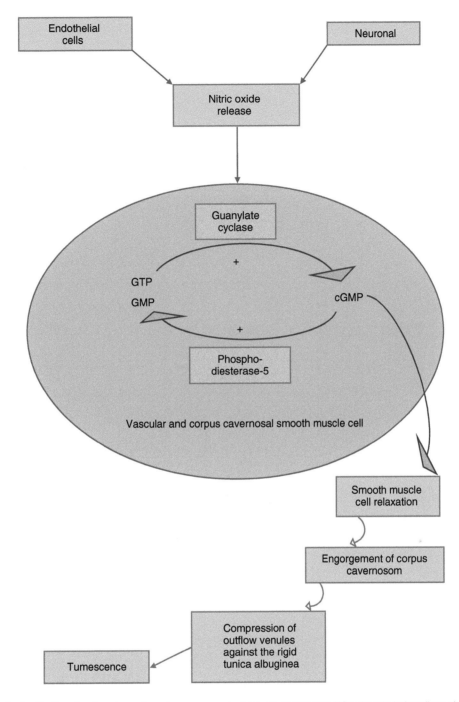

Figure 22.3 Pathways that lead to the relaxation of vascular and corpus cavernosal smooth muscle cells. NO is the principal mediator, via cGMP formation. Intracellular concentrations of cGMP are increased by phosphodiesterase-5 inhibitors.

clinical studies reported that chronic or daily, low dose use of PDE5 inhibitors for ED may significantly improve endothelial dysfunction. The daily dosing of tadalafil, 2.5–5 mg/day, has also been approved by the FDA for treatment of symptoms of Benign Prostatic Hyperplasia. CHD is not an absolute contraindication for PDE5 inhibitors therapy, but particular caution has to be paid in cases of unstable and severe angina pectoris, recent myocardial infarction, certain arrhythmias, poorly controlled hypertension, and concomitant use of

nitrates or nitrate donor oral nitrates because of the risk of excessive reductions in BP.

Another second-line therapy is the use of alprostadil, either intracavernosal or intraurethral. Two products are available for direct injection, Caverject (Pfizer) or Edex (Actient). A small needle is used to inject the medication into the lateral aspect of the penis through a small-gauge needle.

Response is dose related and usually occurs within 10–15 min, and does not require stimulation. The intraurethral

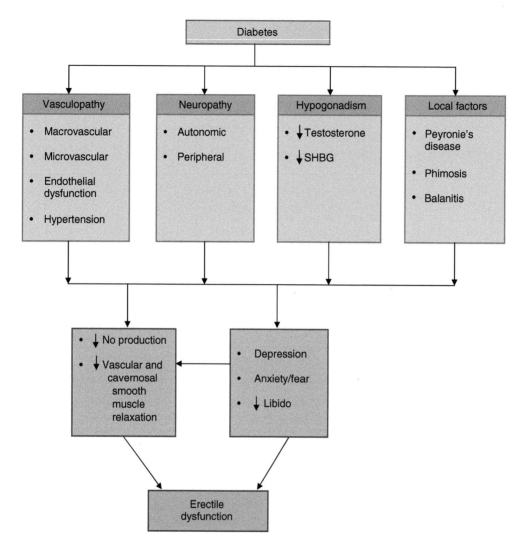

Figure 22.4 Major pathways contributing to ED in diabetic men.

Box 22.1 Key features in the medical history of ED in a diabetic man.

- Onset usually gradual and progressive.
- Earliest feature often inability to sustain erection long enough for satisfactory intercourse.
- Erectile failure may be intermittent initially.
- Sudden onset often thought to indicate a psychogenic cause (but little evidence to support this).
- Preservation of spontaneous and early-morning erections does not necessarily indicate a psychogenic cause.
- Loss of libido consistent with hypogonadism, but not a reliable symptom. Impotent men often understate their sex drive for a variety of reasons.
- Note drug history and smoking.

Box 22.2 The physical examination of a man with ED should consider the following.

- Any features of hypogonadism
- Manual dexterity – if limited, may preclude physical treatment (e.g. intracavernosal injection)
- Protuberant abdomen
- External genitalia
  - Presence of phimosis, balanitis, Peyronie's disease
  - Testicular volume
- Cardiovascular disease (leg pulses, iliac and femoral bruits)

preparation, medicated urethral suppository for erection (MUSE), consists of a tiny pellet of drug inserted into the urethral meatus. Response is also dose related, and onset similar to the cavernosal preparations (Figure 22.6).

Vacuum devices have been in use since the 1970s. A translucent tube is placed over the penis and air pumped out to draw blood into the erectile tissue. A constriction band around the base of the penis then maintains the erection (Figure 22.7). This simple non-pharmacological approach is surprisingly effective, and safe, once patients have become skilled in using the vacuum device. Response rates in diabetic men are around 70%, and the device can work in those who failed to respond to PDE5 inhibitor treatment.

Female sexual dysfunction

Sexual dysfunction seems to be much less common in diabetic women than in men, but there is an increased risk of vaginal dryness and impaired sexual arousal. Menstrual irregularities are also common in diabetic women, particularly in those with obesity and poor glycaemic control. Insulin requirements alter around the time of menstruation in about 40% of diabetic women; the majority need more insulin, but about 10% require less. Type 2 diabetes and impaired glucose tolerance (IGT) are common in women with the polycystic ovary syndrome (PCOS) – features of which include oligomenorrhoea or amenorrhoea, polycystic

Phosphodiesterase type 5 (PDE5) inhibitors	Transurethral or intracavernosal administration of vasoactive compounds
• Sildenafil, tadalafil, vardenafil • Block degradation of cGMP • More effective on an empty stomach • Efficacy rates 60–70% in diabetic men • Contraindicated in men taking oral nitrates	• Papaverine (non-specific PDE inhibitor) • Phentolamine (a-blocker) • Alprostadil (prostaglandin E1) • Transurethral PGE1 via pellets (*Medicated Urethral System for Erection*, MUSE) increases cAMP-mediated smooth muscle relaxation • Intracavernosal injection of PGE1 may be more effective
Vacuum devices and penile implants	Testosterone supplementation
• Non-pharmacological approach using vacuum and a constriction band • Sensation of cold penis and retrograde ejaculation are disadvantages • Vacuum device can be very effective in those failing or unable to use PDE5 inhibitor • Hydraulic, semi-rigid or silicone penile implants are a last resort	• Clinical significance of low testosterone levels in ED is uncertain • Supplementation indicated in symptomatic patients with 9 am total testosterone level <8 nmol/L • Several studies have shown beneficial effect on ED in hypogonadal men • Formulations include gel, patch, implants, injections, tablets

Figure 22.5 Treatment options for diabetic men with ED.

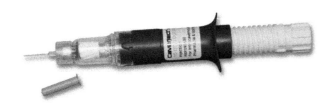

Figure 22.6 Intracavernosal injection of alprostadil, self-injected.

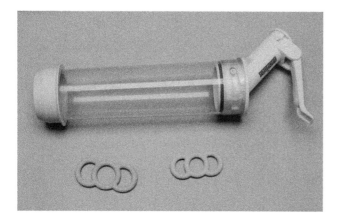

Figure 22.7 A vacuum device with constriction rings.

Gynaecological factors relevant to women
with diabetes or IGT

- Vaginal dryness
- Menstrual irregularities
- Infection
- Contraception
- Hormone replacement therapy
- Pregnancy
- Association with polycystic ovary syndrome (PCOS)

Figure 22.8 Gynaecological factors relevant to women with diabetes or IGT.

ovaries on ultrasound examination, obesity, hirsutism, and raised circulating androgen levels (Figure 22.8). Both type 2 diabetes with IGT and PCOS share an association with insulin resistance. It is thought that hyperinsulinaemia stimulates androgen synthesis and thecal hypertrophy in the ovary.

Genitourinary infections are common in diabetic women. Vaginal candidiasis is especially frequent in poorly controlled subjects; it can be irritating and painful and may interfere with sexual activity. Treatment involves improving control, and local or oral antifungal agents, including fluconazole. Other genital infections, such as genital herpes and pelvic inflammatory disease, occur in diabetic women, but possibly no more frequently than in the general female population. However, urinary tract infections are frequent in patients

with poorly controlled diabetes, and especially in those with autonomic neuropathy and bladder distension (Figure 22.9).

Contraceptive advice is essential in diabetes, because unplanned pregnancies in the poorly controlled patient carry an increased risk of foetal morbidity and mortality. In many countries, the preferred method of contraception for women with diabetes is the oral contraceptive pill – which has the lowest failure rate (apart from sterilisation). On the available evidence, low-dose (<30 μg oestradiol) combined oral contraceptives can be used safely in type 1 and type 2 diabetes; all women who take the pill should have their blood pressure and serum lipids reviewed regularly. As such, according to recent guidelines, these contraceptives must be avoided in case of associated cardiovascular risk factors, cardiovascular disease, or severe microvascular complications such as nephropathy with proteinuria or active proliferative retinopathy. Prescription of combined hormonal contraception in type 2 diabetic women must also be considered with caution due to a frequent association with obesity and vascular risk factors which increase both thromboembolic and arterial risks. In these cases, progesterone-only contraceptives, as well as non-hormonal methods, represent alternatives according to patient wishes, but they may cause menstrual irregularities. As these are not thought to be associated with vascular disease, they are often used more in older women or in those with diabetic complications or risk factors (Figure 22.10).

Genitourinary infections in women with
diabetes

- Vaginal candidiasis
- Vaginal warts, herpes
- Pelvic inflammatory disease
- Urinary tract infections

Figure 22.9 Genitourinary infections in diabetic women.

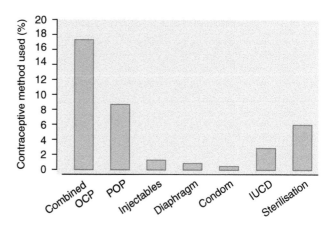

Figure 22.10 Patterns of contraceptive use in women with type 1 diabetes in the UK. OCP, oral contraceptive pill; POP, progesterone-only pill; IUCD, intrauterine contraceptive device. From Lawrensen et al. Diabetic Med 1999; 16: 395 – 399.

CASE HISTORY

A 55-year-old man with a 10-year history of type 2 diabetes attends for annual complications assessment. On routine assessment, he did not volunteer any specific symptoms or problems related to his diabetes, and has no past history of significant micro- or macrovascular complications. However, on direct questioning, he acknowledges a loss of sex drive and frequent difficulties either achieving or maintaining an erection. His BMI is 34, HbA1c 8.1% on metformin 850 mg bid, and Sitagliptin 100 mg od, and BP was 161/90 using lisinopril 20 mg and bendroflumethiazide 2.5 mg daily. He is a non-smoker. The nurse undertaking the complications assessment arranges for him and his wife to attend a follow-up appointment to explore the sexual dysfunction. The history is confirmed, although ED seems to be causing tension and distress in their relationship. Physical examination was unremarkable, but an early morning total testosterone level was low at 6 nmol/L. After discussing the relationship between diabetes and ED (which the patient's wife did not realise), they were better informed and less anxious. The treatment options were discussed, and the couple opted to try a sildenafil 100 mg od, combined with testosterone replacement gel.

Comment: This man has features of the metabolic syndrome, which increases the risk of sexual dysfunction and hypogonadism. There is limited scope to reduce or change his medications; the thiazide diuretic may be worse than a calcium channel blocker in aggravating ED. Patients need to be asked sensitively about sexual dysfunction, they seldom volunteer symptoms unless the health professional gives them an appropriate prompt. Partners and patients need information about the association with diabetes. He is testosterone deficient and symptomatic (loss of libido), so replacement gel is appropriate, with an aim to maintain testosterone levels to a level of >9 nmol/L and not above upper reference range, as it may help with ED. Adequate advice should be provided when starting sildenafil – including to take on empty stomach, to try again on a different day if unsuccessful.

LANDMARK TRIALS

Penson DF, et al. Sexual dysfunction and symptom impact in men with longstanding type 1 diabetes in the DCCT / EDIC Cohort. J. Sex Med. 2009; 6: 1969–1978.

Rosen R, et al. The International Index of Erectile Function (IIEF): A state of the science review. International Journal of Impotence 2002; 14: 226-244.

Bacon CG et al. Association of type and duration of diabetes with erectile dysfunction in a large cohort of men. Diabetes Care 2002; 25:1458-63

Goldstein I et al. Vardenafil, a new phosphodiesterase type 5 inhibitor, in the treatment of erectile dysfunction in men with diabetes: a multicentre double-blind placebo controlled fixed dose study. Diabetes care 2003; 26:777-83

Enzlin P, et al. Sexual dysfunction in women with type 1 diabetes. Long-term findings from the DCCT/EDIC study cohort. Diabetes Care 2009; 32: 780–785.

Vardi M, Nini A. Phosphodiesterase inhibitors for erectile dysfunction in patients with diabetes mellitus. Cochrane Database Syst Rev. 2007:CD002187. [PubMed]

Rendell MS, Rajfer J, Wicker PA, Smith MD. Sildenafil for treatment of erectile dysfunction in men with diabetes: a randomized controlled trial. Sildenafil Diabetes Study Group. JAMA. 1999;281(5):421–426. [PubMed]

KEY WEBSITES

- http://diabetes.niddk.nih.gov/dm/pubs/sup/
- http://www.diabetes.co.uk/diabetes-erectile-dysfunction.html
- http://www.nhs.uk/Pathways/diabetes/Pages/Landing.aspx

FURTHER READING

Malavige LS, et al. Erectile dysfunction in diabetes Mellitus. J. Sex Med. 2009; 6: 1232–1247.

Koudrat Y et al. High prevalence of erectile dysfunction in diabetes: a systematic review and meta-analysis of 145 studies. Diabetic Medicine 2017; 34: 1185–1192

Patel DP et al. Serum biomarkers of erectile dysfunction in Diabetes Mellitus: a systematic review of current literature. Sex med Rev. 2017; 5: 339–348

Penson DF, et al. Do impotent men with diabetes have more severe erectile dysfunction and worse quality of life than the general population of impotent patients? Results from the ExCEED database. Diabetes Care 2003; 26: 1093–1099.

Ucak S et al. Association between sarcopenia and erectile dysfunction in males with type 2 diabetes mellitus. Aging Male 2019; 22: 20–27

Waldinger MD. The neurobiological approach to premature ejaculation. J. Urol. 2002; 168: 2359–2367.

Corona G, et al. NCEP-ATPIII-defined Metabolic syndrome, type 2 diabetes, and prevalence of hypogonadism in male patients with sexual dysfunction. J. Sex Med. 2007; 4: 1038–1045

Wrishko R, et al Safety, efficacy, and pharmacokinetic overview of low-dose daily administration of tadalafil. J Sex Med 2009; 6: 2039–48

Kamenov ZA. A comprehensive review of erectile dysfunction in men with diabetes: 2015; 123: 141–58

Gastrointestinal problems in diabetes

KEY POINTS

- Gastrointestinal symptoms are common in people with diabetes and usually occur in patients with multiple microvascular complications.
- Although associated with autonomic neuropathy, there is often a poor correlation between symptoms and results of objective tests.
- The most troublesome problems are vomiting due to gastroparesis, diarrhoea, and constipation. Symptoms fluctuate and usually remain stable with time.

- The cornerstones of treatment are agents that affect gastrointestinal motility but jejunal feeding is occasionally required for severe cases of gastroparesis.
- Research into the gut microbiota is shedding new light on the cause of glucose intolerance and on the mechanisms of action of treatments for obesity and diabetes such as bariatric surgery and drug therapies.
- Gut microbiota offer a potential new target of therapies for obesity and diabetes.

Disordered gastrointestinal motor function occurs in both type 1 and type 2 diabetes and can result in symptoms of nausea, vomiting, diarrhoea or constipation, malnutrition, poor glycaemic control, and delayed absorption of orally administered drugs (Figure 23.1). Gustatory sweating, typically affecting the head and neck, and postprandial hypotension may also occur. Traditionally, this has been attributed to irreversible autonomic neuropathy, but acute changes in blood glucose also play a role. For example, hyperglycaemia delays gastric emptying by up to 15 minutes, slows gallbladder contraction and small intestinal transit, and inhibits colonic reflexes (Figure 23.2); while hypoglycaemia accelerates gastric emptying (Figure 23.3). The mechanisms are unclear. Every effort should be made to improve glycaemic control in symptomatic patients, including consideration of continuous subcutaneous insulin infusion (CSII).

Symptoms

Gastrointestinal symptoms are common in diabetes, more than in the general population (Table 23.1). However, there is an imprecise relationship between the symptoms and either demonstrable motor dysfunction (e.g. gastric emptying time) or measurements of autonomic neuropathy. Among the additional factors that influence symptoms are hyperglycaemia (which increases the perception of visceral sensation, such as gut fullness); and drugs such as metformin, acarbose and incretins (exenatide and liraglutide), which can cause diarrhoea and faecal incontinence. There is also a link with psychological stress and psychiatric symptoms of anxiety and depression, which doubled the prevalence of GI symptoms in one cross-sectional study. It is important to exclude other endocrine disease which can cause altered gastrointestinal function such as hyper- and hypothyroidism.

Oesophagus

Oesophageal transit is delayed in about 30–50% of subjects with diabetes (mostly because of impaired peristalsis) and is associated with dysphagia, heartburn, and chest pain (Figure 23.4). Endoscopy is required to exclude other disorders, such as carcinoma and candidiasis. Minimal symptoms do not require treatment; indeed, no treatment, including prokinetic drugs, has yet been shown to be effective for more severe symptoms attributable to hypomotility. Consider discontinuation of drugs such as calcium channel blockers which

Handbook of Diabetes, Fifth Edition. Rudy Bilous, Richard Donnelly, and Iskandar Idris.
© 2021 John Wiley & Sons Ltd. Published 2021 by John Wiley & Sons Ltd.

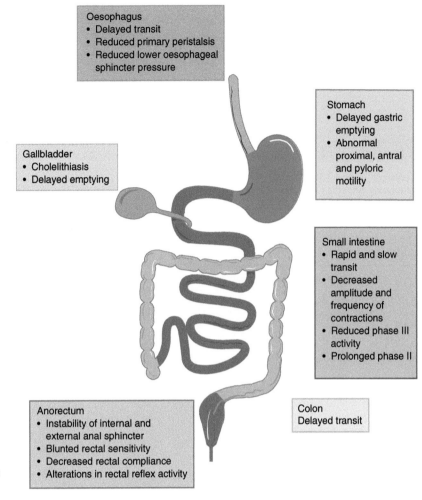

Figure 23.1 Motility disorders associated with diabetes at various levels of the GI tract.

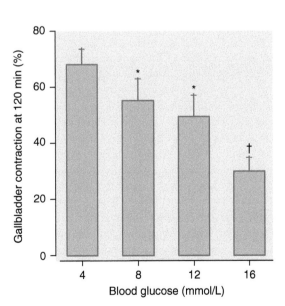

Figure 23.2 Dose-dependent effect of hyperglycaemia on postprandial gallbladder contraction in healthy subjects. $^{\dagger}p < 0.05$ compared with 4 mmol/L; $p < 0.05$ compared with 4, 8 and 12 mmol/L. From Rayner et al. Diabetes Care 2001; 24: 371–381.

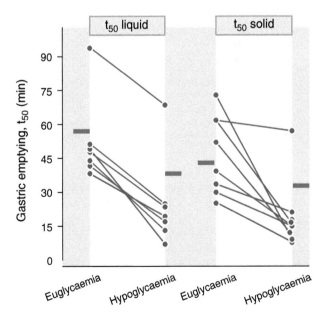

Figure 23.3 Effect of insulin-induced hypoglycaemia on gastric emptying (50% emptying, t50) of 200 g solid (processed beef and vegetables) and liquid (150 mL 100% dextrose in water) in eight subjects with uncomplicated type 1 diabetes (mean ± SD). From Scharcz et al. Diabetic Med 1993; 10: 660–663.

Table 23.1 Prevalence of gastrointestinal symptoms in diabetes mellitus and controls, based on a population-based study of 423 patients with diabetes in Australia (22 type 1, 401 type 2).

	Prevalence rate (%)		
	Controls (*n* = 8185)	Patients with diabetes (*n* = 423)	Adjusted odds ratios with 95% CI
Abdominal pain/discomfort	10.8	13.5	1.63 (1.21–2.20)
Postprandial fullness	5.2	8.6	2.07 (1.43–3.01)
Heartburn	10.8	13.5	1.38 (1.03–1.86)
Nausea	3.5	5.2	2.31 (1.45–3.68)
Vomiting	1.1	1.7	2.51 (1.12–5.66)
Dysphagia	1.7	5.4	2.71 (1.69–4.36)
Faecal incontinence	0.8	2.6	2.74 (1.40–5.37)
Oesophageal symptoms	11.5	15.4	1.44 (1.09–1.91)
Upper dysmotility symptoms	15.3	18.2	1.75 (1.34–2.29)
Any bowel symptom	18.9	26.0	1.84 (1.46–2.33)
Diarrhoea symptoms	10.0	15.6	2.06 (1.56–2.74)
Constipation symptoms	9.2	11.4	1.54 (1.12–2.13)

From Horowitz et al. J Gastroenterol Hepatol 1998; 13: S239–245.

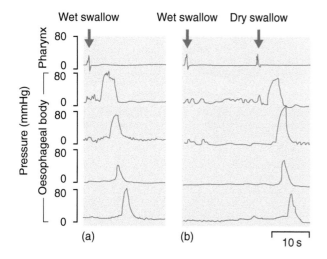

Figure 23.4 Wet swallow-induced oesophageal peristalsis in a healthy subject (a) and in a patient with long-standing insulin-dependent diabetes (b). In the subject with diabetes, the swallow-induced peristaltic wave has insufficient force to propel the water bolus distally (failed peristalsis). A subsequent dry swallow is associated with normal peristalsis, and clears the oesophagus. Adapted from Holloway et al. Am J Gastroenterol 1999; 94: 3150–3157.

can worsen heartburn. Reflux oesophagitis is also exacerbated by obesity. Measures such as propping up the head end of the bed to alleviate nocturnal heartburn and use of alginates may help some patients as may gastric acid reducing treatments such as H2 receptor blockers or proton pump inhibitors (PPI).

Gastroparesis

Delayed gastric emptying (gastroparesis) of a modest extent occurs in up to 50% of people with long-standing diabetes. Symptoms of gastroparesis are characteristically worse postprandially. They include nausea, vomiting, abdominal discomfort and/or fullness, and anorexia, and are reported in 5–12% of all patients with diabetes. In the USA, a 10 year cumulative incidence of symptoms suggestive of gastroparesis has been reported in 5.2% of 269 people with type 1, 1.0% of 409 with type 2 and 0.2% of 735 with no diabetes, and that women were more affected than men. Symptoms are often stable for up to 12 years and do not appear to be associated with mortality. They tend to be worse with solids rather than liquids.

The pathophysiology is complex and probably a combination of vagal neuropathy leading to diminished contractions after a meal, and sympathetic neuropathy leading to a failure of gastric relaxation to accommodate a meal. The former will lead to prolongation of stomach contents and vomiting, the latter to early satiety and fullness. Alterations in GI hormone secretion (such as glucagon) also play a part. There is often a history of long-standing poor glycaemic control, but no direct relationship between HbA1c and development. However, concurrent hyperglycaemia will worsen symptoms.

Examination can reveal epigastric distension and a succussion splash an hour or two after a liquid meal if the stomach is grossly dilated. Radio-isotope scintigraphy is the gold standard method for measuring gastric emptying. Ideally, this should be performed during normoglycaemia and with a dual isotope assessment of both solid and liquid emptying. The drawbacks of this test are its expense and significant radiation exposure. A carbon 13 breath test has acceptable specificity and sensitivity and much less radiation. Other tests include the use of radio-opaque markers to monitor transit time; wireless motility capsules which transmit intraluminal images as well as measures of pH and contractions to an external receiver; and more conventional imaging with ultrasound or MRI. Many of these investigations lack standardisation and have low specificity.

Diagnosis is largely based upon the patient history and in the context of other diabetic complications, especially autonomic neuropathy; investigations should be carried out to rule out other conditions. Of these, oesophagogastroduodenoscopy (OGD) is the most helpful. It is important to remember that some drugs can delay gastric emptying and should be avoided (Box 23.1).

Treatment of symptomatic gastroparesis is difficult; it involves improving glycaemic control, eating small meals often (reducing solid components) and administration of prokinetic drugs such as metoclopramide, domperidone, and erythromycin (possibly best given intravenously or in short oral courses for acute episodes because of tolerance). Use of conventional anti-emetics may also help but have not been subjected to controlled trials. Case reports of the newer agents such as aprepitant have reported benefit in severely affected patients. Endoscopic injection of botulinum toxin into the pylorus has been shown to provide short term benefit in some uncontrolled studies but is no longer recommended for general use. Surgical pyloroplasty has also been shown to help some patients refractory to pharmacological approaches. Severely affected patients may need admission to hospital for intravenous fluids, control of diabetes and possible nasogastric feeding. Placement of a feeding jejunostomy (PEJ) tube to maintain nutrition may be required. Surgical drainage and bypass should be avoided if possible. Trials of gastric electrical stimulation via an implanted pacemaker have been inconclusive, although long-term follow up does suggest symptomatic benefit in some. A stepped approach to the patient with suspected gastroparesis is shown in Table 23.2. It should be remembered that because many of these patients may have diabetic nephropathy and a diminished GFR, care must be taken with doses of drugs in order to avoid side effects.

Box 23.1 List of agents which can exacerbate gastroparesis.

- Opiates
- Anticholinergics (including tricyclics)
- Calcium channel blockers,
- Proton pump inhibitors
- β-Adrenergic antagonists
- Dopaminergic agents
- Nicotine
- Alcohol
- GLP-1 agonists

Small bowel

Autonomic neuropathy and sometimes colonisation of the hypomotile small bowel by colonic bacteria contribute to 'diabetic diarrhoea', but other factors probably play a role. Classically, the diarrhoea is intermittent and worse at night. Bouts that last several days may be followed by remissions. The diagnosis is by exclusion, and other possible causes of diarrhoea, such as drugs (metformin, acarbose, antibiotics, and alcohol), chronic pancreatic insufficiency with malabsorption, and coeliac disease must be considered (Table 23.3).

Table 23.2 Step-wise approach to the patient with suspected gastroparesis.

STEP 1	DIAGNOSIS	Gastric scintigraphy (gold standard) ^{13}C breath test Radiopaque markers Wireless motility capsule Ultrasound MRI
STEP 2	a. EXCLUDE IATROGENIC DISEASE	Drugs (e.g. opioids, GLP 1 agonists, see Box 23.1)
	b. DIETARY	Low fat, low fibre, small particles or fluid based
	c. IMPROVE GLYCAEMIC CONTROL	Consider CSII
STEP 3	MEDICATION	Prokinetic – metoclopramide, domperidone, erythromycin Antiemetics – antihistamines, 5 HT3 antagonists, neurokinin receptor antagonists (aprepitant) Tricyclics
STEP 4	NUTRITION	Enteral feeding
STEP 5	OTHERS	Surgery – venting gastrostomy, jejunostomy, pyloroplasty, gastrostomy Parenteral nutition Gastric electrical stimulator (pacemaker) Acupuncture (Botulinum toxin – no longer recommended)

Based on Camilleri M et al. Am J Gastroenterol 2013.

Table 23.3 A step-wise approach to the patient with suspected autonomic diarrhoea.

STEP 1	EXCLUDE	Coeliac disease (especially type 1 diabetes) Lactose intolerance Pancreatic insufficiency (faecal elastase or calprotectin) Bile salt malabsorption (if cholecystectomy) Microscopic colitis (if watery diarrhoea – consider colonoscopy and biopsy) Medication (e.g. metformin, statins, GLP1 agonists, proton pump inhibitors) Diabetic foods containing sorbitol
STEP 2	CONSIDER	Small intestine bacterial overgrowth (SIBO) – may need hydrogen breath test or trial of antibiotic such as rifaximin for 10–14 days
STEP 3	GENERAL	Improve glycaemic control – may need CSII Correct nutrient, fluid and electrolyte deficiencies
STEP 4	MEDICATION	Loperamide (opioid but does not cross into brain) Codeine – troublesome side effects Diphenoxylate/atropine – opioid crosses into brain Clonidine – troublesome side effects Ondansetron – not licensed Somatostatin analogues – injections and side effects Colestyramine – for suspected bile salt malabsorption

Treatment of diabetic diarrhoea is by opioid derivatives (e.g. loperamide) or a broad-spectrum antibiotic if bacterial overgrowth is suspected or proven by hydrogen breath test. Troublesome diarrhoea, especially when watery, may respond to the α-adrenergic agonist clonidine (unlicensed indication). The long-acting somatostatin analogue octreotide and the 5 HT3 receptor antagonist ondansetron may be helpful when other measures have failed (Table 23.3).

Large bowel

Constipation is also common in patients with diabetes and autonomic neuropathy and poor glycaemic control, though it is usually mild. A thorough history should be taken, including that of drug intake (many narcotics, antihypertensives, and antidepressants can cause constipation). Thyroid function and serum calcium and potassium levels should be assessed to exclude metabolic disorders. Other serious pathology, such as colonic carcinoma, must be excluded, and colonoscopy may be indicated. If constipation requires treatment, fibre and bulking agents are the first choice, and osmotic laxatives (e.g. lactulose) or prokinetic drugs are also usually effective. The 5 HT4 receptor agonist prucalopride is licensed for constipation that does not respond to laxatives, and may also benefit other symptoms such as bloating. Linaclotide binds to bowel wall receptors that activate chloride and water secretion into the gut and is licensed for patients with irritable bowel syndrome and constipation. Finally, there are some preliminary data on the use of the cholinesterase inhibitor pyridostigmine in patients who do not respond to other measures.

Abdominal pain

Pain can be a very troublesome feature of GI autonomic neuropathy and is difficult to treat. It responds best to antidepressant medications such as tricyclics, SSRIs, and SNRIs but these may also have gastrointestinal side effects which may limit dose. Opiates should be avoided in this situation as they are largely ineffective, have the potential for habituation and will certainly worsen nausea and constipation.

Gut microbiota

There is increasing evidence supporting a role for the gut microbiota (defined as the microbes that inhabit the bowel) in diabetes and obesity (Figure 23.5). It is clear that there exists a complex symbiotic relationship between our microbes and their host which contributes to energy metabolism and metabolic signalling. In addition, dietary and health changes in the host have a major impact on the composition of the microbiota.

The fivefold increase in incidence of type 1 diabetes that has been observed in Scandinavia over the last 50 years cannot be due to genetic factors alone. The gut microbiota are possible triggers for the autoimmune process, and there are intriguing data showing subtle differences in its composition in children who either have or are at risk of developing diabetes. A reduction in butyrate and lactate producing bacteria in children who subsequently go on to develop type 1 diabetes suggests more of a role in progression rather than causation, however.

In people with type 2 diabetes, a reduction in butyrate producing bacteria has been described in several studies, but it is unclear whether this might be a primary change or secondary to metformin therapy. A Danish study has found a link

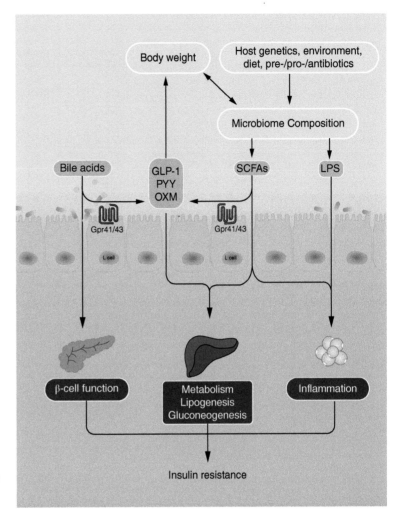

Figure 23.5 Effect of gut microbiota in liver disease, insulin resistance, and type 2 diabetes. GLP-1= glucagon like peptide 1; Gpr41= G-coupled receptor 41; Gpr43 = G-coupled receptor 43; LPS = lipopolysaccharides; OXM = oxyntomodulin; PYY = proteinYY; SCFA = short-chain fatty acids (e.g.butyrate). Reproduced from Aydin et al Current Diabetes Reports(2018) 18: 55 https://doi.org/10.1007/s11892-018-1020-6 with permission and in accordance with the Creative Common License http://creativecommons.org/licenses/by/4.0/

between higher circulating branch chain amino acids and insulin resistance, and the source may be the gut microbiota (Prevotella and Bacteroides spp). Another bacterium linked to obesity and type 2 diabetes is Akkermansia muciniphila, which is found in reduced numbers in people with glucose intolerance and newly diagnosed type 2 diabetes. Higher numbers are associated with better glucose homeostasis.

Alterations in diet, such as increasing complex polysaccharides, change the microbiota but the effects are not uniform in all individuals. Bariatric surgery causes profound change to gut organisms and this may, in part, be due to altered bile acid secretion and enterohepatic circulation. Supplementing diet with probiotics or nutrients such as propionate has been shown to reduce energy intake and improve insulin secretion in short-term studies.

Faecal microbiota transplantation (FMT) can be an effective treatment for severe C. difficile infection in man. A preliminary study of FMT in 18 men who had a range of BMI from lean to overweight showed improvements in insulin sensitivity, which corresponded with an increase in butyrate

producing bacteria in their faeces. These promising data need confirmation and testing in a formal trial.

There is the potential to genetically modify gut bacteria to produce compounds that may improve glycemic control. In mice, Lactococci engineered to produce GLP 1 improved glucose tolerance and such an approach has obvious potential in human therapeutics.

In the past 10 years many hundreds of papers have been published exploring the relationship between gut microbiota and type 2 diabetes and obesity. However, much of this work has been performed in animals, and human studies have been hampered by a lack of standardisation of techniques. Furthermore, much of the data have been derived from faecal samples which may not reflect accurately the microbiology of the small intestine. Nonetheless, manipulation of small bowel flora is an attractive target for interventions in metabolic disease. Future research will undoubtedly shed more light on the complex relationship between gut microbes and their host, with the exciting prospect of novel therapies for obesity and diabetes.

CASE HISTORY

A 32-year-old woman with type 1 diabetes of 20 years' duration with known diabetic nephropathy (eGFR 42 mL/min/1.73 m²) and treated proliferative retinopathy was admitted with a severe pneumonia requiring ventilation and temporary dialysis. Her diabetes control had been poor for many years (HbA1c >108 mmol/mol (12%) and she had suffered bouts of vomiting prior to her admission. Following transfer from the ITU, the vomiting became much worse, requiring regular IV insulin infusion and fluids with highly erratic blood glucose control. She was commenced on CSII. Regular IV metoclopramide then continuous subcutaneous cyclizine infusion were given with little benefit. Nasogastric drainage and then feeding were unsuccessful and were followed by insertion of a percutaneous jejunostomy. Her condition stabilised and she left hospital after a 4-month admission.

Comment: This story is typical of diabetic gastroparesis with an intermittent but more or less stable problem of vomiting made much worse by her acute illness. The protocol used for her IV infusion resulted in intermittent periods of no insulin and undoubtedly contributed to her symptoms and poor glycaemic control.

KEY WEBSITES

- American Gastroenterology Society: www.gastro.org
- American Motility Society: www.motilitysociety.org
- SIGN Guidelines: www.SIGN.ac.uk

FURTHER READING

Azpiroz F, Malagelada C. Diabetic neuropathy in the gut; pathogenesis and diagnosis. Diabetologia 2016; 59: 404–8. doi 10.1007/s00125-015-3831-1

Brunkwall L & Orho-Melander M. The gut microbiome as a target for the prevention and treatment of hyperglycaemia in type 2 diabetes: from current human evidence to future possibilities. Diabetologia 2017; 60: 943–51. doi : 10.1007/s00125-017-4278-3

Bytzer P, Talley MJ, Leeman M, Young LG, Jones MP, Harowitz M. Prevalence of gastrointestinal symptoms associated with diabetes mellitus. A population-based survey of 15,000 adults. Arch Intern Med 2001; 161; 1989–1996.

Camilleri M. Diabetic gastroparesis. N Engl J Med 2007; 356: 820–829.

Camilleri M, Parkman HP, Shafi MA, Abell TL, Gerson L. Clinical guideline: management of gastroparesis. Am J Gastroenterol 2013; 108: 18–37. doi: 10.1038/ajg.2012.373

Knip M, Siljander H. The role of the intestinal microbiota in type 1 diabetes mellitus. Nat Rev Endocrinol 2016; 154: doi 10.1038/nrendo.2015.218

Maisey A. A practical approach to gastrointestinal problems in diabetes. Diabetes Ther 2016; 7: 379–86 doi. 10.1007/s13300-016-0182-y

NICE. Gastroparesis in adults: oral erythromycin. Evidence summary 13; 2013: www.nice.org.uk/guidance/esuom13

Shakil A, Church RJ, Rao SS. Gastrointestinal complications of diabetes. Am Fam Physician 2008; 77: 1697–1702.

Tornblom H. Treatment of gastrointestinal autonomic neuropathy. Diabetologia 2016; 59: 409–13. doi 10.1007/s00125-015-3828-9

Non-alcoholic liver disease (NAFLD)

Introduction

As the obesity epidemic continues to grow, non-alcoholic fatty liver disease (NAFLD) has become the most common cause of chronic liver disease, with an estimated prevalence of between 20% and 30% in the general population. NAFLD represent a disease spectrum which starts with fatty liver, steatosis, and may progress to non-alcoholic steatohepatitis (NASH), hepatic inflammation, and latterly, cirrhosis, where cumulative liver injury result in liver fibrogenesis associated with portal hypertension, hepatic synthesis dysfunction, liver failure, hepatocellular carcinoma, or requirement for liver transplantation. The majority of patients have simple steatosis, but approximately 10–30% develop NASH, while the development of cirrhosis is associated with poor long-term prognosis.

Definition

NAFLD is present when >5% of hepatocytes are steatotic according to histological analysis or by proton density fat fraction in patients who do not consume excessive alcohol consumption (>20g/day for women and >30g/ day for men) and with no secondary cause for steatosis.

Risk factors for NAFLD
Type 2 diabetes mellitus

1. Age – higher risk with increasing age
2. Gender – commoner in men but women are at a higher risk of advanced fibrosis
3. Metabolic syndrome
4. Obesity
5. Ethnicity – higher risk in hispanics and South Asians. Lower risk in blacks
6. Physical inactivity
7. A high-calorie diet, excess saturated fats, refined carbohydrates, sugar-sweetened beverages, a high fructose intake
8. Obstructive sleep apnea.

Natural history of nonalcoholic fatty liver disease

Up to 90% of patients with NAFLD have simple steatosis. This carries a relatively benign prognosis, with no overall increase in mortality. However, 10–30% can progress to NASH which is associated with hepatocellular injury and inflammation. Approximately 25% of patients with NASH will develop progressive liver fibrosis, with an approximate 20–30% of these patients can eventually develop liver cirrhosis. This is often associated with poor long-term prognosis. The Child–Pugh score was developed to classify severity of cirrhosis and prognosis (Figure 24.1).

The largest study to describe the natural history of NAFLD reported the results of a 13.7-year mean follow-up of patients with biopsy proven NAFLD. Mean of patients at diagnosis was 47-years-old. One of the main findings of this study was that survival was reduced by 10% (compared to a general age-matched population) in patients with NASH, but mortality was unaffected in people with simple steatosis. There was a fourteenfold increase in deaths directly attributable to liver disease in patients with an initial diagnosis of NASH compared with individuals without NASH. Thus, NAFLD represents a heterogenous disorder associated with variable risk profiles and require a more precise diagnosis to stratify risk and implement optimal management strategies.

NAFLD and diabetes

NAFLD is long considered to be a metabolic disorder and often co-exists with type 2 diabetes and/or metabolic syndrome. Up to 85% of patients with NAFLD are obese or have been diagnosed with type 2 diabetes (T2D) and the prevalence of NAFLD is approximately 60% in some studies of patients with T2D. Another study estimated the prevalence of advanced fibrosis in asymptomatic patients with T2D to be around 5%–7%. It is difficult to obtain precise estimates of

2 Minute Medicine®	Child-Pugh Score		2minutemedicine.com
Factor	1 point	2 points	3 points
Total bilirubin (μmol/L)	<34	34-50	>50
Serum albumin (g/L)	>35	28-35	>28
PT INR	<1.7	1.71-2.30	>2.30
Ascites	None	Mild	Moderate to Severe
Hepatic encephalopathy	None	Grade I-II (or suppressed with medication)	Grade III-IV (or refractory)
	Class A	Class B	Class C
Total points	5-6	7-9	10-15
1-year survival	100%	80%	45%

Figure 24.1 Child-Pugh score.

the prevalence since establishing a diagnosis is based on the results of a liver biopsy.

Studies have shown that NAFLD may be an important novel cardiovascular risk factor in type 2 diabetes, even after adjusting for conventional cardiovascular risk factors. Cardiovascular events in NAFLD are increased by nearly two-fold in the presence of T2D. NAFLD is also known to increase microvascular complications of diabetes such as chronic kidney disease and retinopathy. Advanced forms of NAFLD such as NASH, advanced fibrosis, cirrhosis, and hepato-cellular cancer is reported to occur more commonly in patients with T2D.

Pathophysiology

Increased adiposity may cause hyperinsulinemia and hyperglycemia, which generates ectopic fat accumulation and insulin resistance in the liver. Subsequent impairment of hepatic function results in the spectrum of hepatic abnormalities described previously.

The pathogenesis of NAFLD has been the subject of intense research in recent years. Excess caloric intake increases fat accumulation in adipose tissue depots, which is typically followed by ectopic fat deposition in the liver and skeletal muscle. Insulin resistance ensues in these tissues which results in a further net increase in the hepatic influx of circulating free fatty acids (FFA) and lipid metabolites. Subsequently, hepatocyte-derived factors (such as cytokines/chemokines) stimulate inflammatory fibrotic response which leads to the development of inflammation and fibrosis in the liver. This is described as the 'multiple-parallel hit' model in the pathogenesis of NASH (Figure 24.2).

Screening

A formal diagnosis of NAFLD and its spectrum of liver abnormality will require a liver biopsy. However, various non-invasive screening tools have been developed to facilitate the identification of patients at high risk of liver fibrosis, which would require further investigation.

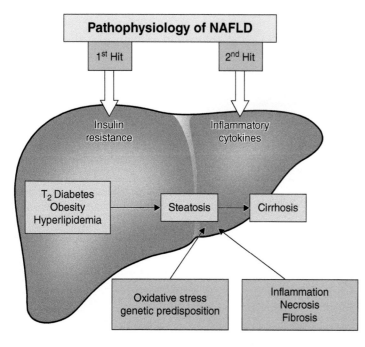

Figure 24.2 Multiple hit model in the pathogenesis of NAFD, NASH and cirrhosis.

Liver enzymes

ALT values do not correlate with histological findings and are unhelpful in both the diagnosis of NAFLD and determining disease severity. Approximately, ~80% of patients have normal-range ALT levels (males <40 IU/L and females <31). If abnormal LFTs are present, these are usually mildly raised transaminases (ALT), aspartate transaminase (AST)) and/or gamma-glutamyltransferase. IU/L).

Non-invasive fibrosis score

Progression to hepatocellular dysfunction and portal hypertension occurs as a result of advanced liver fibrosis. This may be reflected in 'routine' blood tests such as liver function tests (low albumin), full blood count (thrombocytopenia), and coagulation profile (prolonged prothrombin time). These tests provide an indirect measure of fibrosis. With increasing liver fibrosis, the ALT typically falls, and the AST remains stable or rises, and as a result the AST/ALT ratio increases. Previous studies identified a AST/ALT ratio cut-off of >1 as a surrogate marker for increased risk of cirrhosis. A lower cut-off of >0.8 is more sensitive in patients with NAFLD.

For the diagnosis of liver fibrosis, various scores have been developed.

The BARD score is a simple test using the body mass index (BMI), AAR and presence of type 2 diabetes mellitus. A score <2 has a negative predictive value (NPV) of 95–97%, which reliably excludes advanced fibrosis. However, among patients with type 2 diabetes, a large proportion of patients will have a score of ≥2, which limits its utility in clinical practice.

The NAFLD fibrosis score is a validated scoring system that comprises six routinely measured parameters. Advanced fibrosis can be reliably excluded (NPV 93%) using the low cut-off score (<−1.455) and diagnosed with high accuracy positive predictive value (PPV 90%) using the high cut-off score (>0.676).

The FIB-4 score is a widely used non-invasive tests for diagnosing advanced fibrosis in NAFLD. For stage 3–4 fibrosis, a score <1.45 has a 90% NPV and a score >2.67 has an 80% PPV. Various studies have shown that the FIB-4 score is slightly better than other non-invasive tests in diagnosing advanced fibrosis in NAFLD, including in subjects with normal range ALT levels (Figure 24.3).

Score	Indices	Calculation	Interpretation
BARD score	BMI AST/ALT ratio T2DM	Weighted sum: 1.BMI ≥28=1 point 2. AAR ≥0.8=2 points 3.T2DM=1 point	Score ≥2: Sensitivity 0.91, Specificity 0.66, for stage 3–4 fibrosis
NAFLD fibrosis score	Age Hyperglycaemia BMI Platelet count Albumin AST/ALT ratio	$-1.675+0.037\times$age (years)$+0.094\times$BMI (kg/m^2)$+1.13\times$IFG or diabetes (yes=1, no=0)$+0.99\times$AST/ALT ratio$-0.013\times$platelet ($\times10^9$/L)$-0.66\times$albumin (g/dL)	(<−1.455) canreliably exclude liver fibrosis (NPV 93%). A score >0.676 diagnosed with high accuracy (PPV 90%).
FIB-4 score	Age AST ALT platelet	Age$\times$AST (IU/L)/platelet count ($\times10^9$/L)$\times\sqrt{}$ALT (IU/L)	<1.45 has a negative predictive value of over 90% for advanced liver fibrosis. A score of >2.67 has a positive predictive value of 80% for advanced fibrosis.

Figure 24.3 Simple non-invasive tests for fibrosis.

Commercial non-invasive fibrosis tests

The Enhanced Liver Fibrosis (ELF) is an extracellular matrix (ECM) marker set consisting of tissue inhibitor of metalloproteinases 1 (TIMP-1), amino-terminal propeptide of type III procollagen (PIIINP) and hyaluronic acid (HA) showing good correlations with fibrosis stages in chronic liver disease.

- the ELF score combines quantitative serum concentration measurements of three fibrosis markers (TIMP-1, PIIINP, and HA) to a single value.
- The test is best used test in people who have been diagnosed with NAFLD to test for advanced liver fibrosis.
- Diagnose people with advanced liver fibrosis if they have:
  1. an ELF score of 10.51 or above.
  2. NAFLD.

Non-invasive imaging test

Ultrasound. This modality will only highlight the presence of 'fatty liver'. It is not able to differentiate between simple benign steatosis, NASH, and the degree of fibrosis.

Transient elastography (TE, Fibroscan®) Fibrotic livers have reduced elasticity due to the deposition of fibrous tissue in the hepatic parenchyma. Transient Elastography (Fibroscan) gives a 'liver stiffness measurement' (LSM) using pulsed-echo ultrasound as a surrogate marker of fibrosis. In this technique, a 50-MHz wave is passed into the liver from a small transducer on the end of an ultrasound probe that can measure the velocity of the shear wave (in metres per second) as this wave passes through the liver. The shear wave velocity can then be converted into liver stiffness, which is expressed in kilopascals. Due to the high risk of failed acquisition of TE in obese patients, the new XL probe, a larger probe with lower ultrasound frequency and deeper penetration, have been utilised to improve the validity of this technique. A value of <8kPA has a NPV of 96% for ≥stage 3 but only modest PPV (52% at 7.9 kPa and 72% at > 9.6 kPa).

Management
Lifestyle modification

Optimizing metabolic control, dietary and lifestyle modification are the mainstay of treatment for managing NAFLD. A weight loss ≥7% over 12 months was shown to cause NASH regression in 25% and steatosis regression in 40%. Fructose-containing beverages and foods and saturated fatty acids should be avoided as is alcohol intake, which should be maintained below the risk threshold (i.e. <30 g for men; <20 g for women). Increased physical activity is encouraged – a 150–200 min/week of moderate intensity aerobic physical activities in 3–5 sessions such as brisk walking, cycling, and 3 times/week of 45 min of resistance training.

Thiazolidinediones

Pioglitazone versus Vitamin E versus Placebo for the Treatment of Nondiabetic Patients with Nonalcoholic Steatohepatitis (PIVENS) trial, was a phase 3, multicentre, randomised, placebo-controlled, double-blind clinical trial of pioglitazone or vitamin E for the treatment of adults without diabetes who had biopsy-confirmed nonalcoholic steatohepatitis. It concluded that both Vitamin E and pioglitazone were associated with reductions in hepatic steatosis and lobular inflammation but not with improvement in fibrosis scores. In another study, administration of pioglitazone, as compared with placebo, was associated with improvement in histologic findings with regard to steatosis, ballooning necrosis, and inflammation. In addition, subjects in the pioglitazone group had a greater reduction in necroinflammation but the reduction in fibrosis again did not differ significantly from that in the placebo group. In a different randomized controlled trial, Cusi et al also showed that Pioglitazone was associated with a significant reduction of at least two points in the nonalcoholic fatty liver disease activity score in two histologic categories without worsening of fibrosis and 51% had resolution of NASH. In contrast to previous studies, Pioglitazone treatment was also associated with improvement in individual histologic scores, including the fibrosis score. There was also reported improvement in adipose tissue, hepatic, and muscle insulin sensitivity and all 18-month metabolic and histologic improvements persisted over 36 months of therapy. Risk of recurrence however is high, and thus continued treatment is often necessary.

Glucagon-like peptide-1 analogs and DPP-4 inhibitors

Glucagon-like peptide-1 (GLP-1) analogs has been shown to produce an improvement in hepatic steatosis and steatohepatitis by weight loss in multiple animal studies. Subsequent studies in humans have also shown the efficacy of GLP-1 therapy in patients with the NAFLD spectrum. The effect of liraglutide on liver histology was first evaluated in the Liraglutide Efficacy and Action in NASH (LEAN) trial, which compared 48 weeks of liraglutide 1.8 mg versus placebo in 52 patients with biopsy-confirmed NASH (17 subjects had T2DM). A significantly higher proportion of patients on Liraglutide achieved the primary end point of reduced hepatocyte ballooning without impairment of fibrosis (a resolution of NASH) compared with the placebo group. Liraglutide significantly improved steatosis, NAFLD activity score, and hepatocyte ballooning without significant differences in lobular inflammation. The study by Petit et al. (Lira-NAFLD) meanwhile demonstrated that six months of treatment with liraglutide 1.2 mg in 68 patients with poor controlled T2D was associated with a 31% reduction in liver fat content as measured with proton magnetic resonance spectroscopy. The effect was predominantly caused by body weight loss. A further study investigated patients with T2D (HbA1c 6.5%–10%) that have been treated with metformin monotherapy ≥1500 mg/day for at least three months and were diagnosed with NAFLD. 75 patients were randomized to receive either liraglutide 1.8 mg daily, sitagliptin (a DPP4 inhibitor) 100 mg once daily or insulin glargine at bedtime, in addition to their concurrent metformin dose. In the liraglutide and sitagliptin groups, the primary efficacy endpoint, intrahepatic lipid (IHL) measured by magnetic resonance imaging-estimated proton density fat fraction (MRI-PDFF), significantly decreased from baseline. No significant change was observed in the insulin glargine group. Multiple linear regression analysis revealed that change in weight was an independent determinant of change in MRI-PDFF in T2D and NAFLD.

At the time of writing this book, a phase IIb RCT is currently underway to investigate the efficacy and safety of Semaglutide for 72 weeks of treatment in patients with NASH. Individuals were randomized to receive one of three doses (0.1 mg, 0.2 mg, or 0.4 mg) of subcutaneous semaglutide once daily or placebo. At primary analysis, 230 of 320 participants had fibrosis stages F2 to F3. Researchers defined the primary end point as resolution of NASH and no worsening liver fibrosis. Liver biopsies performed at baseline and at the end of the trial revealed that of patients receiving subcutaneous semaglutide 0.4 mg, 33 of 56 patients had NASH resolution compared to 10 of 58 patients on placebo (59% vs 17%). These findings offer hope for the effective management of NAFLD in patients with or without diabetes.

Sodium Glucose cotransporter 2 inhibitors

In experimental animal models of NAFLD, sodium glucose cotransporter 2 inhibitors has been shown to inhibit the development of NAFLD/NASH and improved histological hepatic steatosis or steatohepatitis. However only a few studies have attempted to evaluate the role of SGLT2 inhibitors on liver inflammation and fibrosis histologically in patients with T2D with biopsy-confirmed NAFLD or NASH. A majority of studies with SGLT2 inhibitor in humans have shown improvements in surrogate markers of liver fibrosis such as ALT (Dapagliflozin, Empagliflozin, and Canagliflozin), liver stiffness using transient elastography pressures (Dapagliflozin) or liver fat content, as assessed by MRI (Empagliflozin and Canagliflozin).

In a study by Seko et al. 10 patients with T2D with biopsy-confirmed NASH (hepatic fibrosis stage 1–3) received canagliflozin 100 mg for 12 weeks. The study showed that Canaglflozin was associated with significant improvements in AST and fibrosis-4 index. In a 24-week trial by Cusi et al. canagliflozin 300 mg was shown to decrease intrahepatic triglyceride measured by proton-magnetic resonance spectroscopy compared to placebo (−6.9% vs −3.8%, respectively), and the reduction was strongly correlated with extent of weight loss.

Vitamin E

Oxidative stress occurs in both NAFLD and T2D. As described previously, in the PIVENS trial, 800 IU/day of Vitamin E for 96 weeks improved liver enzymes, steatosis, inflammation, and ballooning (except fibrosis) and induced resolution of NASH in 42% of patients. Consequently, while Vitamin E has been considered as a first-line pharmacotherapy at dose of 800 IU/day for nondiabetic adults with biopsy-proven NASH, it has yet to be recommended in patients with T2D with NASH, NAFLD without liver biopsy, NASH cirrhosis, or cryptogenic cirrhosis due to lack of data in this patient group.

Bariatric surgery

There is mounting evidence that bariatric surgical intervention is associated with significant improvement in liver histology and resolution of NAFLD. However, evidence for safety of bariatric surgery among patients with more advanced liver diseases, such as cirrhosis with portal hypertension, or ascites is still lacking, with some studies reporting little or no postoperative mortality or liver-related complications while other studies have reported complications of bariatric surgery in patients with cirrhosis, including the development of fulminant hepatic failure. Nonetheless, in patients with NASH, regression of NASH has been reported in 85% of patients, and inflammation and fibrosis in 37% and 20%, respectively - attributed to weight loss.

Statins

Clinical trials on statins as treatment for NASH are limited and have shown inconsistent results. However, since NAFLD is considered to be an important CVD risk factor, the use of statins is an important strategy to improve cardiovascular outcomes of patients with NAFLD. The GREACE trial showed the safety of statins in NAFLD/NASH. In dyslipidemia, statins, and other lipid-lowering agents are also considered safe in NAFLD and NASH. Although statin use is warranted in NASH cirrhosis, it should be avoided in decompensated cirrhosis.

CASE STUDY

A 51-year-old patient with type 2 diabetes attended clinic for routine review. His BMI is 30.2kg/m², Hba1c is 8.3% and blood pressure is elevated at 172/90. He is taking metformin 1g BD, Simvastatin 40mg od and Ramipril 10mg od. His liver function showed a slightly raised ALT 51, AST is raised 67 and platelet was reduced at 119. His Fib4 score was 4.02 which suggest that advanced fibrosis is likely. He was therefore referred for a fibroscan investigation. This showed increase pressure of 27 kPA. Subsequent liver biopsy confirmed cirrhosis. The patient was advised to lose weight by undertaking increase exercise and calorie restriction. Therapeutic management should focus on strategies to reduce cardiovascular risk, improve glucose control and improve liver outcomes. This patient was therefore commenced on a GLP-1 analogue treatment Semaglutide 0.5 mg once weekly, and increased to 1mg once weekly. Felodipine was added to his treatment regime in order to achieve optimal blood pressure control.

Comment: Patients with significant liver disease are often asymptomatic. Identifying and assessment of significant liver disease should be undertaken during routine review of all patients with diabetes. The use of a non-diagnostic tool facilitates the identification of patients at high risk of liver fibrosis, so that appropriate further investigation could be implemented.

FURTHER READINGS

Ekstedt M, Franzen LE, Mathiesen UL, et al. Long-term follow-up of patients with NAFLD and elevated liver enzymes. Hepatology 2006; 44: 865–73

Cusi K, Bril F, Barb D, Polidori D, Sha S, Ghosh A, et al. Effect of canagliflozin treatment on hepatic triglyceride content and glucose metabolism in patients with type 2 diabetes. Diabetes Obes Metab. 2018 Nov 16; doi: 10.1111/dom.13584.

Armstrong MJ, Gaunt P, Aithal GP, Barton D, Hull D, Parker R, et al. Liraglutide safety and efficacy in patients with non-alcoholic steatohepatitis (LEAN): a multicentre, double-blind, randomised, placebo-controlled phase 2 study. Lancet. 2016; 387: 679–90

Belfort R, Harrison SA, Brown K et al. A placebo controlled trial of pioglitazone in subjects with nonalcoholic steatohepatitis. N Eng J Med 2006; 355: 2297–307

Harrison SA, Oliver D, Arnold HL, et al Development and validation of a simple NAFLD clinical scoring system for identifying patients without advanced disease. Gut 2008; 57: 1441–7

Angulo P, Hui J, Marchesini G, et al The NAFLD fibrosis score: a noninvasive system that identifies liver fibrosis in patients with NAFLD. Hepatology 2007; 45: 847–54.

Foucher J, Chanteloup E, Verg niol J, et al Diagnosis of cirrhosis by transient elastography (FibroScan): a prospective study. Gut 2006; 55: 403–8

Petit JM, Cercueil JP, Loffroy R, Denimal D, Bouillet B, Fourmont C, et al. Effect of liraglutide therapy on liver fat content in patients with inadequately controlled type 2 diabetes: the Lira-NAFLD Study. J Clin Endocrinol Metab. 2017; 102: 407–15

Bower, G., Athanasiou, T., Isla, A.M., Harling, L., Li, J.V., Holmes, E., et al. (2015). Bariatric surgery and nonalcoholic fatty liver disease. European Journal of Gastroenterology & Hepatology, 27(7): p. 755–768.

Eilenberg M, Langer FB, Beer A, Trauner M, Prager G, Staufer K. Significant Liver-Related Morbidity After Bariatric Surgery and Its Reversal-a Case Series. Obesity surgery. 2018; 28(3): 812–9.

Diabetes and cancer

KEY POINTS

- Type 2 diabetes is definitely associated with an increased risk of cancer of the pancreas, liver, and hepatobiliary tract, uterus, breast (in post-menopausal women) and bowel.
- The associations are confounded by risk factors such as age and body mass that also confer an increased cancer risk.
- There is a reduced incidence of prostate cancer in white Europid men with type 2 diabetes.

- There is no increased risk of cancer in type 1 diabetes.
- There is no proven causative link between specific diabetes treatments and cancer.
- Cancer related mortality rates for some tumours are higher in people with type 2 diabetes.
- Some cancer therapies can cause and/or exacerbate hyperglycaemia.

Introduction

Associations between diabetes and cancer of the pancreas and liver have been appreciated for some time. More recently, links between diabetes and other more common cancers have been confirmed. Recent mortality data from Scotland has suggested that cancer and cardiovascular disease each account for around 25% of deaths in people with diabetes. In 2009, several simultaneously published papers reported an increased incidence of cancer in patients with type 2 diabetes who were using long-acting insulin analogues. There followed extensive research into the relationship between cancer incidence, diabetes, and its treatment. This chapter will review the current state of knowledge, but as this is a fast-moving field new data are likely to become available in the next few years.

Epidemiology

A recent meta-analysis of the data linking diabetes and cancer confirms a positive association between diabetes and cancer of the liver, pancreas and biliary tract (Table 25.1). There is an increased risk of endometrial cancer (two-fold); and colorectal and post-menopausal breast cancers (20–40%). Stomach cancer may be more common in Japanese people

with diabetes. Previously reported associations between bladder, kidney, and non-Hodgkin's lymphoma were not confirmed as statistically significant. Prostate cancer seems to be less common, at least in white, Europid men with type 2 diabetes. A recent study has modelled the impact of a BMI >25 kg/m² and diabetes on global cancer incidence and concluded that diabetes alone may have accounted for approximately 2% of all cancers in 2012 (Figure 25.1). There are no significant reported associations between cancer and type 1 diabetes.

Possible biological mechanisms

Type 2 diabetes is associated with several pathophysiological changes that may pre-dispose to cancer development (Table 25.2). Firstly, at the time of diagnosis, and for at least 8 years preceding this, many patients are hyperinsulinaemic and have higher circulating levels of IGF1 (insulin-like growth factor), both of which stimulate cell growth. Secondly, there are also changes to IGF binding proteins that may result in higher tissue exposure to free, unbound IGF1. Thirdly, circulating concentrations of pro-inflammatory cytokines are also raised which may facilitate carcinogenesis. Finally, hyperglycaemia may in itself encourage cancer growth as malignant

---

Handbook of Diabetes, Fifth Edition. Rudy Bilous, Richard Donnelly, and Iskandar Idris.
© 2021 John Wiley & Sons Ltd. Published 2021 by John Wiley & Sons Ltd.

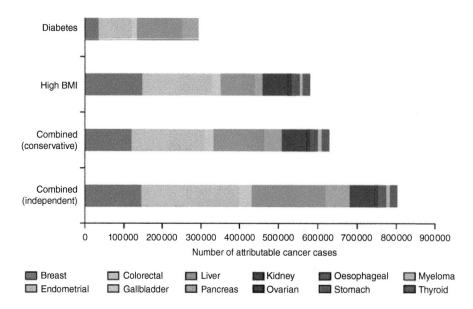

Figure 25.1 Global cancer cases in 2012 due to diabetes and BMI ≥ 25 kg/m² separately and combined. The independent combined estimate assumes diabetes and raised BMI act as independent risk factors for cancer. The conservative estimate assumes overlap of pathophysiology of diabetes and raised BMI with cancer. From Pearson-Stuttard et al. Lancet Diabetes Endocrinol 2018 with permission.

cells are heavily glucose dependent for energy provision. However, the lack of an increased cancer incidence in type 1 diabetes makes this latter mechanism less likely.

One of the difficulties in exploring the link between diabetes and cancer is the fact that both diseases share some common risk factors and associations. Both are more common in the elderly, in those who are overweight, in people with poor diet and who are physically less active, in those who smoke, and in those from poorer socio-economic backgrounds.

The situation is further complicated by the problem that the precise dates of onset of cancer and/or diabetes in an individual are almost impossible to ascertain. For example, it has been estimated that cancerous change in a bowel adenoma may have occurred 20 or more years before presentation.

A person developing diabetes during this time period may therefore be recorded as having a positive association but there may be little or no causative link.

Another potential bias is the phenomenon of reverse causality in that the cancer itself may cause diabetes. This is perhaps most likely with liver and pancreatic cancers, but the long duration of known diabetes prior to the cancer diagnosis in many of these patients means that such bias cannot explain all of the observed association. Ascertainment bias may also occur in people with newly diagnosed diabetes. Contact with health care professionals and routine surveillance may expose a previously undiagnosed cancer, and there are some data that suggest that a cancer diagnosis is more common in the first 12 months after diabetes is confirmed.

Effect of diabetes on cancer mortality and treatment

The impact of diabetes on cancer mortality is complex and reported data are subject to bias. In particular, it is important

Table 25.1 List of cancers and the strength of their reported association with type 2 diabetes.

Cancer type	Strength of association
Liver	Definite
Pancreas	Definite
Hepatobiliary	Definite
Uterine	Twofold
Breast (post menopausal)	20–40 %
Colorectal	20–40 %
Bladder	Possible
Kidney	Possible
Non-Hodgkin's lymphoma	Possible
Stomach	Possible (in Japanese)
Prostate	Reduced (in white Europid)

Table 25.2 Potential mechanisms linking diabetes and cancer.

Diabetes specific	Non-diabetes specific
Hyperinsulinaemia	Age
Raised bioavailable IGF1	Weight
Increased inflammatory cytokines	Poor diet
Hyperglycaemia	Physical inactivity
	Smoking
	Socio-economic deprivation

to distinguish between all-cause and cancer specific mortality. People with diabetes have an approximately twofold increased cardiovascular mortality which is likely to increase reported overall mortality in those who also have cancer. However, it does seem that diabetes is linked to an increase in cancer specific mortality in those with colorectal cancer, and in women with breast and endometrial cancers. This does not seem to be the case in people with liver or pancreatic cancers, perhaps because of the often rapid progression of these tumours following diagnosis; nor in those with lung or ovarian cancer. Both all-cause and cancer specific mortality are increased in men with diabetes who develop prostate cancer, despite the reported lower incidence.

Women with diabetes tend to present later with breast and endometrial cancer than those without, partly because they have lower attendance rates for mammography and cervical screening. This behaviour is probably not diabetes specific and may be confounded by other associations such as socio-economic deprivation.

Cancer treatment patterns in people with diabetes differ from those without. For example, younger women with breast cancer are more likely to undergo surgery if they have diabetes, whereas the reverse is true for older women. Reported rates of complications following surgery or other cancer treatments are higher in people with diabetes, but there are wide variations by both cancer type and by treatment centre and country. Patients with diabetes have been reported to respond less well to chemotherapy for bowel cancer than those without.

Effects of cancer therapy on diabetes

High dose glucocorticoid therapy is widely used to reduce cerebral oedema in people with primary and secondary brain tumours; to reduce pain from metastatic tumours in the liver and elsewhere; and as a primary therapy for some haematological malignancies. In people without diabetes, 30% will develop hyperglycaemia in the diabetic range, and some will remain with diabetes long-term. People with diabetes receiving glucocorticoids will require at least a 50% increase in their insulin dose, and those on oral hypoglycaemic agents will often need a switch to insulin until the steroid dose is reduced.

Men with prostate cancer receiving androgen deprivation therapy are more likely to develop diabetes, and those with pre-existing diabetes will often require an escalation of their glucose lowering therapy. Oestrogen receptor modulator treatments have the same effects in women.

Some newer, more experimental therapies specifically target cell signalling pathways that affect glucose metabolism. mTOR inhibitors such as sirolimus can cause both a reduction in insulin secretion and an increase in insulin resistance resulting in hyperglycaemia in 12–50% of recipients. Anti IGF1 receptor antibodies are an experimental therapy often used with sirolimus and this combination has reported rates of hyperglycaemia of >70%.

Effects of diabetes therapies on cancer incidence and progression

Metformin use has been linked to both lower incidence rates of some cancers (such as colorectal) as well as improved overall survival (in breast and lung cancer). However, there are several areas of potential bias in these reports. Metformin is first line therapy and is more likely to be used in people with newly diagnosed diabetes or those with less severe hyperglycaemia, both situations where cardiovascular mortality and cancer risk may be lower. Metformin is contraindicated in those with chronic kidney disease stages 4 and 5 and those with severe heart failure and liver disease, all of whom would be expected to have a higher mortality rate. An immortality bias has been proposed as a possible explanation of the apparent positive benefit of metformin on cancer incidence and progression. For example, people with diabetes are initially treated with non-pharmacological therapies and then go on to receive metformin if their glucose control is not to target. If they develop cancer beforehand, they are often included in the comparator group for those who go on to receive metformin, thus introducing a bias. The correct comparison needs to start from the same observation period (Figure 25.2). Large prospective trials of metformin on cancer prevention are currently ongoing and may shed more light on this issue.

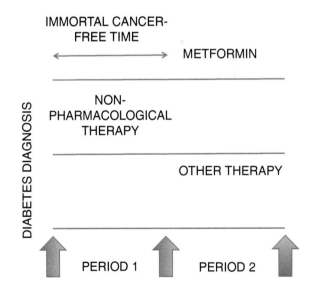

Figure 25.2 Immortality bias with metformin treatment. Cancer rates recorded in period 1 will not be associated with metformin use thus introducing an immortal time bias. This is particularly important as there is an increase in cancer detection following diagnosis of diabetes. The correct design should only compare cancer rates in period 2.

As mentioned in the introduction, a putative link between insulin use (notably long-acting analogues) and cancer incidence was proposed in 2009. The lack of any increase in cancer incidence and insulin use in people with type 1 diabetes implies that insulin itself is unlikely to be carcinogenic. Moreover, the lack of any reports of subcutaneous cancers at insulin injection sites does not support a direct effect on tumour genesis, despite the often observed lipohypertrophy. Newer insulin analogues have different binding properties to the insulin receptor, and some appear to also have a stimulating effect on the IGF1 receptor, at least in vitro. Some tumours overexpress insulin receptor A and hybrid insulin-IGF1 receptors providing a plausible hypothesis for enhanced tumour growth. However, the indications for insulin therapy are related to both diabetes duration (and thus age) and hyperglycaemia (thereby by implication with both insulin resistance and obesity), both of which increase cancer risk. As many people with diabetes are on multiple glucose lowering therapies, usually introduced in a stepwise pattern with insulin as the last step, then any cancer risk is likely to be more associative than causative. At the time of writing there is no conclusive or consistent link between insulin analogue use and cancer incidence and progression.

Pioglitazone (but not rosiglitazone) was linked to bladder cancer in experimental diabetes and carries a warning to this effect on its use in humans. Prolonged use or its initiation in those deemed to be of high risk of bladder cancer, are not recommended. The reports of increased bladder cancer in people using pioglitazone have been hotly debated and the positive links disputed.

More recently, incretin related treatments have been linked to pancreatic and other cancers. GLP-1 agonists have been associated with thyroid C cell tumours in animals, but no cases have been reported in man. The small series of pancreatic tumours that were published a few years ago have prompted an extensive retrospective review of all published randomised controlled trials (RCTs) of these agents, as well as including such cancers as a prospective end point in on-going studies. No significant associations have been confirmed, although there are serious limitations in using therapeutic RCTs in this way as they were not designed to answer such questions. The incidence rate of all cancers in people over 70 is around 20/1000/year, so in order to collect a sufficient number of relatively rare pancreatic tumours, many thousands of patients would need to be studied for many years, using specific tests for identification, in order to settle this question definitively.

FURTHER READING

Johnson JA et al. Diabetes and cancer (1): evaluating the temporal realtionship between type 2 diabetes and cancer incidence. Diabetologia 2012; 55: 1607–18 Doi: 10.1007/s001 25-012-2525-1

Pearson-Stuttard J, Zhou B, Kontis V, Bentham J, Gunter MJ, Ezzati M. Worldwide burden of cancer attributable to diabetes and high body-mass index: a comparative risk assessment. Lancet Diabetes Endocrinol 2018; 6: e6–e15 doi: 10.1016/S2213-8587 (18)30150-5

Renehan AG et al. Diabetes and cancer (2): evaluating the impact of diabetes on mortality in patients with cancer. Diabetologia 2012; 55: 1619–32 Doi: 10.1007/s001 25-012-2526-0

Shlomai G et al Type 2 diabetes mellitus and cancer: the role of pharmacotherapy. J Clin Oncol 2016; 34; 4261–9 Doi: 10.1200/ JCO.201667.4044

Tsilidis KK et al. Type 2 diabetes and cancer: umbrella review of meta analyses of observational studies. BMJ 2014; 350; g7607 doi: 10.1136/bmj.g7607

Chapter 26

Skin and connective tissue disorders in diabetes

Diabetes affects the cellular biochemistry of skin and connective tissues, in particular collagen synthesis and structure, as well as cutaneous microvascular blood flow. Several non-infective skin conditions are associated with type 1 and/or type 2 diabetes. Microangiopathy of the dermal vessels is thought to play an important role in the pathogenesis of lesions such as diabetic dermopathy ('shin spots') or necrobiosis lipoidica diabetocorum, The former is relatively common (reportedly present on the legs in up to 10–15% of patients) whereas the latter is rare (<0.3% of patients) and occurs mostly in the 40 to 60 year age group. Whether granuloma annulare is associated with diabetes is unclear, but the strongest evidence suggests a link with type 1 diabetes. The presence of disseminated granuloma annulare or necrobioisis lipoidica should precipate an investigation for the presence of diabetes, in patients who are not known to have diabetes. In addition, there are also a number of skin or nail infections (fungal and bacterial) which are more commonly associated with diabetes, e.g paronychia (Box 26.1).

Diabetic dermopathy

Diabetic dermopathy (also known as spotted leg syndrome or 'shin spots') is characterised by hyper-pigmented, atrophic macules, a few millimetres in diameter, which typically occur as clusters on the shins (Figure 26.1). They are more common in older patients with diabetes, especially those over the age of 50 years (one or two such lesions also occur in up to 3% of non-diabetic people). The spots slowly become well-circumscribed, atrophic, brown, and scaly scars. The usual site is the pretibial region, but forearms, thighs, and bony prominences may be involved. There is no effective treatment and the degree of glycaemic control has no effect on disease severity. The spots tend to resolve over 1–2 years.

Necrobioisis lipoidica diabetocorum

Necrobiosis lipoidica diabeticorum (NLD) is found in only 0.3% of patients with diabetes, but occurs almost exclusively in patients with diabetes, typically in the 40 to 60 year age group, and it is more common in women. NLD appears as bilateral red–brown papules on the anterior surface of the shins (Figure 26.2). The lesions gradually enlarge to form yellow, atrophic plaques with a translucent lustre and stippled with telangiectasia. Ulceration occurs in about 25%. The lesions are partially or completely anaesthetic. The aetiology of NLD is unknown, and treatment options include topical or systemic steroids, antiplatelet therapy, niacinamide, photodynamic therapy, or anti-TNF drugs (eg infliximab). In patients with protracted lesion with ulceration, surgical intervention may be necessary.

Acanthosis nigricans

This skin lesion is typically associated with insulin resistance, and therefore is seen in obese patients, those with lipodystrophy, polycystic ovarian syndrome and in those with rare insulin resistance syndrome due to a defect in insulin receptor or antibodies against the insulin receptor. Typically, acanthosis nigricans appear as dark patches of skin with a thick, velvety

---

> **Box 26.1** Non-ulcerative, non-infective skin conditions associated with diabetes.
>
> Diabetic dermopathy
> Necrobioisis lipoidica diabetocorum
> Acanthosis nigricans
> Diabetic bullae
> Granuloma annulare

Handbook of Diabetes, Fifth Edition. Rudy Bilous, Richard Donnelly, and Iskandar Idris.
© 2021 John Wiley & Sons Ltd. Published 2021 by John Wiley & Sons Ltd.

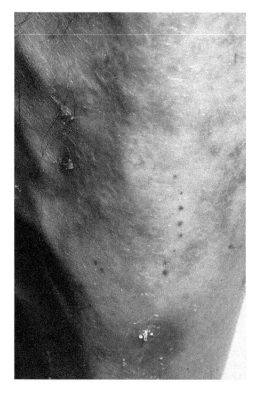

Figure 26.1 Diabetic dermopathy or 'shin spots'. Source: Courtesy of Professor J Verbov, University of Liverpool, Liverpool, UK.

texture, commonly on skin folds and the arm pits, neck, elbows, knees, and knuckles (Figure 26.3). Its development and growth is triggered when Increased circulating insulin levels act via insulin-like growth factor-1 (IGF-1) receptors in the skin to stimulates rapid growth of epidermal skin cells.

Diabetic bullae

Diabetic bullae (or bullosis diabeticorum) are painless blisters which appear spontaneously anywhere on the feet in patients with diabetes (Figure 26.4). The lesions are rare, but occur most often over the toes and heels and seem to be more common among adult males. The blisters can range in size from a few millimetres to centimetres in diameter. There may be an association with neuropathy and retinopathy. Histologically, the lesions usually arise as intra-epidermal blisters containing clear fluid, but occasionally the blisters are sub-epidermal. Immunofluorescent studies have failed to identify a cause. Treatment involves decompression of the bullae by draining its fluid and allowing the roof of the bullae to remain intact as a protective covering.

Granuloma annulare

The extent of the lesion varies from discrete papules to annular erythematous plaques and these have a predilection for the distal extremities. The underlying pathogenesis is unclear but some suggest trauma as a trigger. Treatment

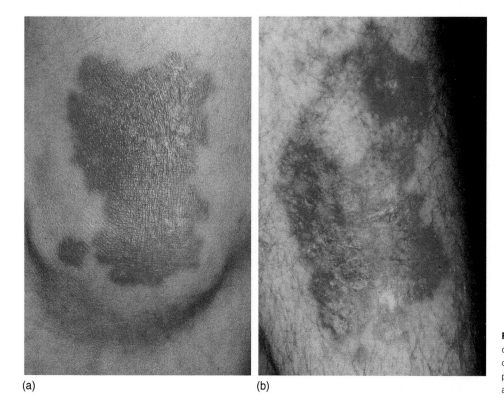

(a)   (b)

Figure 26.2 Necrobiosis lipoidica diabeticorum (NLD). (a) An early lesion on the ankle, and (b) a longstanding patch of NLD illustrating a yellow atrophic appearance with telangiectasia.

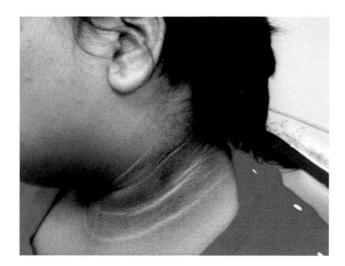

Figure 26.3 In children, acanthosis nigricans is associated with obesity (± type 2 diabetes), insulin resistance, and hyperinsulinaemia. Reproduced with permission from Marimuthu et al. Arch. Dis. Child 2009; 94: 477.

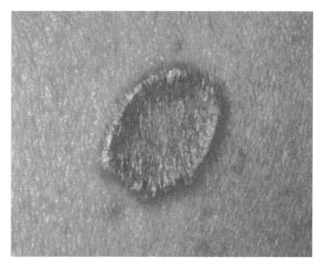

Figure 26.5 Granuloma annulare. Taken from http://healthool.com/granuloma-annulare/.

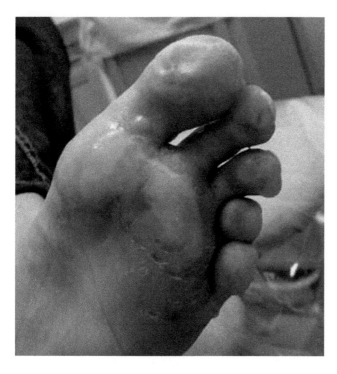

Figure 26.4 Diabetic bullae – blistering of the foot. Reproduced with permission from Bristow. Diab. Metab. Res. Rev. 2008; 24 (Suppl. 1): S84–S89.

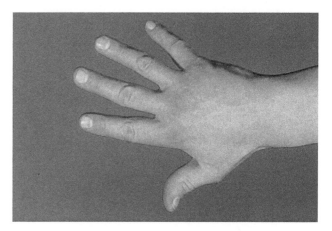

Figure 26.6 Garrod's knuckle pads.

of the localised form of granuloma annulare includes topical steroids but more disseminated lesions are treated by niacinamide or by PUVA therapy (Figure 26.5).

Skin thickening, waxy skin, and stiff joints

The skin is generally thickened in diabetes, probably because of glycation of dermal collagen and cross-linking to form advanced glycation end products (AGEs). Usually, this is clinically insignificant, but the combination of thickened, tight, and waxy skin with limited joint mobility (cheiroarthropathy) is present in 30–40% of type 1 diabetic patients and a third of patients with joint stiffness have waxy, tight skins on the dorsum of the hands. This can lead to stiff and painful fingers. It is important to recognise these changes because of the possible correlation with microvascular complications. Thickening over the dorsum of the fingers is termed 'Garrod's knuckle pads' (Figure 26.6).

A typical sign of the 'diabetic hand syndrome' is the 'prayer sign', where patients are unable to oppose the palmar surfaces of the hand (Figure 26.7), due to limited joint mobility because of thickened and waxy skin.

Dupuytren's contracture occurs in up to half of diabetic patients, especially in the elderly and those with long-standing disease; it often co-exists with cheiroarthropathy (Figure 26.8).

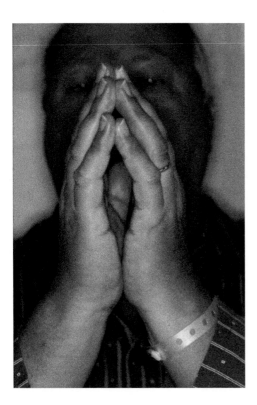

Figure 26.7 The 'prayer sign', another feature of cheiroarthropathy.

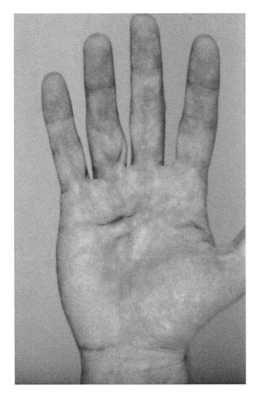

Figure 26.8 Dupuytren's contractors. Courtesy of Dr G Gill, University of Liverpool, Liverpool, UK.

'Trigger finger' occurs when there is intermittent locking of the finger due to stenosing flexor tenosynovitis (Figure 26.9). It is often associated with diabetes. Nodular swelling and thickening of the tendon sheath can often be palpated. It responds to steroid injection. Adhesive capsulitis of the shoulder (more often called 'frozen shoulder') is another non-articular fibrosing disorder that occurs more commonly in patients with diabetes than in the general population; it results in pain and limitation of movement.

Other skin conditions

Various other skin problems are associated with longstanding diabetes, but are not specific to diabetes. These include bacterial infections (e.g. boils and sepsis caused by Staphylococcus aureus), Candida albicans infections (e.g. vulvovaginitis, balanitis, intertrigo, and chronic paronychia) and tinea (dermatophyte fungal infections) (Figure 26.10).

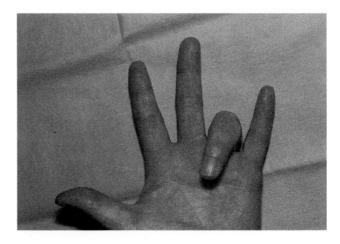

Figure 26.9 Trigger finger in a diabetic patient.

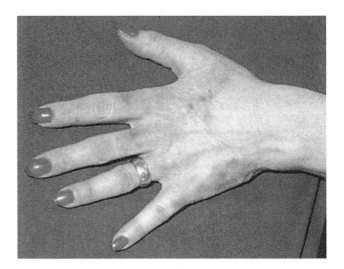

Figure 26.10 Tinea manus, showing the characteristic erythematous, scaly margin.

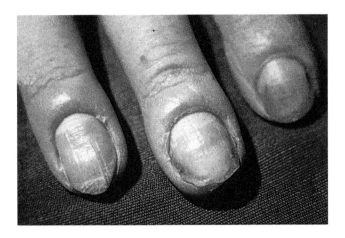

Figure 26.11 Chronic paronychia caused by Candida albicans.

The Sodium glucose transport-2 (SGLT2) inhibitor treatment is associated with an increased risk for developing genitourinary tract infection. Note also the occurrence of neuropathic and ischaemic foot ulcers in diabetes and the dry skin caused by decreased sweating with autonomic neuropathy.

Chronic paronychia presents with swelling and erythema around the nail folds, with a discharge (Figure 26.11). Severe involvement may produce oncholysis. Treatment is by keeping the fingers dry and the use of antifungal drugs; systemic drugs such as terbinafine, as well as topical medications, may be necessary.

CASE HISTORY

A 58-year-old woman with type 2 diabetes of 15 years duration presented to his family doctor with a skin lesion over the front of his left shin and joint stiffness. The plaque lesion had been present for 8–months and was gradually enlarging. It was giving few, if any symptoms. Examination confirmed an 8 cm irregular atrophic patch with yellowish pigmentation, which the family doctor first thought was a fungal infection. There were no other skin rashes, and the feet and lower limb circulation were generally good. Topical anti-fungal cream had no effect and the patient was referred to the dermatologist, who diagnosed Necrobiosis Lipoidica diabeticorum. A punch skin biopsy confirmed a chronic granulomatous dermatitis, typical of NLD. Further examination revealed presence of the prayer sign. This triggered further assessment of microangiopathy risks, which confirmed the presence of diabetic nephropathy (based on increased albumin creatinine ratio and widespread changes of background diabetic retinopathy).

Comment: NLD can be confused with fungal infection. If there is diagnostic uncertainty, a skin biopsy should be performed, as in this case. The differential diagnoses histologically include sarcoid and cutaneous lymphoma. NLD is typical in this age group, and this location; it may occur bilaterally on the legs. Secondary ulceration is not uncommon. The lesion may not improve with better glycaemic control. Rarely, squamous cell carcinoma can arise from NLD. Steroids (topical cream or intra-lesional injection) are the mainstay of treatment, but photodynamic therapy and anti-TNF drugs have been used with some success.

The presence of diabetic cheiroarthropathy may be associated with increased risk of microvascular complications.

LANDMARK TRIALS

Wang YR, et al. The prevalence of diagnosed cutaneous manifestations during ambulatory diabetes visits in the United States, 1998–2002. Dermatology 2006; 212: 229–234.

Horton WB et al. Diabetes Mellitus and the Skin: Recognition and Management of Cutaneous Manifestations. South Med J. 2016; 109: 636–646

Min MS et al. Treatment of recalcitrant granuloma annulare (GA) with adalimumab: A single-center, observational study. J Am Acad Dermatol. 2016; 74(1): 127–33.

Zeichner JA, et al. Treatment of necrobiosis lipoidica diabeticorum with the tumour necrosis factor antagonist etanercept. J. Am. Acad. Dermatol. 2006; 54: 120–121.

Hu S, et al. Treatment of refractory ulcerative necrobiosis lipoidica diabeticorum with infliximab. Arch. Dermatol. 2009; 145: 437–439.

Berking C, et al. Photodynamic therapy of necrobiosis lipoidica – a multicentre study of 18 patients. Dermatology 2009; 218: 136–139.

Statham B, et al. A randomised double–blind comparison of aspirin dipyridamole combination versus placebo in the treatment of necrobiosis lipoidica diabeticorum. Acta. Derm. Venereol. 1981; 61: 270–271.

Jennings MB, et al. Treatment of toe nail onychomycosis with oral terbinafine plus aggressive debridement: IRON-CLAD, a large randomised, open-label, multicentre trial. J. Am. Podiatr. Med. Ass. 2006; 96: 465–473.

KEY WEBSITES

- http://diabetes.webmd.com/guide/skin-problems
- http://www.diabetes.org/type-1-diabetes/skin-complications.jsp
- http://www.telemedicine.org/dm/dmupdate.htm

FURTHER READING

De Macedo GM et al. Skin disorders in diabetes mellitus: an epidemiology and physiopathology review. HYPERLINK "https://www.ncbi.nlm.nih.gov/pubmed/27583022" \o "Diabetology & metabolic syndrome."Diabetol Metab Syndr. 2016; 8(1): 63.

Marimuthu S, et al. Acanthosis nigricans. Arch. Dis. Child 2009; 94: 477.

Erfurt-Berge C et al. Updated results of 100 patients on clinical features and therapeutic options in necrobiosis lipoidica in a retrospective multicentre study. Eur J Dermatol. 2015; 25(6): 595–601.

Matsuoka LY, et al. Spectrum of endocrine abnormalities associated with acanthosis nigricans. Am. J. Med. 1987; 83: 719–725.

Piette EW et al. Granuloma annulare: Pathogenesis, disease associations and triggers, and therapeutic options. J Am Acad Dermatol. 2016; 75(3): 467–79.

Harth W, et al. Topical tacrolimus in granuloma annulare and necrobiosis lipoidica diabeticorum. Br. J. Dermatol. 2004; 150: 792–794.

Bristow IR, et al. Topical and oral combination therapy for toenail onychomycosis: an updated review. J. Am. Podiatr. Med. Ass. 2006; 96: 116–119.

Psychological and psychiatric problems in diabetes

KEY POINTS

- As with any chronic disease diagnosis, children and adults with newly diagnosed diabetes can develop adjustment disorders.
- Adults with both type 1 and type 2 diabetes have around twice the prevalence of depression as the age-matched non-diabetic population. Anxiety is also common and can exacerbate glycaemic control.
- Diabetes distress is now a recognised phenomenon with origins in the communication with health care professionals.

- Cognitive dysfunction can be demonstrated in children and adults with diabetes and is related to chronic hyperglycaemia.
- Hypoglycaemia can cause short-term memory loss but there are no conclusive data relating severe episodes to long-term cognitive dysfunction.
- Eating disorder is a particular problem for girls with type 1 diabetes but abnormal eating behaviours are also common in type 2 diabetes.

Diabetes is associated with increased rates of psychological disorders such as depression and anxiety. In addition, there is over-representation of people with type 2 diabetes in patients with serious mental illnesses. Incidence and prevalence vary with gender, recent or longstanding diagnosis, age of diagnosis, and type of diabetes. There is also a greater understanding of the links between diabetes and cognitive function, with subtle changes in children and young adults and cognitive impairment in the elderly. Over the last decades, the concept of diabetes distress has been proposed. Eating disorders are also more common, in both type 1 and type 2 diabetes. Each of these areas will be dealt with in turn but it is important to recognise that they are often co-related, and it is sometimes hard to categorise patients into a single diagnosis.

Depression and anxiety

A sorrowful personality type in people with diabetes was originally described by Thomas Willis in the 17th century. There is a bidirectional relationship between diabetes and depression and anxiety disorders. Adults with depression are 37% more likely to develop type 2 diabetes, whilst those with established diabetes have an OR of 1.34 for developing incident depression. Estimates of prevalence vary greatly and are usually based on self-administered questionnaires. Consequently, it can be difficult to distinguish between a formal diagnosis of depression and depressive symptoms. About 9% of adults with diabetes have a formal diagnosis of depression, a much wider range has been reported for children (9–45%). Another study diagnosed depressive disorder in 6% of people recently diagnosed with type 1 diabetes and 14% developed worsening symptoms over the subsequent five years. Depressive symptoms are more common at around 30% for children, 12% for adult type 1 (vs ~3% for age matched people without diabetes) and 19% (vs ~11%) for type 2 diabetes.

The associated risk factors for depression in people with diabetes are the same as for the general population (female gender, marital status, childhood adversity, and socio-economic deprivation) but with the addition of more specific, diabetes-related associations. These include insulin use (in type 2 diabetes), the development of complications (particularly foot infections and nephropathy), sexual dysfunction, hypoglycaemia, and poor diabetes control. The possible mechanisms linking the two conditions have been

---

Handbook of Diabetes, Fifth Edition. Rudy Bilous, Richard Donnelly, and Iskandar Idris.
© 2021 John Wiley & Sons Ltd. Published 2021 by John Wiley & Sons Ltd.

Box 27.1 Potential shared (common ground) and diabetes specific mechanisms linking depression and diabetes.

Common ground
1. Overactivity of the immune system and chronic inflammation
2. Dysfunction of the hypothalamic-pituitary-adrenal axis
3. Shared genetics (not a great deal of evidence so far)

Diabetes specific
1. Burden of disease
2. Lifestyle and adherence (depression makes this harder to achieve)
3. Antidepressant medications (no concrete evidence to date)
4. Alterations to brain structure & function secondary to hyper and hypoglycaemia
5. Sleep dysfunction (associated with insulin resistance)
6. Environmental factors (intrauterine (Barker) hypothesis and socio-economic deprivation)

Box 27.2 Depressive symptoms.

Symptoms must be present for at least 2 weeks to make the diagnosis
- Depressed mood most of the day, nearly every day (also anxiety, irritability)
- Loss of interest or enjoyment
- Decreased appetite and weight loss
- Loss of libido
- Insomnia (early morning wakening, initial insomnia or interrupted sleep) or hypersomnia
- Fatigue or loss of energy
- Psychomotor retardation
- Poor concentration
- Reduced self-esteem and confidence
- Thoughts of hopelessness, worthlessness or guilt
- Suicidal ideas or attempts

Box 27.3 Diagnostic tools for the diagnosis of depression.

Primary Care Health Questionnaire (PHQ 9)
Self-reported measure by answering 9 questions relating to depressive symptoms
Correspond to criteria for major depressive disorder
Can use for diagnosis and response to intervention
Highest specificity

Beck Depression Inventory (BDI-11)
21 items self-reporting of somatic and cognitive symptoms over previous 2 weeks

Centre for Epidemiological Studies – Depression Scale (CESD)
20 items assessing depressive symptoms over the last week
Highest sensitivity

Hospital Anxiety and Depression Scale (HADS)
Brief self-report over last week
7 questions around depression; 7 around anxiety
In-patient use

categorised into so-called 'common ground' and diabetes specific (Box 27.1).

Diagnosis of depression can be difficult as many symptoms overlap with those associated with diabetes such as weight change, lethargy, and diminished libido (Box 27.2). Several tools have been developed and meta analysis has suggested that the Primary Care Health Questionnaire (PHQ 9) has the highest specificity and the Centre for Epidemiological Studies – Depression Scale (CESD) the highest sensitivity (Box 27.3). These tools should only be used as part of a structured care programme and not for survey purposes. A simple enquiry asking if the person has felt down or depressed or lost interest should suffice as a basic screening tool.

Anxiety also has a bidirectional relationship with diabetes but is less well studied and has an even greater overlap with diabetes distress (see below). The OR for baseline anxiety with incident diabetes is 1.47 and is associated with being overweight or obese, concurrent cardiovascular disease or symptoms, unhealthy lifestyle behaviours, and sleep disturbance. Of people recently diagnosed with type 1 diabetes 8% were found to have an anxiety disorder; and people with type 1 diabetes diagnosed at an average age of 9 years had a two-and-a-half-fold increased risk of developing an anxiety disorder over 26 years of follow-up. Similar risks have been noted in people with type 2 diabetes but after only 5–6 years follow-up. A meta-analysis of studies in people with diabetes of >16 years duration found a pooled OR of 1.25 (95% CI 1.10, 1.39) for anxiety disorder and symptoms, compared to age and gender matched people without diabetes.

There are few high-quality trials of interventions of psychological therapy or medication in people with diabetes and depression, and even fewer for anxiety. A stepped care plan is recommended for depression and needs to be integrated with educational support to help diabetes management. Mindfulness, motivational interviewing, and cognitive behavioural therapy have all been shown to help. If the depressive symptoms do not improve, they should be combined with medical therapy. SSRIs are recommended as first line as they are well tolerated and have fewer side effects than tricyclics.

Sertraline may have some benefits in terms of glycaemic control and avoidance of weight gain. For anxiety symptoms a combined approach with education is also recommended and there is significant overlap with strategies for diabetes distress (see below). Positive affect approaches improve well-being in the short-term and reduce stress. Psychological interventions have been shown to have only a modest effect on glycaemic control. A meta-analysis of 70 controlled trials involving 14,796 individuals with type 2 diabetes found a pooled mean reduction in HbA1c of −3.7 mmol/mol (0.19%). The greatest benefit was seen with self-help materials, CBT, and counselling.

Diabetes distress

Diabetes distress was first described by the Joslin Clinic in 1995 as 'negative emotional or affective experience resulting from the challenge of living with the demands of diabetes' and is thought to result from a combination of increasing demands on the patient to manage their disease and the development of complications. The incidence has been estimated as 38–48% over the 18 months post diagnosis, and the prevalence as 18–45%. It can be confused with depression and anxiety, there is a shared variance of around 20–30%. Using the Problem Areas in Diabetes (PAID) tool around 20–40% of people with type 1 and type 2 diabetes will experience distress at some time. Associated features are shown in Box 27.4. Although some of the concerns about complications and control could be motivational, the relationship between distress and self care concerns is usually negative.

The development of diabetes distress is thought to be linked to communication, particularly around the time of diagnosis. Patients report that an emphasis on biomedical explanations is unhelpful and many feel that opportunities are missed to explore the relevance of the information to their personal circumstances. They also felt that more time should be spent on problem-solving and identifying goals that are relevant and realistic. Finally, they said their concerns and worries should be better validated and that warnings of future negative medical consequences often exacerbated the problem. The use of language in interactions between members of the diabetes team and people with diabetes and their carers can contribute to diabetes distress. A recent guide on how to avoid negative concepts during consultations has been produced by NHS England following a collaboration between providers and users of diabetes services and is available on their website (see useful websites at the end of this chapter).

Many national guidelines now recommend that symptoms and signs of diabetes distress should be explored on a regular (perhaps annual) basis using PAID or the Diabetes Distress Scale (DDS) tools. Different formats of the DDS are available for type 1 and type 2 diabetes, younger and older people with diabetes, and for carers and parents. However, as for depression and anxiety, these tools are only useful as part of a structured programme addressing some of the communication and educational issues mentioned above. These tools should not be used for survey purposes alone as they may inadvertently contribute to or exacerbate distress. A focus on the professional relationships with the diabetes care team using a person-centred approach incorporating motivational techniques and emotional support is recommended. Care teams need to demonstrate empathy by acknowledging distress, exploration of exacerbating factors, initiation of problem solving and setting of realistic goals, and affirmation of success. Research suggests that some patients respond well to group sessions, particularly if they are facilitated by a non specialist. A minimum of six sessions spread out over 3 or 4 months is suggested. Regrettably, patient surveys suggest that only a minority of services (at least in the UK) have adopted such an approach, and health care professional team surveys imply that part of the reason lies in their lack of confidence, knowledge and skills in these techniques.

Box 27.4 Features of diabetes distress revealed using the PAID tool.

Non-diabetes related
More common in women
More common with lack of social support
More common in ethnic minority groups
Low self esteem
Poor dietary and lifestyle behaviours

Diabetes related
Shorter duration of diabetes
Worries about complications and the future
Feeling of powerlessness
Feeling burnt out with diabetes information especially blood glucose data
Fears of hypoglycaemia
Overwhelmed with management responsibilities and new technologies
Associated with poor glycaemic control

Cognitive changes

Cognitive changes have been described at all stages of diabetes (Box 27.5). Some studies have found that children diagnosed under the age of 5 or 6 years are most at risk of cognitive dysfunction with lower cognitive scores in mental efficiency and IQ, visuospatial ability (copying, solving jigsaws), and executive functioning (Figure 27.1). Meta-analysis has suggested that the effect size is low and did not confirm sustained effects on learning and memory, but did show a greater effect in those with a younger onset of diabetes. Links have been made with number of episodes of severe hypoglycaemia implying that the developing brain might be more vulnerable to insult, but others have found stronger associations with chronic hyperglycaemia. Social

Box 27.5 Cognitive changes seen in people with diabetes.

Type 1 diabetes – lower scores in the following :
Intelligence (IQ)
Academic achievement
Attention span
Psychomotor speed
Executive functioning

All more prominent in those with worse glycaemic control and/or younger age of onset.

Type 2 diabetes – lower scores in the following
Attention span
Psychomotor speed
Executive functioning and planning
Learning
Memory

All more prominent in those with worse glycaemic control

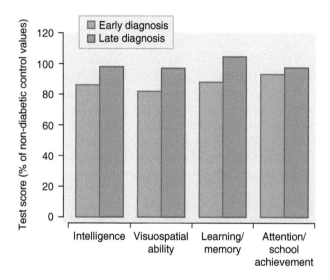

Figure 27.1 The impairment of cognitive ability in 125 adolescents with type 1 diabetes diagnosed at <5 years of age (early diagnosis), compared with those diagnosed at >5 years of age (late diagnosis). From Ryan et al. Pediatrics 1985; 75: 921–927.

factors such as school attendance (which might be affected in those having recurrent hypo- and hyperglycaemia), and home problems (including psychosocial) have to be taken into account and are sometimes neglected in earlier studies.

In the DCCT/EDIC study, those participants with an HbA1c > 73 mmol/mol (8.8%) had a moderate decrease in motor speed and psychomotor efficiency compared to those with a value < 58 mmol/mol (7.4%), but they found no evidence of deterioration over time. The Pittsburgh Study of

97 middle-aged people with type 1 diabetes found a prevalence of cognitive dysfunction of 28%, a similar value to that seen in people without diabetes aged > 85 years, and more than five times that seen in control subjects without diabetes (5%). These workers estimated a doubling in prevalence rates from adolescence based upon previously published data. They suggest that one reason for the difference between the Pittsburgh and DCCT studies may be the age of onset of diabetes; all of the Pittsburgh subjects had onset in childhood, whereas the DCCT subjects were more likely to be diagnosed in early adulthood or late adolescence when brain development is mostly complete.

Cognitive impairment is said to be 1.5–2.5 times more prevalent in adults with type 2 diabetes than age-matched controls. Older adults with type 2 diabetes, experiencing chronic hyperglycaemia may have deficits in psychomotor tasks, attention, learning and memory (Box 27.5). MRI studies have shown a greater loss in grey matter in the cerebrum, putamen, medial temporal, and frontal lobes. There is also an increased prevalence of small vessel disease and lacunar infarcts. Dementia overall is 73% more likely in people with type 2 diabetes, with a 56% increase in Alzheimer's disease and a 1.27-fold increase in vascular dementia. The reasons are probably multiple: microvascular damage to central nervous system neurones in response to chronic hyperglycaemia, macrovascular (cerebrovascular) disease, amyloid deposits as in Alzheimer's (Apo ε 4 deficiency), and insulin resistance. There are no data conclusively linking hypoglycaemia alone to cognitive dysfunction in adults with diabetes, and, like depression, the relationship is likely to be bidirectional – those with dementia are more prone to hypoglycaemia due to forgetfulness with therapy or diet, whilst severe hypoglycaemia may also damage the ageing brain.

Severe Mental Illness

Severe mental illness (SMI) comprises major psychiatric disorders including schizophrenia, psychotic depression, and bipolar disorder. People with SMI are at increased risk of developing type 2 diabetes (Table 27.1), and the prevalence

Table 27.1 Relative risks (95% CI) for type 2 diabetes in people with serious mental illness from different ethnic groups in London.

Ethnicity	Age 18 – 34 yrs	35 – 54 yrs	>55 yrs
White British	**8.77** (4.69,16.40)	**2.54** (2.13, 3.02)	**1.08** (0.96, 1.21)
Indian	**5.20** (2.01, 13.41)	**1.78** (1.36, 2.34)	**1.02** (0.99, 1.53)
Pakistani	**4.54** (1.49, 13.99)	**1.81** (1.33, 2.47)	**1.11** (0.88, 1.39)
Bangladeshi	**6.18** (4.62, 8.28)	**1.71** (1.48, 1.98)	**1.12** (1.03, 1.23)
Black Caribbean	**7.32** (3.66, 14.63)	**2.06** (1.74, 2.44)	**1.04** (0.94, 1.15)
Black African	**3.00** (1.34, 6.73)	**1.85** (1.48, 2.31)	**0.99** (0.81, 1.22)

Data from 189 GP practices. Adjusted for gender, area deprivation level and anti-psychotic medications. Adapted from Das-Munshi et al Diabetic Medicine 2017; 34: 916-24 with permission.

of diabetes in people with SMI is 10–15%, a rate 2–3 times higher than that seen in the matched general population. Up to 70% of cases of type 2 diabetes in people with SMI may be undiagnosed. This increase in risk for type 2 diabetes is likely to be multifactorial. People with SMI are more likely to be sedentary, smoke, and to have a diet higher in saturated fat and refined sugars and lower in fruit and vegetables than the general population. There are also likely to be genetic factors. Both SMI and type 2 diabetes are highly heritable, and a number of genes have been identified which are associated with an increased risk of both conditions. Direct metabolic effects of SMI such as abnormalities of the hypothalamic–pituitary–adrenal axis may also play a part, and the metabolic effects of anti-psychotic medications including weight gain are also likely to be contributory. People with SMI have poorer outcomes from their diabetes, with higher rates of microvascular and macrovascular complications and a higher mortality rate when compared with people with type 2 diabetes without SMI. In spite of this, they are less likely to be screened for microvascular and macrovascular complications, less likely to be prescribed cardiovascular preventative medication, and less likely to receive diabetes self-management education. It is therefore important that services are designed to consider the specific needs of people with SMI. For example, lifestyle education programmes which encompass the principles of dietary modification and increased physical activity have been shown to be deliverable in people with SMI, and are effective in reducing weight and improving cardiovascular risk factors. Pharmacological agents such as metformin and orlistat may be helpful in mitigating weight gain associated with the use of anti-psychotic medications. A key problem is often the fragmented care that people are offered, an integrated approach with multidisciplinary involvement of diabetes and mental health care professionals is ideal but all too often unavailable.

Eating disorders

Girls with type 1 diabetes are 2.4 times more likely to have a clinical eating disorder and 1.9 times more likely to engage in subclinical disordered eating behaviours. These figures are estimates based upon definitions that do not take account of the fundamental elements of diabetes care which requires balancing diet and insulin. There is also a considerable overlap with depression, anxiety, and diabetes distress. Despite these confounding factors, it seems that bulimic behaviours are more common in type 1 diabetes, but there is no increased risk of anorexia nervosa. Notwithstanding, the consequences are severe with an estimated 35% 10-year mortality in young women with diabetes and a clinical eating disorder diagnosis.

Insulin omission behaviours are much more common (20–25% in some surveys) and are exhibited by both sexes (although still more common in girls and women). The

long-term effects of these behaviours are unclear, but they do seem to persist in the medium term and are associated with poorer glycaemic control, more frequent episodes of DKA, and increased microvascular complications. There is thought to be a three-fold increased mortality in young women with these behaviours.

In adults with type 2 diabetes a small increase in binge eating disorders has been described. For children and young adults, a much greater proportion show disordered eating behaviours and clinical eating disorders compared to their age and gender matched controls with type 1 diabetes.

The causes are multifactorial. The societal pressures to achieve and maintain a 'perfect' body image are the same as for all young people and do not explain the observed increase in people with diabetes. Many youngsters with newly diagnosed diabetes lose weight beforehand and then gain it after insulin is initiated and this may lead to an association of the diabetes onset (and all of its stress) and body weight. Young people soon realise that omitting insulin does not cause an immediate medical crisis and can avoid weight gain with eating so there is no requirement for calorie restriction. Omitting insulin may be a way of 'regaining control'. Carbohydrate counting and dietary awareness may induce a preoccupation with food. The burdensome nature of diabetes, the need to monitor blood glucose, the unpredictability of glycaemia, and the need to balance treatment, exercise, and social life all pose an increased risk for the adoption of challenging dietary behaviours.

The use of routine screening tools for the detection of eating disorders in people with diabetes is not recommended because of the potential of encouraging abnormal eating behaviours. They also lack any diabetes specific context.

There is no specific therapy for people with diabetes and eating disorder, but a multi disciplinary and multi specialty approach is even more important in these complex cases of established eating disorder and type 1 diabetes than for other psychological problems. Less severe disordered eating behaviours respond to the types of interventions that are used for alleviating diabetes distress.

Published guidance.

Both NICE and the ADA have published guidance on the detection and management of psychological problems in people with diabetes. The detailed recommendations for children and young adults in the UK are reproduced in Box 27.6. For adults, NICE suggests that diabetes teams should be alert to the possibility of the development of depression and/or anxiety and have appropriate skills for their initial management. Both guidelines stress the importance of the multidisciplinary and multi specialist approach.

Box 27.6 NICE Guidance for the detection and management of psychological and social problems in children and young adults.

Diabetes teams should be aware that children and young people with type 1 diabetes have a greater risk of emotional and behavioural difficulties.

Offer children and young people with type 1 diabetes and their family members or carers (as appropriate) emotional support after diagnosis, which should be tailored to their emotional, social, cultural and age-dependent needs.

Assess the emotional and psychological wellbeing of young people with type 1 diabetes who present with frequent episodes of diabetic ketoacidosis (DKA).

Be aware that a lack of adequate psychosocial support has a negative effect on various outcomes, including blood glucose control in children and young people with type 1 diabetes, and that it can also reduce their self-esteem.

Offer children and young people with type 1 diabetes and their family members or carers (as appropriate) timely and ongoing access to mental health professionals with an understanding of diabetes because they may experience psychological problems (such as anxiety, depression, behavioural and conduct disorders and family conflict) or psychosocial difficulties that can impact on the management of diabetes and wellbeing.

For the treatment of depression and antisocial behaviour and conduct disorders in children and young people with type 1 diabetes see the NICE guidelines on depression in children and young people and antisocial behaviour and conduct disorders in children and young people.

Diabetes teams should have appropriate access to mental health professionals to support them in psychological assessment and the delivery of psychosocial support.

Offer children and young people with type 1 diabetes who have behavioural or conduct disorders, and their family members or carers (as appropriate), access to appropriate mental health professionals.

Offer specific family-based behavioural interventions, such as behavioural family systems therapy, if there are difficulties with diabetes-related family conflict.

Consider a programme of behavioural intervention therapy or behavioural techniques for children and young people with type 1 diabetes in whom there are concerns about psychological wellbeing in order to improve:
- health-related quality of life – for example, counselling or cognitive behavioural therapy (CBT), including CBT focused on quality of life
- adherence to diabetes treatment – for example, motivational interviewing or multisystemic therapy
- blood glucose control in children and young people with high HbA1c levels (HbA1c above 69 mmol/mol [8.5%]) – for example, multisystemic therapy.

Offer screening for anxiety and depression to children and young people with type 1 diabetes who have persistently suboptimal blood glucose control.

Diabetes teams should be aware that children and young people with type 1 diabetes may develop anxiety and/or depression, particularly when difficulties in self-management arise in young people and children who have had type 1 diabetes for a long time.

Refer children and young people with type 1 diabetes and suspected anxiety and/or depression promptly to child mental health professionals.

Diabetes teams should be aware that children and young people with type 1 diabetes, in particular young women, have an increased risk of eating disorders. For more guidance on assessing and managing eating disorders, see the NICE guideline on eating disorders.

Be aware that children and young people with type 1 diabetes who have eating disorders may have associated difficulties with:
- suboptimal blood glucose control (both hyperglycaemia and hypoglycaemia)
- symptoms of gastroparesis.

For children and young people with type 1 diabetes in whom eating disorders are identified, offer joint management involving their diabetes team and child mental health professionals.

From NG18 Diabetes (type 1 and type 2) in children and young adults: diagnosis and management. With permission.

CASE HISTORY

A 17-year-old girl with type 1 diabetes of 6 years' duration was referred to our clinic for further management of her insulin pump therapy. Her family had bought the pump after a local appeal for funds because her diabetes control was so erratic, and she had had multiple admissions for DKA. She was needle phobic and admitted she disliked blood glucose tests so much that she only performed them very occasionally. She had to spend an hour or so before each pump cannula change in order to will herself to insert it. Consequently, she changed the cannulae infrequently. Her BMI was 19 kg/m² and her HbA1c was 108 mmol/mol (12%). She had poor dentition with active periodontal disease, enamel ero-

sion, and caries. She did not wish to see the dietitian. Interrogating her pump showed that she did not give mealtime boluses often and there were occasions when the pump was disconnected for long periods.

When this was pointed out she became very defensive and left the clinic. It later transpired that she was very concerned about her body image and was worried about the potential for weight gain with glycaemic correction. She disconnected the pump when she went to night clubs because she did not want others to notice it and it would not fit under her clothes discretely. For all these reasons, an agreement was reached to discontinue CSII on safety grounds. She agreed to a single daily injection of long-acting and occasional short-acting analogues. Her glycaemic control remains poor with HbA1c levels above 97 mmol/mol (11%). She would not acknowledge any problem with diet and declined to see a psychologist.

Comment: This girl has a difficult combination of needle phobia and almost certain eating disorder, probably at the anorexia part of the spectrum, although her poor dentition raises the possibility of bulimia (stomach acid corrodes tooth enamel). Insulin pump therapy is fraught with hazard in this situation; without regular blood monitoring, it is hard to set basal rates and detect metabolic decompensation which can occur more quickly on CSII. She is at risk of this because she is not changing the cannula frequently, raising the likelihood of local infection which will block insulin absorption, and she is disconnecting the pump for long periods. For these reasons, CSII had to be discontinued on safety grounds. Addressing the eating disorder and needle phobia requires active engagement from the patient and until she was willing to do this, there was little prospect of any improvement in her diabetes. At present, she attends clinic once or twice a year on her terms. She has since undergone two successful pregnancies although one baby was small for gestational age, and the other large. Her control was much better during the pregnancies but has since returned to her previous level and she continues to engage only infrequently.

KEY WEBSITE

- www.nice.org.uk (NG 17 and NG 18)
- SIGN Guidelines: www.SIGN.ac.uk
- ADA www.diabetes.org
- Use of language: www.england.nhs.uk/publication/language-matters-language-and-diabetes

---

FURTHER READING

American Diabetes Association. Standards of medical care in diabetes – 2020. Diabetes Care 2020; 43: Suppl 1: S163–82

Broadley MM, Zaremba N, Andrew B et al. 25 years of psychological research investigating disordered eating in people with diabetes: what have we learnt. Diabetic Med 2020; 37: 401–8

Cukierman T, Gerstein HC, Williamson JD. Cognitive decline and dementia in diabetes – systematic overview of prospective observational studies. Diabetologia 2005; 48: 2460–2469.

Das-Munshi J, Ashworth M, Dewey ME et al. Type 2 diabetes mellitus in people with severe mental illness: inequalities by ethnicity and age. Cross sectional analysis of 588,408 records from the UK. Diabetic Med 2017; 34: 916–24.

Holt RIG, de Groot M, Hill Golden S. Diabetes and depression. Curr Diab Rep 2014; 14:

Kodl C, Seaquist ER. Cognitive dysfunction and diabetes mellitus. Endo Rev 2008; 29: 494–511.

Kubiak T, Priesterroth L, Barnard-Kelly KD. Psychosocial aspects of diabetes technology. Diabetic Med 2020; 37: 448–54

Nunley KA, Rosano C, Ryan CM et al. Clinically relevant cognitive impairment in middle-aged adults with childhood-onset type 1 diabetes. Diabetes Care 2015; 38: 1768–76

Pouwer F, Schram MT, Iversen MM et al. How 25 years of psychosocial research has contributed to a better understanding the links between depression and diabetes. Diabetic Med 2020; 37: 383–92

Skinner TC, Joensen L, Parkin T. Twenty-five years of diabetes distress research. Diabetic Med 2020; 37: 393–400

Smith KJ, Beland M, Clyde M et al. Association of diabetes with anxiety: A systematic review and meta- analysis. J Psychosom Res 2013; 74: 89–99

Smith KJ, Deschendes SS, Schmitz N. Investigating the longitudinal association of diabetes and anxiety: a systematic review and meta-analysis. Diabetic Med 2018; 35: 677–93

Winkley K, Upsher R, Stahl D et al. Psychological interventions to improve glycaemic control in patients with type 2 diabetes: a systematic review and meta-analysis BMJ Open Diabetes Res Care 2020; 8: e001150.doi.10.1136/bmjdrc-2019-001150

Young-Hyman D, de Groot M, Hill-Briggs F et al. Psychosocial care for people with diabetes: a position statement of the American Diabetes Association. Diabetes Care 2016; 39: 2126–40

Part 3

The spectrum and organisation of diabetes care

Chapter 28

Intercurrent situations that affect diabetes control

KEY POINTS

- Regular exercise is a key component of good diabetes self-management, although the impact on HbA1c is modest; walking is the most practical form of exercise.
- Long-term mortality is lower among people with diabetes who take regular exercise.
- Drugs that may worsen hyperglycaemia include steroids, diuretics and β-blockers. These may unmask type 2 diabetes at times of concomitant illness, e.g. chest infection.
- Infections are common in patients with diabetes and may be asymptomatic.
- Managing patients with diabetes during planned or emergency surgical procedures requires care to avoid hypo- or hyperglycaemia.
- Risk stratification of patients with diabetes undergoing surgery helps guide their management in the peri and postoperative period.

Exercise

Regular exercise can be considered as a preventative measure in people at high risk of developing type 2 diabetes, whereas it is widely accepted as an important component of therapy for established disease. In type 1 diabetes, exercise is also important for long-term cardiovascular health, but poses unique problems for the patient who has to balance insulin dose and energy intake and expenditure.

During aerobic exercise in people without diabetes, insulin secretion from the pancreas is suppressed and glucagon release is enhanced. This leads to increased glucose release from the liver, initially from glycogenolysis, and subsequently from gluconeogenesis. As exercise continues or during more intense anaerobic exercise, other counter-regulatory hormones are released leading to increased lipolysis, which can provide an energy source directly as well as contributing to gluconeogensis. Because of this balance of responses, blood glucose levels remain stable. Glycogen stores in the liver and muscle are replenished after exercise and this process may take up to 24 hours depending upon its' duration and intensity.

In type 1 diabetes, insulin levels are not suppressed and may even be increased if it is injected into an exercising limb or secondary to increased subcutaneous blood flow. Moreover, glucagon responses can be blunted, particularly in those individuals with a duration of diabetes >5 years. Both of these factors increase the risk of hypoglycaemia. With more intense or prolonged exercise, the catecholamine and cortisol response tend to cause hyperglycaemia. Delayed hypoglycaemia may occur during the period post-exercise. Hypoglycaemia is much less of a problem in people with type 2 diabetes unless they are insulin deficient, but hyperglycaemia may occur with prolonged exercise.

The person with type 1 diabetes therefore has to take into account their blood glucose level at the start of exercise; the likely duration and intensity of the exercise; the quantity, timing, and quality of their last carbohydrate intake; and the quantity, timing and type of their last insulin dose. Dealing with all of these variables is complicated and many patients find them a real barrier to undertaking regular exercise. Many have to embark on a guided path of trial and error in order to discover the best regimen. Nonetheless, the benefits are well established, and all patients should be encouraged to exercise regularly. There are many examples of athletes and sportspersons with type 1 diabetes that have competed at the highest level.

Handbook of Diabetes, Fifth Edition. Rudy Bilous, Richard Donnelly, and Iskandar Idris.
© 2021 John Wiley & Sons Ltd. Published 2021 by John Wiley & Sons Ltd.

Current guidance suggests that blood glucose levels should be between 5.0 and 13.9 mmol/L at the start of exercise. Below this range, extra carbohydrate should be taken (10–20g is suggested); above 14.0 mmol/L a blood or urine ketone test is recommended and moderate exercise is discouraged if the blood level is >1.5 mmol/L. Continuous glucose monitoring may help and certainly can provide reassurance for patients, particularly in the overnight period following exercise. However, there are potential problems with the lag response of interstitial glucose concentrations during exercise, as well as pootential physical displacement of the sensor.

Moderate exercise up to 30 minutes should require a modest increase in carbohydrate intake of between 10 – 20g/hour, for periods over 1 hour the requirement is likely to be 75 – 90g/hour. For endurance sports or mixed intensity exercise (such as team games) insulin adjustment is also necessary (see below).

Exercise pre-meal or after an overnight fast is least likely to lead to hypo or hyperglycaemia, but this timing is not always convenient. Post-prandial exercise requires either an increase in mealtime carbohydrate, or a reduction in insulin dose, or both. Observational studies suggest that exercise within an hour of a meal is least likely to cause hypoglycaemia. There are also data to suggest that low glycaemic index (GI) carbohydrates are associated with less hypoglycaemia. It is also important to consider the other components of the meal since fat and protein may slow carbohydrate absorption; and the time of day. Hypoglycaemia post-exercise is more of a problem in the afternoon and evening than in the morning, possibly as a result of higher circulating levels of counter regulatory hormones earlier in the day (the dawn phenomenon).

Insulin dose adjustment for exercise is easier for those on CSII (see Chapter 10) than on multiple daily injections (MDI) because of the ability to vary the basal or background insulin level on an hourly basis, and the lack of a subcutaneous depot of long-acting insulin. Reductions in basal insulin infusion rates of 20–50%, 30–60 minutes beforehand are suggested. A 20% reduction in basal insulin dose the night before planned moderate exercise is suggested for those on MDI. A 25 – 75% reduction in pre-meal dose is suggested for those undertaking post-prandial exercise for both CSII and MDI. In order to prevent delayed hypoglycaemia, particularly if the exercise has been performed later in the day or evening, a reduction in overnight basal insulin infusion, or night time long-acting insulin, of around 20% together with a night-time snack of low GI carbohydrate is recommended.

Individuals undertaking endurance exercise, such as triathlons or long-distance running, will need specialist advice. For all forms of exercise in type 1 diabetes there is helpful web-based guidance (www.runsweet.com).

Exercise has many benefits for people with both types of diabetes (Box 28.1). In particular, there are improvements in insulin sensitivity (Figure 28.1), glycaemia (Figure 28.2), and mortality (Figure 28.3). Meta-analysis has shown a reduction

---

Box 28.1 Benefits of aerobic activity.

Cellular
Increased mitochondrial density
Increase in oxidative enzymes
Improved immune function
Increased insulin sensitivity

Microvascular
Increased compliance and reactivity

Cardiovascular
Increased cardiac output
Lowered blood pressure
Reduced mortality
Respiratory
Improved lung function and capacity

Metabolic
Reductions in HbA1c
Reduced LDL cholesterol
Increased HDL cholesterol
Reduced triglycerides

---

in HbA1c of 5–6 mmol/mol (0.5%) for regular combined anaerobic and aerobic exercise. The greatest benefit in cardiovascular risk factor reduction is seen with sustained, regular, and supervised combined aerobic and resistance exercise programmes. For older people with diabetes, flexibility and balance exercise (such as Yoga and Tai Chi) is also important, although there is less evidence in terms of improvement in cardiovascular risk factors. The ADA has produced recommendations for exercise, and these have been widely adopted (Box 28.2). Unfortunately, surveys of people with diabetes show that very few (<50% in some studies in the UK) are undertaking exercise on a regular basis. Education, provision, encouragement, and engagement are critical.

Drugs

Numerous drugs can affect diabetic control and cause hyper– or hypoglycaemia by interfering with insulin secretion or action or both, or by interacting with diabetes therapies (Table 28.1). Hyperglycaemia can be caused or worsened by many drugs. Oral contraceptives rarely worsen diabetic control; the risks of hyperglycaemia are highest with the now obsolete high–dose oestrogen pills, combined pills that contain the progestogen levonorgestrel, and in women with a history of gestational diabetes. High-dose thiazide diuretics (e.g. 5 mg/day of bendroflumethiazide) cause insulin resistance and impair insulin secretion, whereas lower dosages (2.5 mg/day bendroflumethiazide), which are still effective in controlling blood pressure, do not. Diabetogenic drugs that damage the β cell include pentamidine (an antiprotozoal agent) and cyclosporin.

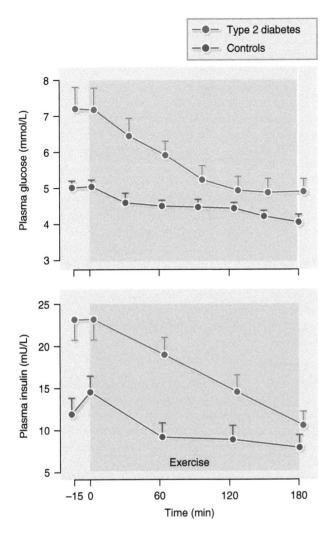

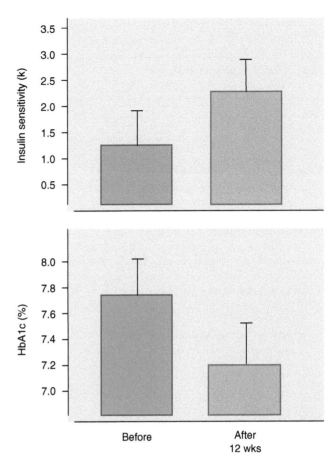

Figure 28.1 Changes in plasma glucose and insulin concentrations during prolonged low-intensity exercise in non-obese patients with type 2 diabetes. The exercise (30–35% of maximal) was performed after an overnight fast. The fall in endogenous insulin secretion diminishes the risk of hypoglycaemia during exercise in type 2 diabetes. From Devlin et al. Diabetes 1987; 36: 434–439.

Steroids can induce diabetes in those at risk and will certainly exacerbate glycaemia in people with established diabetes. It is estimated that 10% of UK hospital in-patients are prescribed steroids, the majority for respiratory disease. The goals of treatment are to prevent symptoms of thirst, polyuria and lethargy and current guidelines recommend a target blood glucose range of 6–10 mmol/L (although this can be relaxed in the context of frailty, multiple co-morbidities, or terminal illness). The physiological equivalence of prescribed steroids is around 20 mg hydrocortisone (4–5 mg prednisolone) per day. Any prescription in excess of this dose is likely to increase blood glucose. Monitoring of capillary blood glucose is essential, once daily in those deemed to be at risk and at least four times daily in those with known diabetes. The duration of glucocorticoid action ranges from 8 hours

Figure 28.2 Progressive resistance exercise training, supervised over 12 weeks (three sessions per week), leads to increases in insulin sensitivity and decreased HbA1c in patients with type 2 diabetes. Adapted from Misra et al. Diabetes Care 2008; 1282–1287.

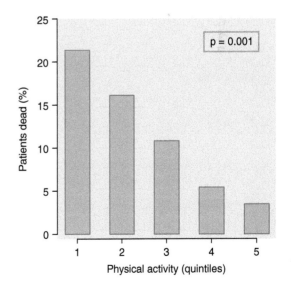

Figure 28.3 Proportion of men who died during a 7-year follow-up period among 548 patients with type 1 diabetes, stratified according to their physical activity quintile. Quintile cut-offs were 398, 398–1000, 1000–2230, 2230–4228 and more than 4228 kcal/week. From Moy et al. Am J Epidemiol 1993; 137: 74–81.

(hydrocortisone), 16–36 hours (prednisolone) and 18–54 hours (methylprednisolone, dexamethasone and betamethasone). The peak glycaemic action is 4–8 hours after oral dosing (shorter if intravenous).

Box 28.2 Recommendations for exercise for people with diabetes.

1. Adults with diabetes should engage in 150 minutes of moderate – vigorous activity per week spread over 3 days. Ideally there should be no more than 2 consecutive days with no activity
2. In addition, there should be 2 – 3 sessions per week of resistance activity on non-consecutive days
3. Children and young adults should participate in 60 minutes per day of moderate – vigorous aerobic exercise, and undertake muscle and bone strengthening exercise 3 times a week
4. Older adults should consider flexibility exercises and balance training 2 – 3 times a week
5. Supervised, regular, sustained and combined training programmes are recommended for maximum benefit

Adapted from Colberg et al Diabetes Care 2016; 39: 2065–79.

Table 28.1 Drugs that may exacerbate or provoke hyperglycaemia.

Hormonal preparations
Corticosteroids
High dose oestrogens
Gonadorelin analogues
Somatostatin analogues (in type 2 diabetes)
Growth hormone

Cardiovascular therapies
High dose thiazides
Loop diuretics
Non-selective β-adrenoceptor blocking agents
Statins

β$_2$ adrenoceptor agonists
Salbutamol
Ritodrine

Anti-psychotic agents
Clozapine
Olanzapine
Quetiapine
Risperidone

HAART
Anti-rejection therapies
Cyclosporine
Sirolimus
Tacrolimus

Others
Fluoroquinolones
Pentamidine
Diazoxide
Streptozotocin
Isotretinoin

For newly provoked hyperglycaemia or for people with diabetes on diet and/or metformin, a short acting sulfonylurea such as gliclazide may be enough to control blood glucose. If the patient is insulin naive, then an initial dose of 10 units NPH is suggested, given at the same time as the steroids. If they are already on insulin, then an increase of up to 40% of their usual dose may be required. The increase should be continued for up to 24 hours after the steroid course is complete. For long-term steroid use, the insulin increase may need to be sustained and gradually tapered as the steroid dose is reduced.

Several drugs apart from sulfonylureas, glinides and insulin can cause or exacerbate hypoglycaemia. Important examples are alcohol, sulphamethoxazole (combined with trimethoprim in co-trimoxazole), quinine, mefloquine, non-selective β-adrenoceptor blocking agents, aspirin and paracetamol (acetaminophen) in overdosage; and the numerous drugs that enhance the action of sulfonylureas (e.g. probenecid, sulphonamides, monoamine oxidase inhibitors, chloramphenicol, fluconazole). (See also Chapter 8)

Infections

Diabetes can be associated with a wide range of infections (Box 28.3), some of which are more frequent than in the general population such as urinary tract infections. Others occur almost exclusively in subjects with diabetes (e.g. malignant otitis externa) or run a different or more aggressive course in the host with diabetes (e.g. respiratory tract infections). Defects in immunity in diabetes may explain the susceptibility to infection, including impaired polymorphonuclear leukocyte function. Other contributory causes in some patients include frequent hospitalisation, delayed wound healing, and concomitant chronic kidney disease.

About 25% of women with diabetes have asymptomatic bacteriuria (this is four times more common than in the

---

Box 28.3 Classification of infections in diabetes mellitus.

Common infections with increased incidence in patients with diabetes:
- Urinary tract infections
- Respiratory tract infections
- Soft tissue infections

Infections predominantly occurring in patients with diabetes:
- Malignant otitis externa
- Necrotizing fasciitis
- Fournier's gangrene
- Emphysematous infections
- Cholecystitis
- Perinephric abscess
- Foot infections

population without diabetes). *Escherichia coli* is the most common pathogen. Urinary tract infections (UTI) may be asymptomatic or present with dysuria, frequency or urgency (lower UTI, cystitis); or flank pain, fever and vomiting (upper UTI, pyelonephritis). Perinephric abscess and renal papillary necrosis are rare complications of upper UTI and may be more common in people with diabetes.

Respiratory infections caused by certain micro-organisms, including *Staphylococcus aureus*, gram-negative bacteria, *Mycobacterium tuberculosis,* and Mucor, are more common in people with diabetes. Respiratory infection with Streptococcus, Legionella, and influenza virus is associated with increased morbidity and mortality in people with diabetes. Cough and fever are the usual presenting complaints, although ketoacidosis can be the first manifestation. People with diabetes seem to be more prone to serious infection with the Sars Cov-2 virus (COVID-19), representing up to 25% of patients requiring ventilation in the UK. Mortality is also greater and seems linked to ethnicity and co-existing obesity, hypertension, and cardiovascular disease. The reasons are unclear, although the impaired immune responses caused by hyperglycaemia, and the up-regulated cytokine activity seen in those with microvascular complications may play a part.

Deep soft tissue infections with bacteria (e.g. pyomyositis, a muscle abscess caused by *Staph. aureus* that occurs after trauma and haematoma) and fungi (e.g. cutaneous mucormycosis) are more common in diabetes. Polymicrobial necrotising fasciitis is more common in people with diabetes. A particular type of perineal fasciitis called Fournier's gangrene is also more common and has been associated with the use of SGLT2 inhibitors in some case reports. This condition affects predominantly older men and starts with pain in the pubic area which rapidly develops into a necrotising lesion involving the genitalia and anterior abdominal wall. Early and sometimes extensive surgery is required together with broad spectrum antibiotics.

Some rare infections occur predominantly in patients with diabetes. Malignant otitis externa is a life-threatening condition in elderly patients with diabetes, usually due to *Pseudomonas aeruginosa* (Figure 28.4). Patients present with ear discharge, severe pain, and hearing impairment, with oedema, cellulitis, and polypoid granulation of the auditory canal. Cranial osteomyelitis and intracranial spread of infection may occur.

Rhinocerebral mucormycosis is a rare infection caused by fungi of the Rhizopus or Mucor species, which grow best in acid media; ketoacidosis is a predisposing factor. About 50% of cases are in diabetic patients. The fungi have a predilection to invade blood vessels. Onset may be with nasal stuffiness, epistaxis, and facial and ocular pain. A characteristic black necrotic eschar (scab) occurs on the nasal turbinates or palate (Figure 28.5). Complications include cavernous sinus thrombosis, cranial palsies, visual loss, frontal lobe abscesses,

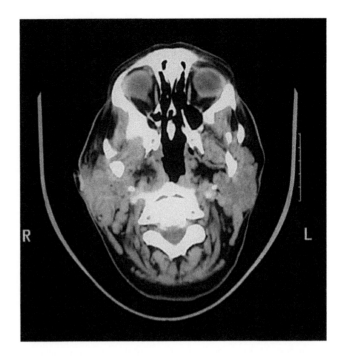

Figure 28.4 Necrotizing ('malignant') otitis externa. This magnetic resonance scan shows extensive soft tissue necrosis and swelling on the right, with early involvement of the underlying bone. The patient was a 28-year-old woman with long-standing diabetes. Courtesy of Professor G Williams, University of Bristol, Bristol, UK.

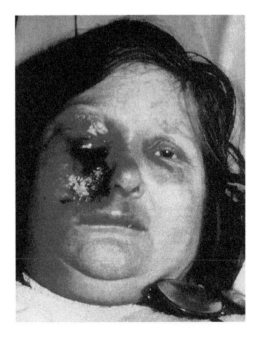

Figure 28.5 Rhinocerebral mucomycosis. Typical appearance, in a 45-year-old woman with poorly controlled type 1 diabetes. Periorbital and facial swelling had been present 3–4 days before admission. Major reconstructive surgery was required. From Rupp. N Engl J Med 1995; 333: 564.

and carotid artery or jugular vein thrombosis, which causes hemiparesis. Mortality is very high.

Many of these serious infections will cause stress related hyperglycaemia which will likely require intravenous insulin, at least in the acute phase. Once the patient is well enough to eat and drink then an MDI regimen is likely to provide the most flexible approach. Regular blood glucose monitoring 4–7 times a day will be required.

Enteral feeding

Stroke is a common complication of diabetes, and hyperglycaemia may occur de novo at presentation. The increasing use of enteral feeding in patients with stroke and/or cognitive impairment poses management challenges for teams looking after people with diabetes. Regular blood glucose monitoring is essential to guide treatment and recent UK guidelines suggest a target range of 6–12 mmol/L. In people with type 2 diabetes on diet and/or metformin alone, then metformin solution is available and can be given before the feed starts and at intervals thereafter. If this does not suffice, or the person is on multiple oral agents, then insulin will be required in a regimen similar to that used for steroid therapy (see above). NPH or premixed insulin should be given at the start of the infusion and after 4–8 hours if required. For those on insulin therapy such as MDI, then basal insulin should be continued and boluses of short acting insulin given at the beginning, and at intervals during the feed. Multidisciplinary team consultation between elderly care, dietetic and diabetes teams is essential.

Surgery and critical intercurrent illness

The physiological stress associated with surgery causes secretion of counter-regulatory hormones such as cortisol and catecholamines, which decrease insulin sensitivity and inhibit insulin release. In insulin-deficient patients, this may cause significant hyperglycaemia and ketosis. In general, the metabolic disturbance is more pronounced in people with type 1 diabetes. Hypoglycaemia is the other major risk of surgery. After preoperative assessment to confirm fitness for anaesthesia, optimisation of control (recommended HbA1c <69 mmol/mol (<8.5%) and liaison with the surgical and anaesthetic teams; management plans depend on whether or not the patient is insulin treated and the nature and duration of surgery (Boxes 28.4 and 28.5).

Management of diabetes throughout the perioperative period depends upon the patient's background therapy and glycaemic control; the nature, timing, and duration of the procedure, and the likely speed of recovery in terms of regaining normal dietary intake (Box 28.6 and Figure 28.6)

Box 28.4 Patients with diabetes undergoing surgery, endoscopy or interventional radiological procedure: general principles of management.

- Good glycaemic control before and after the procedure reduces risk of complications.
- The main risk to anaesthetised or sedated patients is unrecognised hypoglycaemia.
- Put patients first on morning, or first on afternoon list where possible.
- Anaesthetic and procedural management should minimise risks of vomiting, anorexia and sedation.
- When emergency procedures are required, resuscitation, fluid replacement and correction of hyper- or hypoglycaemia should be addressed preoperatively.
- Careful selection of cases for day-case or elective procedures.

Box 28.5 Risk stratification of patients with diabetes undergoing a surgical procedure.

Low risk
- Well-controlled patients on 'diet alone' or oral hypoglycaemia.
- Minor procedures or procedures where anaesthesia, sedation and procedure itself lasts no longer than 45 mins, and not likely to need IV fluids postoperative.

Medium risk
- Well-controlled insulin-treated patients (HbA1c < 69 mmol/mol <8.5%)
- Not ketotic
- Likely to need IV fluids for <24 hours
- Postoperative problems unlikely

High risk
- Any patient with diabetes undergoing major surgery and/or likely to need IV fluids for >24 hours postoperatively
- Patient ill, septic or ketotic
- Patients with chronic poor glycaemic control (HbA1c >69 mmol/mol (>8.5%)
- Potential to become unstable due to condition or as a result of special preparations, procedure or anaesthesia.

A variable rate intravenous insulin infusion (VRIII) is only necessary for 'high risk' patients.

There is no high-quality evidence to inform the ideal choice of IV fluid for a VRIII. There are many different local regimens and a recent Cochrane review was unable to make a firm recommendation. In the UK, the Joint British

---

Box 28.6 Management of diabetes during the perioperative period (See also Figure 28.6).

Low-risk patients (no need for VRIII)
- Omit oral hypoglycaemic drugs on the day of the procedure, or on the day of fasting for special preparations if this is before the day of the actual procedure.
- If patient is on the afternoon list and allowed to eat, give a light breakfast (tea and toast).
- Restart usual medication as soon as patient starts eating normally.
- However, patients due to receive IV contrast medium should omit metformin 48 hours beforehand if their eGFR is ≤ 44 ml/min/1.73m2 or on the day of the procedure if it is urgent, and should not restart for 48 hours.

Well-controlled medium-risk patients (VRIII not usually needed)
Consider reduction of 20% of overnight (long acting) insulin the night before.
Morning surgery
- Omit the morning dose of insulin and record blood glucose.
- Post procedure: immediately prior to eating **normal** meal, give SC insulin (generally the usual dose).
Afternoon surgery patients
- If patient is not allowed to eat, omit the morning insulin.
- If they are allowed to eat, give patient ½ of their usual insulin dose before eating a light breakfast (tea and toast). Monitor blood glucose.
- Post procedure, once able to eat **normally**, resume usual insulin dose.

High-risk patients
Morning surgery patients
- At 07.30 record blood glucose and commence VRIII via a syringe driver, with a separate infusion of 5% glucose + 0.45% sodium chloride + either 0.15% or 0.30% potassium chloride OR 4% glucose + 0.18% sodium chloride + 0.15% or 0.30% potassium chloride 1 litre/8 hours (less for elderly or those with heart failure).
Afternoon surgery patients
- If they are allowed to eat, give patients ½ their usual insulin dose before a light breakfast.
- 1 hour before procedure, record blood glucose and commence VRIII and IV fluid infusion, as above.
Both morning and afternoon patients
- Prescribe VRIII on the 'variable dose' section of the drug chart.
- As soon as patients are eating **normally**, resume usual SC insulin, then **1 hour later** discontinue the continuous insulin and IV infusions.
NB: Patients on insulin undergoing extended fasting due to their condition, or for special preoperative preparation, should omit insulin at time of fasting and commence VRIII with separate infusion of glucose containing fluid as above.
VRIII = Variable rate Intravenous Insulin Infusion (Figure 28.7).

Diabetes Societies recommend a solution of 5% Glucose, 0.45% Sodium Chloride with either 0.15% or 0.30% Potassium Chloride. Unfortunately, this is not widely available, and 4% Glucose with 0.18% Sodium Chloride with 0.15% or 0.30% Potassium Chloride fluid is usually substituted. Either way, the infusion rate is set at 1L/8hrs, and a parallel infusion of insulin is delivered using 50 units of soluble (such as Actrapid or Humulin S) added to 50 ml 0.9% Sodium Chloride and delivered by a syringe driver at a variable rate according to the blood glucose (Figure 28.7). The target range is 6–10 mmol/L. Some centres still use the original Glucose–Potassium–Insulin regimen and, although this does have the potential side effect of hyponatraemia in prolonged use, it is still very convenient requiring a fixed infusion rate and avoids the need for a separate syringe driver.

The management of critically ill patients with diabetes has been the subject of intense research in recent years, but the early studies suggesting a benefit of really tight glycaemic control have not been confirmed and may actually cause harm through hypoglycaemia. Current advice is to maintain blood glucose in the range 6.0–10.0 mmol/L (140–180 mg/dL in the USA) using a VRIII. For patients experiencing an acute coronary syndrome there is now thought to be no benefit of a VRIII unless the patient's blood glucose is >11.0 mmol/L.

Insulins	Day prior to admission	Day of surgery / whilst on a VRIII		
		Patient for a.m. surgery	**Patient for p.m. surgery**	**If a VRIII is being used***
Once daily (evening) (e.g. Lantus*or Levemir* Tresiba* Insulatard* Humulin I*) Insuman Basal*)	Reduce dose by 20%	Check blood glucose on admission	Check blood glucose on admission	Continue at 80% of the usual dose
Once daily (morning) Once daily (morning) (Lantus* or Levermir* Tresiba* Insulatard* Humulin I*) Insuman Basal*)	Reduce dose by 20%	Reduce dose by 20% Check blood glucose on admission	Reduce dose by 20% Check blood glucose on admission	Continue at 80% of the usual dose
Twice daily (e.g. Novomix 30*, Humulin M3* Humalog Mix 25* Humalog Mix 50* Insuman* Comb 25, Insuman* Comb 50 twice daily Levemir* or Lantus*)	No dose Change	Halve the usual morning dose. Check blood glucose on admission Leave the evening meal dose unchanged	Halve the usual morning dose. Check blood glucose on admission Leave the evening meal dose unchanged	Stop until eating and drinking normally
Twice daily- separate injections of short acting (e.g. animal neutral, NovoRapid* Humulin S*) Apidra* **and intermediate acting** (e.g. animal isophane Insulatard* Humulin* Insuman*	No dose Change	Calculate the total dose of both morning insulins and give half as intermediate acting only in the morning. Check blood glucose on admission Leave the evening meal dose unchanged	Calculate the total dose of both morning insulins and give half as intermediate acting only in the morning. Check blood glucose on admission Leave the evening meal dose unchanged	Stop until eating and drinking normally

Figure 28.6 Suggested modifications of existing insulin regimens for people with diabetes undergoing surgical or other procedures requiring fasting. VRIII = Variable rate Intravenous Insulin Infusion. Reproduced from JBDS for In-patient Care. Management of adults with diabetes undergoing surgery and elective procedures 2016. With permission.

Glucose mmol/L	Insulin Rates (ml/hr)						
	Standard Rate (Start on standard rate unless indicated)		Reduced Rate (for use in insulin sensitive patients i.e needing less than 24 units/day)		Increased Rate (for use in insulin resistant patients i.e needing more than 100 units/day)		Customised scale
	if no basal insulin	if basal insulin continued	if no basal insulin	if basal insulin continued	if no basal insulin	if basal continued	
<4	0.5 ml/hr and administer 100 ml iv 20% glucose	0 ml/hr and administer 100 ml iv 20% glucose	0.2 ml/hr and administer 100 ml iv 20% glucose	0 ml/hr and administer 100 ml iv 20% glucose	0.5 ml/hr and administer 100 ml iv 20% glucose	0 ml/hr and administer 100 ml iv 20% glucose	
4.1–6	0.5 ml/hr and consider 50 ml iv 20% glucose*	0 ml/hr and consider 15 ml iv 20% glucose*	0.2 ml/hr and consider 50 ml iv 20% glucose*	0 ml/hr and consider 50 ml iv 20% glucose*	0 ml/hr and consider 50 ml iv 20% glucose*	0 ml/hr and consider 15 ml iv 20% glucose*	
6.1–8	1	1	0.5	0.5	2	2	
8.1–12	2	2	1	1	4	4	
12.1–16	4	4	2	2	6	6	
16.1–20	5	5	3	3	7	7	
20.1–24	6	6	4	4	8	8	
>24.1	8	8	6	6	10	10	
>24.1	Ensure insulin is running, and not measuring an artefact						

Figure 28.7 Suggested VRIII rates in patients undergoing surgery or prolonged fasting. VRIII = Variable rate Intravenous Insulin Infusion. Reproduced from JBDS for In-patient Care. Management of adults with diabetes undergoing surgery and elective procedures 2016. With permission.

CASE HISTORY

An 84-year-old woman developed urinary incontinence. She had early dementia and type 2 diabetes treated with metformin. Her family doctor noted an area of cellulitis affecting the lower leg, spreading from a superficial abrasion. Her HbA1c was 76 mmol/mol (9.1%).

Comment: Infections are common in patients with diabetes, especially if glycaemic control is poor. It is likely that this woman has both a urinary tract infection (a urine culture is important) and a spreading cellulitis that require antibiotic therapy. It is also possible that her incontinence is secondary to hyperglycaemia and polyuria. She requires treatment of her cellulitis and additional diabetes therapy but avoiding an SGLT2 inhibitor because of her urinary symptoms. Incontinence in elderly patients should always prompt enquiry into diabetes control and raise suspicion of asymptomatic lower urinary tract infection.

LANDMARK CLINICAL TRIALS

Alberti KGMM and Thomas DJB. The management of diabetes during surgery. Br J Anaesthesia 1979; 51: 693–710. doi.org/10.1093/bja/51.7.693

This paper reviewed the metabolic responses to surgery in people with diabetes and the current literature on management regimens. They proposed a simple glucose–potassium–insulin (GKI) infusion which was the basis of management in the UK until its current iteration in the JBDS guidelines. It is still widely used because of its simplicity.

KEY WEBSITES

- UK NHS website: www.nhs.uk/Diabetes
- Diabetes UK website with a link to JBDS guidelines: www.diabetes.org.uk
- Joint British Societies for Diabetes websites with excellent guidelines: www.diabetologists–abcd.org.uk/JBDS/JBDS.htm
- Scottish guidelines website: www.SIGN.ac.uk
- ADA Website with annually updated Clinical Practice Guidelines: www.diabetes.org
- Website on exercise for people with diabetes and health care professionals: www.runsweet.com
- NG 17 and 18 Type 1 diabetes: www.nice.org.uk

FURTHER READING

Colberg SR, Siberg RJ, Yardley JE et al. Physical activity/exercise and diabetes: a position statement of the American Diabetes Association. Diabetes Care 2016; 39: 2065–79

Colunga-Lozano LE, Gonzalez Torres FJ, Delgado-Figueroa N et al. Sliding scale insulin for non-critically ill adults with diabetes mellitus. Cochrane Database of Systematic Reviews 2018; Issue 11: Art.No.:CD011296.doi:10.1002/14651858.CD011296.pub2

Houlder SK, Yardley JE. Continuous glucose monitoring and exercise in type 1 diabetes: past, present and future. Biosensors 2018; 8: 73–85

JBDS-IP The use of variable rate intravenous insulin infusion VRIII in medical inpatients. 2014. www.diabetologists-abcd.org.uk/JBDS/JBDS.htm

JBDS-IP Management of hyperglycaemia and steroid (glucocorticoid) therapy. 2014. www.diabetologists-abcd.org.uk/JBDS/JBDS.htm

JBDS-IP Glycaemic management during the inpatient enteral feeding of stroke patients with diabetes. 2018. www.diabetologists-abcd.org.uk/JBDS/JBDS.htm

JBDS-IP. The management of adults with diabetes undergoing surgery and elective procedures. 2016. www.diabetologists-abcd.org.uk/JBDS/JBDS.htm

Misra A, Alappan NK, Vikram NK, et al. Effect of supervised progressive resistance-exercise training protocol on insulin sensitivity, glycaemia, lipids and body composition in Asian Indians with type 2 diabetes. Diabetes Care 2008; 31: 1282–1287.

Pan B, Ge L, Xun Y-Q et al. Exercise training modalities in patients with type 2 diabetes mellitus: a systematic review and network meta-analysis. Int J Behavioural Nutrition and Physics Activity 2018; 15: 72–86

Riddell MC, Gallen IW, Smart CE et al. Exercise management in type 1 diabetes: a consensus statement. Lancet Diabetes Endocrinol 2017; 5: 377–90

Scott S, Kempf P, Bally L et al. Carbohydrate intake in the context of exercise in people with type 1 diabetes. Nutrients 2019; 11: 3017–38

Stevens DL, Bryant AE. Necrotizing soft-tissue infections. N Engl J Med 2017; 377: 2253–65

Vadstrup ES, Frolich A, Perrild H, et al. Lifestyle intervention for type 2 diabetes patients: trial protocol of the Copenhagen Type 2 Diabetes Rehabilitation Project. BMC Public Health 2009; 9: 166.

Venmans LM, Hak E, Gorter K, Rutten G. Incidence and antibiotic prescription rates for common infections in patients with diabetes in primary care over the years 1995 to 2003. Int J Infect Dis 2009; 13(6): 344–351.

Wu N, Bredin SSD, Guan Y et al. Cardiovascular health benefits of exercise training in persons living with type 1 diabetes: a systematic review and meta–analysis.J Clin Med 2019; 8: 253–79

Chapter
29

Pregnancy and diabetes

KEY POINTS

- Maternal type 1 and 2 diabetes is the most common medical problem that complicates pregnancy, affecting around 1 in 250 births in the UK.
- Increased rates of maternal complications in pregnant women with diabetes include pre-eclampsia, polyhydramnios, pre-term delivery and Caesarean section.
- Pregestational diabetes is associated with a nearly 4-fold increase in major congenital malformations, a 4-fold increase in perinatal mortality and 3-fold increase in stillbirth rate compared to age- and parity-matched non-diabetic women. These complications are closely related to glycaemic control in early pregnancy.
- Women with type 2 diabetes have a similar complication rate to those with type 1.

- Preconception and antenatal strict glycaemic control reduces the risk of congenital malformation and maternal complications.
- Macrosomia (large-for-dates foetus) is at least twice as common in women with pre-gestational and gestational diabetes, and can lead to complications during delivery including shoulder dystocia.
- Babies born to mothers with diabetes are more prone to neonatal hypoglycaemia, jaundice and hypocalcaemia, and some need admission to the neonatal unit post-delivery.
- Gestational diabetes affects 4–16% of pregnancies in the UK and is more common in women from ethnic minorities. The glycaemic criteria for diagnosis remain controversial with no universal consensus.
- Good glycaemic control in women with gestational diabetes can reduce complications for both mother and child.

Pregestational diabetes is the most common medical problem that complicates pregnancy, affecting around 1 in 250 births (0.4%) in the UK. The National Diabetes in Pregnancy (NDIP) audit has been running in England and Wales since 2014 and, whilst the data are not complete for all pregnancies in women with diabetes, the latest report for 2018 comprised 4400 datasets and provides essential information on the quality and standards of care, and the outcomes for mother and baby. This showed for the first time that pregnancies in women with type 2 diabetes now exceed those in type 1, which is a more than two-fold increase from the 25% reported by the CEMACH (Confidential Enquiry into Maternal and Child Health) report in 2002/3. The prevalence of diabetes in pregnancy is increasing; using a primary care database of over 440,000 pregnancies, the prevalence of type 1 diabetes has risen from 1.56 per 1000 pregnancies

in 1995 to 4.09 in 2015. For type 2 diabetes the rates have increased from 2.34 per 1000 in 1995, to 5.09 in 2008 and 10.62 in 2012. Prevalence rates for gestational diabetes (GDM) have also increased, but this is partly due to changes in diagnostic criteria and screening practice. This means that all primary care antenatal services are likely to have to care for women with varying degrees of glucose intolerance. Diabetes can cause problems for both the mother and foetus and, despite recent advances in antenatal care, the outcome in terms of perinatal health and survival remains significantly less good than for pregnancy in the absence of diabetes. Gestational diabetes usually occurs in the second half of pregnancy and is becoming more common because of increasing maternal obesity and age, although absolute rates are highly dependent on the population under study and reflect the background risk of type 2 diabetes.

Handbook of Diabetes, Fifth Edition. Rudy Bilous, Richard Donnelly, and Iskandar Idris.
© 2021 John Wiley & Sons Ltd. Published 2021 by John Wiley & Sons Ltd.

Effects of pregnancy on the woman with diabetes

In women with pre-existing diabetes, insulin sensitivity is increased in the first trimester increasing their risk of hypoglycaemia. After 16 weeks gestation, blood glucose levels rise and insulin requirements usually increase, on average by 40% after the 18th week (range 0–300%) (Box 29.1). This is because pregnancy induces insulin resistance through the diabetogenic effects of placental hormones, cytokines such as TNF-α, and progesterone; the effects of which are maximal in the second and third trimesters. Hyperglycaemia as a result of insulin resistance and consequent enhanced lipolysis is probably favourable in the woman without diabetes as it encourages nutrient transfer to the growing foetus, but in the woman

---

Box 29.1 Effects of pregnancy on the woman with pre-existing diabetes.

Susceptible to hypoglycaemia in early pregnancy due to increased insulin sensitivity and changes in eating due to nausea and need for tight glycaemic control

Increasing insulin requirements in later pregnancy due to decreased insulin sensitivity induced by pregnancy related hormones

Potential hypoglycaemia in later pregnancy due to delayed gastric emptying and/or oesophageal reflux

Risk of deterioration of retinopathy and nephropathy

Risk of DKA increased due to renal bicarbonate loss and pro-ketotic metabolism in later pregnancy

Risk of urinary tract infection due to increased glycosuria secondary to a reduction in the renal threshold for reabsorption

---

with diabetes it can be seen as a form of accelerated starvation and predisposes to ketosis. As pregnancy progresses and the diaphragm is pushed upwards, there is a relative increase in alveolar ventilation with a consequent respiratory alkalosis and compensatory renal tubular loss of bicarbonate. There is a fall in serum bicarbonate and loss of acid-buffering capacity, which partly explains why DKA can occur in pregnancy at relatively modest hyperglycaemia or even normoglycaemia.

Because of the stringent glycaemic targets in pregnancy, there is a real risk of hypoglycaemia; 41% of 323 women with diabetes in The Netherlands who were pregnant in 1999–2000 reported at least one severe episode, and one died in a road traffic accident almost certainly as a result of hypoglycaemia. Women who are driving should be advised to follow guidance on blood glucose monitoring carefully (see Chapter 32). The NDIP 2015 report found a >3 fold increase in hospital admissions for hypoglycaemia in pregnant women with type 1 and type 2 diabetes compared to their non-pregnant counterparts aged 20–39 years, and the 2018 report found that 12% of women with type 1 diabetes reported hospital care for hypoglycaemia.

Effects of maternal diabetes on the pregnancy

Maternal diabetes can affect the foetus adversely by causing developmental malformations, altered islet cell development (increased insulin secretion) due to hyperglycaemia and by accelerating growth (macrosomia) (Figure 29.1, Box 29.2). Pre-eclampsia is more common in pregnancies with diabetes (particularly in women with nephropathy); there was a reported >12-fold increase compared to pregnancy without diabetes in The Netherlands in 1999–2000. Maternal mortality is also significantly higher than in non-diabetic

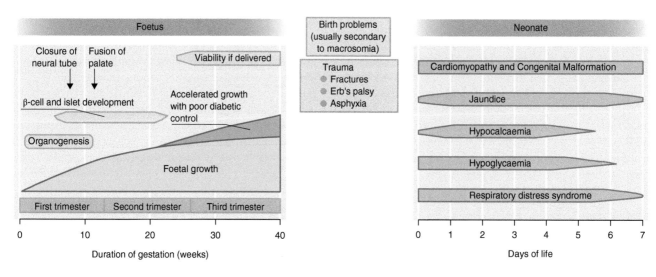

Figure 29.1 Impact of maternal diabetes on the foetus and neonate by gestational and neonatal age.

Box 29.2 Effects of maternal diabetes on pregnancy.

Need for pre-conceptual care and planning
Increased risk of congenital malformation with poor glycaemic control in early pregnancy
Increased risk of an SGA infant with poor glycaemic control in early pregnancy
Increased risk of an LGA infant with poor glycaemic control in later pregnancy
Increased risk of polyhydramnios
Increased risk of miscarriage, late intra-uterine death and stillbirth
Increased risk of pre-eclampsia
Increased risk of birth trauma with an LGA infant
Increased risk of induction of labour and Caesarean section
Increased maternal and neonatal morbidity and mortality

SGA = Small for Gestational Age. LGA = Large for Gestational Age

pregnancies; there were two deaths in the Dutch cohort (0.6% of 323) and five within 1 year of delivery in the CEMACH cohort of 3733, but only three of these may have had a diabetes link.

Diabetes is teratogenic, particularly in the first 8 weeks' gestation when the major organs are forming. Major congenital malformations occurred in 144 of the CEMACH cohort, about twice the non-diabetic rate, and there was no difference by type of diabetes; the major defects affected the heart (42%), musculoskeletal (17%), and nervous (13%) systems. Malformation rate is closely related to hyperglycaemia in early pregnancy. In the North of England diabetes in pregnancy survey (NorDiP) from 1996–2008, women with pre-gestational diabetes had a relative risk of 3.8 (95% CI 3.2,4.5) for non-chromosomal major congenital anomalies compared to women without diabetes. In this cohort, the adjusted odds ratio was 1.3 per 11 mmol/mol (1%) linear increase in peri conception HbA1c ≥45 mmol/mol (6.3%). Pre-existing nephropathy was also a significant risk factor. NPID 2018 report a congenital anomaly rate of 48/1000 for type 1 and 40/1000 type 2 diabetes affected pregnancies, which is unchanged from 2014. Preconception care and tight glycaemic control are associated with lower rates (for obvious reasons, there are no randomised controlled trials in this area). 84% of the Dutch cohort pregnancies were planned and 75% achieved a first-trimester HbA1c <53 mmol/mol (<7.0%), despite which their congenital malformation rates remained over three times those seen in non-diabetic women. Part of the problem is that HbA1c is only a measure of average glycaemia; peak blood glucose or variation may be more important, and very few women have complete normoglycaemia before or at conception, or during embryogenesis. Nonetheless, the Dutch researchers

reported an odds ratio of 0.34 (95% CI 0.13–0.88) for major malformations in women with diabetes with a planned versus an unplanned pregnancy.

Perinatal mortality rate has fallen in recent years but is still 3–4 times that in non-diabetic pregnancy (32/1000 in the CEMACH 2002-3 report). Stillbirth rates remain about 3 times those of the non-diabetic population (13.7 vs 4.2/1000 births in the NDIP 2019 report), and are linked to standard of glycaemic control throughout pregnancy; in the CEMACH enquiry less than 50% of women with a stillbirth ever achieved an HbA1c < 53 mol/mol (<7.0%) at any time during their pregnancy, whereas >70% of women with a normal pregnancy outcome recorded an HbA1c <53 mmol/mol at some stage. NDIP 2018 showed that < 45% of women with type 1 and <75% with type 2 diabetes achieved an HbA1c ≤48 mol/mol (6.5%) indicating that glycemic control is still less than ideal. Rates of stillbirth and congenital anomaly are similar for women with type 1 and type 2 diabetes.

Accelerated foetal growth, which leads to a macrosomic, large-for-gestational-age infant (Figure 29.2), is caused by enhanced delivery of glucose and other nutrients to the foetus. This stimulates the islets and induces foetal

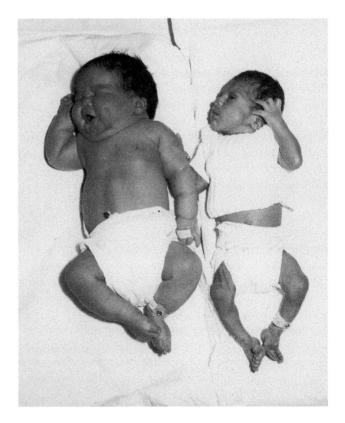

Figure 29.2 (*Left*) A macrosomic baby born to a mother with diabetes. (*Right*) A normal baby of similar gestation born to a mother without diabetes.

hyperinsulinaemia, which promotes abdominal fat deposition, skeletal growth and organomegaly. Complications for these large babies include birth trauma and neonatal hypoglycaemia and hypocalcaemia. Despite being large for gestational age, the macrosomic foetus tends to be dysmature and is prone to the respiratory distress syndrome at birth. Rates of macrosomia depend upon the definition; in the NDIP 2018 report the overall proportion of babies ≥ 90th centile birth weight was 54% for type 1 and 26% for type 2 diabetic pregnancies, but this figure was significantly greater for those whose third trimester HbA1c ≥48 mmol/mol (6.5%) (61 vs 48% for type 1; 50 vs 18% for type 2 diabetes). The NorDiP study found an average increase in birthweight of 310g per 11 mmol/mol (1%) increase in third trimester HbA1c ≥53 mmol/mol (7.0%), with an increasing probability of an LGA infant from 27% in mothers with an HbA1c of 37 mol/mol (5.5%) to 66% in those with an HbA1c of 70 mol/mol (8.5%), emphasising the importance of glycaemic control in the later stages of pregnancy for preventing macrosomia.

Less well documented is the prevalence of small for gestational age (SGA) infants which occurs more frequently in type 2 diabetes (13% type 2 vs 5% type 1 in NDIP 2018). This may reflect the older age of women with type 2 diabetes, as well as the increased prevalence of hypertension and obesity. NorDIP found that higher periconception HbA1c, maternal smoking and the presence of microvascular complications were associated with the likelihood of an SGA infant.

Management of pregnancy in diabetes
Pre-pregnancy counselling

Management of pregnancy in women with diabetes begins with preconception advice and counselling (Box 29.3). This includes an explanation of the risks of pregnancy and the requirements for a successful pregnancy, including frequent clinic visits beginning as soon as possible after conception, optimised metabolic control, stopping both smoking and drinking alcohol, and a folate-rich and supplemented diet (5 mg/day – a higher dose than usually recommended for non-diabetic pregnancy). Potentially teratogenic drugs should be replaced with safer alternatives – ACE inhibitors and statins are contraindicated, for example. Women should undergo retinal screening and urinalysis for an albumin:creatinine ratio (ACR). Outpatient preconception care of women with diabetes is thought to reduce congenital anomalies by about two-thirds. Regrettably, only a minority of women in the UK attend for pre-pregnancy counselling. The NDIP report for 2018 revealed that <45% of women with type 1 and <25% with type 2 diabetes were taking 5mg folic acid prior to pregnancy, and <20% of women with type 1 and <40% with type 2 diabetes had a first trimester HbA1c level in the recommended target range of ≤48 mmol/mol (6.5%). Achieving tight glycaemic control

---

Box 29.3 Pre-pregnancy care. Adapted from NICE Guidance NG 3.

Give advice and information on:
- the risks of diabetes in pregnancy and how to reduce them with good glycaemic control
- structured diabetes education programmes such as DAFNE
- achieving a target HbA1c of ≤48 mmol/mol (6.5%) without significant hypoglycaemia
- avoiding pregnancy if HbA1c ≥86 mmol/mol (10.0%)
- maintaining contraception until glycaemic control optimised
- diet, bodyweight and exercise, including weight loss for women with a BMI over 27 kg/m², smoking cessation and alcohol avoidance
- hypoglycaemia and hypoglycaemia unawareness and avoidance
- pregnancy-related nausea/vomiting and strategies for maintaining good glycaemic control
- retinal and renal assessment
- taking folic acid supplements (5 mg/day) from preconception until 12 weeks of gestation
- review of, and possible changes to, medication (stop statins and any antihypertensive medication contraindicated in pregnancy), glycaemic targets and self-monitoring routine
- use of blood ketone monitoring to detect DKA
- frequency of appointments and local support, including emergency telephone numbers.

---

prior to pregnancy can pose real challenges for family and employment. In this regard it must be emphasised that any improvement in glycaemia confers benefit and reduces the risks of complications for both the mother and foetus, even if the recommended HbA1c target is not achieved. Overall, only one in eight women could be said to be well prepared for pregnancy and this has not changed materially during the five years of the audit. NICE recommends that women with an HbA1c level ≥ 86 mmol/mol (10%) should not try to conceive because of the high risk of an adverse outcome.

Management of established pregnancy

NICE guidance for the management of pregnancy in pregestational diabetes includes optimisation of glycaemic control, aiming for a fasting plasma glucose concentration 4–5.3 mmol/L, a 1-hour postprandial peak ≤7.8 mmol/L or a 2-hour post prandial peak < 6.4 mmol/L. There is no target for HbA1c but women should be advised that the risk of an adverse outcome increases with levels ≥ 48 mmol/mol (6.5%) (Box 29.4). The ADA Guidelines suggest similar glycaemic targets (the 2-hour post prandial is 6.7 mmol/L (120 mg/dL)) but an HbA1c ≤ 42mmol/mol (6.0%) where it is safe to do so. Virtually all women with type 1 diabetes require a basal-bolus insulin injection regimen to achieve strict glycaemic control, with at least four times daily blood glucose

Box 29.4 Suggested antenatal care for women with pre-gestational diabetes.

Appointment	Care for women with diabetes during pregnancy*
Booking appointment (Joint diabetes and antenatal care) – ideally by 10 weeks	Discuss information, education and advice about how diabetes will affect the pregnancy, birth and early parenting (such as breastfeeding and initial care of the baby).
	If the woman has been attending for preconception care and advice, continue to provide information, education and advice in relation to achieving optimal blood glucose control (including dietary advice).
	If the woman has not attended for preconception care and advice, give information, education and advice for the first time, take a clinical history to establish the extent of diabetes-related complications (including neuropathy and vascular disease), and review medicines for diabetes and its complications.
	Offer retinal assessment for women with pre-existing diabetes unless the woman has been assessed in the last 3 months.
	Offer renal assessment for women with pre-existing diabetes if this has not been performed in the last 3 months.
	Arrange contact with the joint diabetes and antenatal clinic every 1–2 weeks throughout pregnancy for all women with diabetes.
	Measure HbA1c levels for women with pre-existing diabetes to determine the level of risk for the pregnancy.
	Offer self-monitoring of blood glucose or a 75 g 2-hour OGTT as soon as possible for women with a history of gestational diabetes who book in the first trimester.
	Confirm viability of pregnancy and gestational age at 7–9 weeks.
16 weeks	Offer retinal assessment at 16–20 weeks to women with pre-existing diabetes if diabetic retinopathy was present at their first antenatal clinic visit.
	Offer self-monitoring of blood glucose or a 75 g 2-hour OGTT as soon as possible for women with a history of gestational diabetes who book in the second trimester.
20 weeks	Offer an ultrasound scan for detecting foetal structural abnormalities, including examination of the foetal heart (4 chambers, outflow tracts and 3 vessels).
28 weeks	Offer ultrasound monitoring of foetal growth and amniotic fluid volume. Offer retinal assessment to all women with pre-existing diabetes.
	Women diagnosed with gestational diabetes as a result of routine antenatal testing at 24–28 weeks enter the care pathway.
32 weeks	Offer ultrasound monitoring of foetal growth and amniotic fluid volume. Offer nulliparous women all routine investigations normally scheduled for 31 weeks in routine antenatal care.
34 weeks	No additional or different care for women with diabetes.
36 weeks	Offer ultrasound monitoring of foetal growth and amniotic fluid volume. Provide information and advice about: • timing, mode and management of birth • analgesia and anaesthesia • changes to blood glucose-lowering therapy during and after birth care of the baby after birth • initiation of breastfeeding and the effect of breastfeeding on blood glucose control • contraception and follow-up.
37^{+0} weeks to 38^{+6} weeks	Offer induction of labour, or caesarean section if indicated, to women with type 1 or type 2 diabetes; otherwise await spontaneous labour.
38 weeks	Offer tests of foetal wellbeing.
39 weeks	Offer tests of foetal wellbeing.
	Advise women with uncomplicated gestational diabetes to give birth no later than 40^{+6} weeks.

*Women with diabetes should also receive routine care according to the schedule of appointments in the NICE guideline on antenatal care, including appointments at 25 weeks (for nulliparous women) and 34 weeks, but with the exception of the appointment for nulliparous women at 31 weeks.

OGTT = oral glucose tolerance test.

Taken from NICE Guidance NG3 Diabetes in pregnancy: management from preconception to the post natal period: www.nice.org.uk/guidance/ng3.

self-monitoring (NICE recommends seven tests per day). The choice of insulin is controversial. There are no prospective trials that establish the safety of the new long-acting analogues, but neither are there many for older insulins. Current guidance suggests that long-acting analogues should not be started in pregnancy but may be continued after discussion with the pregnant woman. Neutral protamine Hagedorn (NPH) should be used if a change is requested or a new longer acting preparation is started. The short-acting analogues aspart and lispro are safe to continue. Updated NICE guidance states that continuous subcutaneous insulin infusion (CSII – insulin pump therapy) can now be offered as an alternative option in those who have difficulty achieving good control on multiple injections without unacceptable hypoglycaemia, although meta-analysis has shown no advantage over multiple injection therapy in terms of pregnancy outcome. Suitably powered prospective trials are required in order to determine optimum management of glycaemia in pregnancy.

There have been several studies of the use of continuous glucose monitoring (CGM) in pregnancy with some minor benefit in terms of overall diabetes control, and a positive (if modest) impact on pregnancy outcome when compared with multiple daily injections. The largest of these, CONCEPTT, reported in 2017 and showed significant benefit to the foetus in terms of fewer LGA infants, less neonatal hypoglycaemia and a 1-day shorter hospital stay. Updated NICE guidance states that continuous glucose monitoring should be offered to all pregnant women with type 1 diabetes, as well as to any with type 2 on insulin who have severe hypoglycaemia and/or who have unstable blood glucose levels causing concern.

Screening for complications is necessary, since pregnancy can worsen renal function in women with established nephropathy (defined as serum creatinine >124 μmol/L or estimated GFR (eGFR), <45 mL/min/1.73 m²). Consequently, blood pressure should be controlled carefully (e.g. with labetalol, methyldopa or nifedipine) and the ADA recommends treatment to maintain BP <135/85 but > 120/80 mmHg. Increasing proteinuria and hypertension are common in worsening nephropathy but can be difficult to distinguish from pre-eclampsia in later pregnancy (see below). eGFR equations are not validated in pregnancy so timed creatinine clearances are sometimes necessary to monitor declining renal function. Retinopathy may also deteriorate rapidly during diabetic pregnancy, especially when glycaemic control is improved suddenly. Increased frequency of surveillance and early photocoagulation should be considered in high-risk patients during pre-conception care and early pregnancy.

Obstetric assessment includes regular ultrasound scans for estimation of gestational age, detecting major malformations, monitoring foetal growth and assessing the volume of amniotic fluid. The maternal complications of diabetic pregnancy include pre-eclampsia (hypertension, proteinuria, oedema and foetal compromise), polyhydramnios, urinary tract infections, vaginal candidiasis, carpal tunnel syndrome, reflux oesophagitis and preterm labour. Careful monitoring

of blood pressure is also necessary as the odds ratio for pre-eclampsia is 1.65 for each increase of 11 mmol/mol (1%) in HbA1c level and is also much more likely in those with established albuminuria prior to conception.

Insulin requirements usually increase gradually through the second trimester, coinciding with increasing insulin resistance and food intake, and may continue to increase until 34–36 weeks' gestation. HbA1c is less precise as an estimate of glycaemic control in later pregnancy because of altered red cell survival, possible pregnancy related iron deficiency, and increased circulating blood volume leading to a dilutional fall in haemoglobin concentration. Estimated average blood glucose derived from HbA1c is 7.4–7.7 mmol/L for an HbA1c of 64 mmol/mol (8.0%) in pregnancy, which is around 2.6 mmol/L lower than in the non-pregnant population.

In the UK, NICE recommends women with diabetes are delivered between 37 and 38+6 weeks, because of the risk of late stillbirth. In 2018 45% of type 1 and 25% type 2 diabetic pregnancies were delivered before 37 weeks. The NDIP audit also found that just 12.6% of type 1 and 13.8% of type 2 diabetic pregnancies went into spontaneous labour in 2017, with a Caesarean section rate of over 60% for women with type 1 and 54% with type 2 respectively. Emergency Caesarean section rates were 30.0% in 2013 compared to 37.6% 10 years earlier in CEMACH, these data were not provided in the 2018 NPID report.

If an early delivery is anticipated, then antenatal corticosteroids in high dose are often given in order to facilitate foetal lung maturation. This will inevitably cause hyperglycaemia and may even provoke DKA. For these reasons careful monitoring, preferably in hospital, is required and insulin doses increased by 50% or more for 48 hours in order to prevent metabolic decompensation. Some guidelines recommend a glucose and insulin IV infusion to maintain glycaemic control during during steroid administration.

During labour, diabetes should be controlled by continuous intravenous infusions of insulin (typically 2–4 U/h) and glucose. The target blood glucose is 4–7 mmol/L. Women on CSII can often be managed with adjustments in their infusion rates without the need for intravenous glucose. After delivery, insulin requirements return almost immediately to pre-pregnancy values or less, and doses should be reduced in order to avoid hypoglycaemia. Elective Caesarean section is indicated if mechanical problems with vaginal delivery are anticipated (e.g. malpresentation or disproportion), or for foetal compromise and severe pre-eclampsia. Breastfeeding requires a further 10–20% reduction in insulin dose but should be encouraged as it helps prevent neonatal hypoglycaemia and promotes maternal weight loss post delivery.

Neonates are more likely to need admission to the special care baby unit post delivery, although there is no need for this to be routine. They are, however, more prone to develop hypoglycaemia, especially if the mother is on insulin treatment, but they should only require admission if they are symptomatic (usually at a capillary blood glucose ≤ 2mmol/L). Babies are also more prone to hyperbilirubinaemia, polycythaemia and hypocalcaemia, especially if they are LGA, and LGA infants are more prone to birth trauma.

The numbers of pregnant women with type 2 diabetes are increasing, especially in the developing world where this type of diabetes predominates, but they also comprised 51.4% of pregnancies in the NDIP 2018 report. As a group, these UK women were older and much more likely to be of Afro-Caribbean, Asian or other ethnic minority background than those with type 1 diabetes, and to have come from more socioeconomically deprived backgrounds. Women with type 2 diabetes more often present later in pregnancy, and have other risk factors for poor outcome, such as obesity, hypertension, and greater age and parity. However, outcome in terms of complications appears no different than for women with type 1.

Management of pregnancy in type 2 diabetes is the same as that for type 1 diabetes. In general, women should change to insulin before conception or early in the first trimester. Oral hypoglycaemic agents may not achieve sufficiently good glycaemic control; moreover, some cross the placenta, may aggravate foetal hyperinsulinaemia, and are potentially teratogenic (although evidence is conflicting). Metformin crosses the placenta and, although it is not licensed for use in pregnancy, there is increasing experience of its use (particularly in gestational diabetes) such that it is currently supported by NICE (but not the ADA). So far there have been no reported safety concerns except for an association with increased childhood body weight in some studies, although this finding has many other confounding factors. Glibenclamide is no longer recommended for use in NICE Guidance.

Gestational diabetes

Gestational diabetes mellitus (GDM) is glucose intolerance first recognised in pregnancy. It will therefore include women with impaired glucose tolerance, those with previously unrecognised type 2 diabetes, and those who develop type 1 diabetes when pregnant. The earlier in pregnancy it is diagnosed, the more likely it is to be type 1 or 2 diabetes. The pathophysiology is a combination of pregnancy-induced insulin resistance and diminished insulin secretory capacity. Some studies suggest that women who develop GDM have demonstrable deficiencies in β cell function prior to pregnancy. The Hyperglycaemia and Adverse Pregnancy Outcomes (HAPO) Study showed a linear relationship between fasting and post-glucose load plasma glucose for birthweight (OR for birthweight >90th centile is 1.32 for each 0.4 mmol/L increase in fasting plasma glucose and 1.38 for each 1.3 mmol/L increase in 2-hour post 75 g oral glucose load). There was no cut-off point. An expert panel has reviewed the data and produced an international consensus on diagnostic plasma glucose levels for GDM based upon a 75% increase in odds for the development of the study outcomes (Table 29.1). The implication of these

Table 29.1 Diagnostic values of plasma glucose for Gestational Diabetes following a 75g Oral Glucose Tolerance Test from NICE and WHO/IADPSG. Overt diabetes is diagnosed with a fasting plasma glucose ≥ 7.0mmol/L (≥ 126 mgdL) ± HbA1c ≥48 mmol/mol (≥ 6.5%).

	NICE	NICE	WHO/IADPSG	WHO/IADPSG
Fasting	5.6 mmol/L	100 mg/dL	5.1 mmol/L	92 mg/dL
1 hr post 75g OGTT			10.0 mmol/L	180 mg/dL
2 hr post 75g OGTT	7.8 mmol/L	140 mg/dL	8.5 mmol/L	153 mg/dL

> **Box 29.5** Maternal risk factors for development of gestational diabetes from NICE Guidance NG3.
>
> BMI ≥ 30 kg/m²
> Previous macrosomic baby (birthweight ≥ 4.5 kg)
> Previous gestational diabetes
> Family history of diabetes in a first degree relative
> Minority ethnic family origin with a high prevalence of diabetes

new criteria was that up to 18% of pregnant women would now meet the diagnostic criteria for GDM. The WHO have adopted these criteria in 2013 but recognised that they will have to be reviewed as more data become available. Partly in response to the lack of consensus in diagnostic criteria, NICE undertook a cost and clinical effectiveness analysis for GDM using outcome data from the Australian Carbohydrate Intolerance Study in Pregnant Women (ACHOIS) and other intervention trials. They concluded that a fasting blood glucose of ≥5.6 and a 2-hour post 75g oral glucose load blood glucose of ≥7.8 mmol/L met current NICE thresholds for cost effectiveness. Other national bodies (including SIGN) have adopted the WHO 2013 criteria, whereas other specialist groups (such as the American College of Obstetrics and Gynecology–ACOG) have not. The ADA supports both the WHO 2013 and also the Carpenter–Coustan two step diagnostic procedure recommended by ACOG (a 50g oral glucose challenge followed by a 100g 3-hour OGTT). Different diagnostic criteria are used in Canada, Australia and New Zealand, and India. It is worth pointing out that not all foetal macrosomia is determined by maternal blood glucose, a significant proportion is maternal obesity related and some authors have argued for a much less glucose-centred focus on trying to prevent LGA infants.

Because of the lack of agreed diagnostic criteria, true prevalence is hard to ascertain but WHO estimates that 10–25% of all pregnancies worldwide are complicated by GDM. In the UK and Ireland, a GDM prevalence of 4–16% is reported and is dependent upon the screening test and background population risk of diabetes. The publication of ACHOIS demonstrated for the first time that intervention with intensive glucose control could reduce complications for the mother and child, and this finding was confirmed by the trial reported by Landon et al. As a result, there is now an intensive debate about the benefit of screening, its timing, diagnostic criteria, and treatment. WHO and ADA recommend universal screening but not all agree and NICE did not find this cost effective so they (and SIGN) continue to recommend a targeted approach (Box 29.5). There is simply no consensus on either the sampling strategy or screening test. Further research in this area is desperately needed and several large studies are ongoing or planned.

Treatment is controversial, but glycaemic targets are similar to those for established diabetes (Table 29.2). Many women with GDM will achieve these targets with diet and lifestyle change. Obese women can safely restrict calorie intake in pregnancy, but this should be under the direction of a dietitian. There is no hard evidence supporting any particular dietary strategy for GDM. Other lifestyle advice in terms of increasing exercise should be given and a 2-week trial of both with home blood glucose monitoring is recommended. If glycaemic targets are not achieved, then treatment with metformin (up to 1500 mg/d but starting at 500 mg/d) should be considered. If targets are still not reached, then insulin should be started. Timing is important and NICE guidance suggests earlier insulin use if maternal fasting blood glucose during the OGTT is >7mmol/L.

There is no evidence-based guidance on preferred mode of delivery but because many of the babies are large there is a risk of birth trauma and inevitably the Caesarean section rate is high. Neonates have a similar risk for the same medical problems as for the offspring of mothers with pregestational diabetes. Moreover, macrosomic infants have a two-fold risk for childhood obesity and increased odds for developing diabetes and cardiovascular disease in adulthood. It is not known if prevention of macrosomia will reduce these risks; prospective and long-term studies will be required to settle this question. Follow-up studies of the ACHOIS and Landon studies have not demonstrated differences in glycaemia and obesity rates in offspring from the intensive vs the conventional treatment arms.

Diabetes usually resolves after delivery (except in those with newly diagnosed type 1 or 2 diabetes) so all hypoglycaemic therapy should be stopped. It is recommended that capillary blood glucose monitoring be continued for 24–48 hours postpartum to confirm a return to normal glucose tolerance. NICE guidance suggests screening with a fasting blood glucose at 6–13 weeks or an HbA1c at >13 weeks postpartum to exclude persistent glucose intolerance. The ADA recommend postpartum testing with a 75g OGTT with repeat diabetes screening for the mothers every 3 years. GDM is very likely to recur in subsequent pregnancies, and all women planning to have another baby should be advised to seek preconception assessment.

Table 29.2 Recommended blood glucose targets pre- and during pregnancy for both pre-gestational and gestational diabetes. Women are recommended to test at least 4 times per day and either 1 hour OR 2 hours post meals.

	Pre pregnancy blood glucose [mmol/L (mg/dL)]	Pre pregnancy HbA1c [mmol/mol (%)]	Pregnancy blood glucose [mmol/L (mg/dL)]	Pregnancy HbA1c [mmol/mol (%)]
NICE				
Waking	5 – 7.0 (90 – 126)	≤ 48 (6.5)		
Pre meal	4 – 7.0 (72–126)		4 – 5.3 (72-96) if on insulin ≤ 5.3 (96) if on diet or metformin	
1h post meal	5 – 9.0 (90 – 160) [up to 90 mins]		≤ 7.8 (≤ 140)	
2h post meal			≤ 6.4 (≤ 115)	
SIGN				
Pre meal	4 – 6.0 (72 – 110)	≤ 53 (≤ 7.0)	4 – 6.0 (72 – 110)	
1h post meal	≤ 8.0 (≤ 144)		≤ 8.0 (≤ 144)	
2h post meal	≤ 7.0 (≤ 126)		≤ 7.0 (≤ 126)	
Bed time	≥ 6.0 (≥ 108)		≥ 6.0 (≥ 108)	
ADA				
Fasting		42 – 48 (6 – 6.5)	≤ 5.3 (≤ 96)	≤ 42 (≤ 6.0) optimal in 3rd trimester if no hypoglycaemia
1h post meal			≤ 7.8 (≤ 140)	
2h post meal			≤ 6.7 (≤ 120)	≤ 53 (≤ 7.0) if hypoglycaemia

NICE = National Institute for Health and Care Excellence. SIGN = Scottish Intercollegiate Guidelines Network. ADA = American Diabetes Association.

The lifetime risk of developing type 2 diabetes over the subsequent 10 years in women with GDM is linear at 35–60%, depending on the background risk of the population, making GDM one of the strongest predictive risk factors for the future development of diabetes. Women who have had GDM therefore need health education about reducing weight, increasing exercise and improving their cardiovascular risk profile. NICE recommends annual screening for diabetes in women who were diagnosed with GDM.

CASE HISTORY

A 28-year-old woman with type 1 diabetes of 20 years' standing and poor overall control was commenced upon CSII prior to planning a pregnancy. Her HbA1c gradually improved over 6 months from 84 to 54 mmol/mol (9.8% to 7.1%). During this time, she had careful retinal surveillance and there was no change in her mild background retinopathy. Her urine ACR was normal at <2 mg/mmol and she was normotensive (BP 118/78 mmHg). Shortly thereafter she conceived a singleton pregnancy and her control further improved to an HbA1c of 48 mmol/mol (6.5%). Her progress was uneventful until the 32nd week when she developed increasing proteinuria > 2 g/day. Her blood pressure rose to 138/96 mmHg and she reported blurred vision. Foetal growth was satisfactory. Ophthalmological exam revealed ischaemic changes with multiple cotton wool spots but no new vessels. Her discs appeared normal. Over the next week, she developed headache and sickness with photophobia and worsening blurred vision. An MRI scan was normal, a lumbar puncture revealed normal pressures and CSF. Over the next week BP rose further to 144/102 mmHg, proteinuria increased to >4 g/d and she developed significant peripheral oedema. She was commenced on methyldopa and labetalol. The next foetal scan showed a diminished growth velocity, and she was admitted for antepartum corticosteroids. Following these, her BP settled but her proteinuria continued to worsen, creatinine clearance declined, and her visual symptoms deteriorated. Because of this she was delivered at just over 35 weeks' gestation of a live baby girl who spent 3 weeks on the neonatal unit, but then did very well with no adverse sequelae. The woman's visual symptoms and headache rapidly resolved. Her ischaemic retinopathy improved without the need for photocoagulation. She remained significantly proteinuric, however. Because of this and her completely normal renal function before pregnancy, she underwent a renal biopsy six months later. This showed classic features of diffuse diabetic glomerulosclerosis. She is now managed with an angiotensin receptor blocker (she developed a cough on lisinopril) and still has microalbuminuria (ACR 8 mg/mmol). BP is 130/78 mmHg.

Comment: There are several learning points arising from this case. Firstly, although pregnancy can worsen established nephropathy, it is unusual for it to appear *de novo* antenatally. Secondly, she developed pre-eclampsia, and this might have been responsible for both the retinal changes (secondary to vasoconstriction and hypertension) and the development of nephropathy. It is interesting that the eye changes resolved almost immediately after delivery, but she remained albuminuric. Transient retinal ischaemia is described in diabetic pregnancy but is unusual; early delivery is strongly recommended in this situation. Pre-eclampsia is more common in diabetic pregnancy, particularly in women with nephropathy. Monitoring renal function is difficult where pre-eclampsia is superimposed on nephropathy and requires repeated, timed urine collections to estimate creatinine clearance. Lastly, the temporary improvement in blood pressure with steroids is a well-recognised feature of pre-eclampsia and should be a prompt to consider the diagnosis.

Contraception

There are no strong data to support any particular method of contraception in women with diabetes and current NICE guidance refers to the UK Medical Eligibility Criteria for Contraceptive use (UKMEC). All women with diabetes including GDM should have the opportunity to discuss contraception postpartum and this should be recorded in the patient record.

LANDMARK CLINICAL TRIALS

Crowther CA, Hiller JE, Moss JR, et al, for the ACHOIS Trial Group. Effect of treatment of gestational diabetes mellitus on pregnancy outcomes. N Engl J Med 2005; 352: 2477–2486.

The ACHOIS Trial has completely revolutionized our thinking and approach to GDM. Prior to its publication, there were no data to suggest that GDM was of any clinical significance because there were no properly powered intervention studies to show that management influenced outcome. Six hundred women were randomised to routine care or an intensive programme of dietary advice, blood glucose monitoring and insulin therapy, in order to maintain pre- and post-prandial levels <5.5 and <7.0 mmol/L respectively. The postprandial target was relaxed to <8.0 mmol/L after 35 weeks' gestation. There was a relative risk of 0.33 (95% CI 0.14–0.75) for serious perinatal complications (death, shoulder dystocia, bone fracture, or nerve palsy) in the intensively treated women. However, there was also an increased rate of induction of labour and more of the infants required admission to the neonatal unit. Caesarean section rates were the same between groups, but postpartum mood and quality of life were better in the intensive arm.

There has been an extensive critique of these findings and the complication rate in the routine care women seems higher than in many published series. There has also been some concern over the definition of shoulder dystocia. The subsequent study of Landon et al. also showed the benefit of intensive management of GDM and the debate has shifted to its definition and diagnosis.

With the publication of HAPO and evidence from ACHOIS that glycaemic intervention is of benefit, the management of GDM will never be the same.

KEY WEBSITES

- NICE 2015 Diabetes in pregnancy : management from preconception to the post natal period : www.nice.org.uk/guidance/ng3
- SIGN Guidelines: www.sign.ac.uk/assets/sign116.pdf
- Healthcare Quality Improvement Partnership National Diabetes Audit digital.nhs.uk/data-and-information/publications/statistical/nationl-pregnancy-in-diabetes-audit/national-diabetes-in-pregnancy-audit-annualreport-2018 (NDIP Audit Report)

FURTHER READING

American Diabetes Association. Standards of medical care in diabetes – 2020. Diabetes Care 2020; 43: Suppl 1: S183–S192.

Bell R, Glinianaia SV, Tennant PWG et al Peri-conception hyperglycaemia and nephropathy are associated with risk of congenital anomaly in women with pre-existing diabetes: a population-based cohort study. Diabetologia 2012; 55: 936–47doi: 10.1007/s00125-012-2455-y

Bellamy L, Casas J-P, Hingorani AD, Williams D. Type 2 diabetes after gestational diabetes: a systematic review and meta-analysis. Lancet 2009; 373: 1771–1779.

Chu SY, Callaghan WM, Kim SY, et al. Maternal obesity and risk of gestational diabetes mellitus. Diabetes Care 2007; 30(8): 2070– 2076.

Coton SJ, Nazareth I, Petersen I. A cohort study of trends in the prevalence of pre gestational diabetes in pregnancy recorded in UK general practice between 1995 and 2012. BMJ Open 2016; 6: e009494 doi: 10.1136/bmjopen-2015-009494

Cundy T, Holt RIG. Gestational diabetes: paradigm lost? Diabetic Med 2017; 34 : 8–13 doi: 10.1111/dme.13200

Crowther CA, Hiller JE, Moss JR, et al, for the ACHOIS Trial Group. Effect of treatment of gestational diabetes mellitus on pregnancy outcomes. N Engl J Med 2005; 352: 2477–2486.

Evers I, de Valk H, Visser G. Risk of complications of pregnancy in women with type 1 diabetes: nationwide prospective study in the Netherlands. BMJ 2004; 328: 915–918.

Farrar D et al Continuous subcutaneous insulin infusion versus multiple daily injections of insulin for pregnant women with diabetes. Cochrane Database System Rev 2016 CD 005542 doi: 10.1002/14651858.CD005542.pub3

Farrar D et al Different strategies for diagnosing gestational diabetes to improve maternal and infant health. Cochrane Database System Rev 2017 CD007122 doi: 10.1002/14651858.CD007122.pub4

Feig DS, Donovan LE, Corcoy R et al Continuous glucose monitoring in women with type 1 diabetes (CONCEPTT): a multi-centre international randomised controlled trial. Lancet 2017; http://dx.doi.org/10.1016/S0140-6736(17)32400-5

Glinianaia SV, Tennant PWG, Bilous RW et al HbA1c and birthweight in women with pre-conception type 1 and type 2 diabetes: a population-based cohort study. Diabetologia 2012; 55: 3193–3203 doi: 10.1007/s00125-012-2721-z

HAPO Study Cooperative Research Group. Hyperglycaemia and adverse pregnancy outcomes. N Engl J Med 2008; 358: 1991–2002.

International Association of Diabetes and Pregnancy Study Groups Consensus Panel. Recommendations on the diagnosis and classification of hyperglycaemia in pregnancy. Diabetes Care 2010; 33: 676–682.

Joint British Diabetes Societies for Inpatient Care JBDS 12 2017. Management of glycemic control in women with diabetes on obstetric wards and delivery units www.diabetologists-abcd.org.uk/JBDS/JBDS.htm

Tennant PWG, Glinianaia SV, Bilous RW et al Pre-existing diabetes, maternal glycated haemoglobin and the risks of fetal and infant death: a population-based cohort study. Diabetologia 2014; 57: 285–94 doi: 10.1007/s00125-013-3108-5

Chapter 30

Diabetes in childhood and adolescence

The vast majority of cases of diabetes in children are type 1 diabetes (T1D), caused by autoimmune destruction of β-cells in the pancreatic islets. Two peaks of T1D presentation occur in childhood and adolescence – one between 5 and 7 years of age, and the other occurring at or near puberty. While the underlying aetiological causes remains unclear, both genetic and environmental triggers are thought to be involved. A steady increase in the incidence of type 1 diabetes has been reported worldwide (average increase 2.5–3% per year worldwide with significant geographical variations). The incidence of T1D varies considerably between countries with more than 350-fold variation in incidence among reporting countries. For example, the lowest incidence is in China, India, and Venezuela where the incidence is only 0.1% per 100,000 per year. In contrast, pooled analysis showed that the increase in the incidence of type 1 diabetes in Europe is approximately 3.4% per annum, with a maximum rate of increase of 6.6% per annum in a Polish centre. Several centres in high-incidence countries, including Finland and Norway, along with two centres in the UK, showed reducing rates of increase in more recent years. Intriguingly, with some exceptions, the incidence of T1D is positively related to distance north of the equator (i.e. the so-called North–South Gradient). As such, an estimated 24% of all children with type 1 diabetes live in the European region, followed close by South East Asia (23%), with North America and the Caribbeans accounting for 19% of case worldwide.

The explanation for the considerable geographical variation in the incidence of T1D within Europe and the increasing trend towards younger age at diagnosis is unclear. The maternal and infant environment, as well as dietary factors, may be important. Data are inconsistent with respect to breastfeeding, and the introduction of cow's milk and cereals. An emerging dietary risk factor may be the early consumption of root vegetables (potatoes, carrots, etc)

between 3 and 4 months of age, and it is interesting that per-capita consumption of potatoes correlates with the incidence of type 1 diabetes in different countries. Other possible triggers for type 1 diabetes in early life include placental transmission of enteroviruses, food toxins, and cereals, which could activate autoimmune pathways during pregnancy. This evidence supports changes in environmental factors that operate early in life as a potential cause (Figures 30.1 and 30.2).

When diagnosing diabetes in a child or a young person, clinicians should assume T1D. However there are also rarer causes of diabetes in childhood which needs to be considered such as cystic fibrosis (which usually requires insulin), monogenic such as the neonatal forms of diabetes or maturity-onset diabetes of the young (MODY, see Chapter 8) and various other genetic syndromes such as Down's syndrome, Wolfram or DIDMOAD syndrome (diabetes insipidus, diabetes mellitus, optic atrophy and deafness), lipoatrophic diabetes, and Mitochondrial diabetes (see Chapter 8). There is also a rise in the incidence of Type 2 diabetes presenting in childhood (Box 30.1).

Childhood diabetes usually presents acutely with polyuria (including nocturia and incontinence), thirst, and polydipsia; about 40% have diabetic ketoacidosis (DKA). Other symptoms are weight loss, fatigue and abdominal pain. A simultaneous febrile illness is noted in about 20% of cases, particularly in younger children. Other possible presenting features include muscle cramps, infections (e.g. boils, urinary tract infections), behaviour disturbance, and poor school performance (Table 30.1).

DKA is a medical emergency that requires urgent admission to hospital, intravenous rehydration and insulin infusion. While DKA is often associated with plasma glucose level above 11mmol/L, children and young people taking insulin for diabetes may develop DKA with normal blood

Handbook of Diabetes, Fifth Edition. Rudy Bilous, Richard Donnelly, and Iskandar Idris.
© 2021 John Wiley & Sons Ltd. Published 2021 by John Wiley & Sons Ltd.

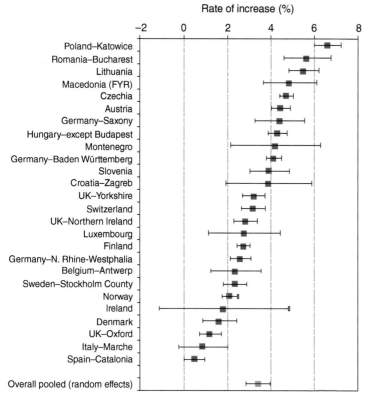

Figure 30.1 Trends and cyclical variation in the incidence of childhood type 1 diabetes in 26 European centres in the 25-year period 1989–2013: a multicentre prospective registration study. Patterson. *Diabetologia* 2019; 62(3): 408–417.

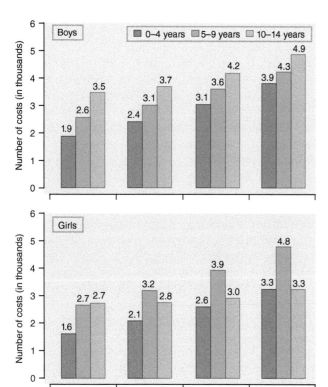

Figure 30.2 Predicted numbers of newly diagnosed cases of childhood-onset type 1 diabetes in Europe for boys and girls in three age bands: 0–4 years, 5–9 years, and 10–14 years. Adapted from Patterson et al. *Lancet* 2009; 373: 2027–2033.

Box 30.1 Consider Type 2 diabetes in children and young people if individuals have the following features.

- a strong family history of type 2 diabetes
- are obese at presentation
- are of black or Asian family origin
- have no insulin requirement (or insulin requirement of <0.5units/kg/day after the partial remission phase
- if they show evidence of insulin resistance (e.g. acanthosis nigricans)

Adapted from NICE guideline 2015 https://www.nice.org.uk/guidance/ng18?unlid=4816099252016917124749

Table 30.1 Symptoms before diagnosis in 1260 children with type 1 diabetes.

	Symptom noted *n* (%)	First symptom noted by the family *n* (%)
Polyuria	1159 (96%)	854 (71%)
Weight loss	731 (61%)	104 (9%)
Fatigue	630 (52%)	82 (7%)
Abdominal pain	277 (23%)	31 (3%)
Changes in character	137 (11%)	22 (2%)
Others	238 (19%)	36 (3%)
No symptom/ unspecified	16 (1%)	78 (6%)

glucose levels. Severe DKA (pH<7.1) is life-threatening (Boxes 30.2 and 30.3; Figure 30.3).

The most common cause of death during DKA in children is cerebral oedema, which leads to herniation of the brain stem, extension of the cerebellar tonsils into the foramen magnum, and respiratory arrest. Risk factors for developing cerebral oedema include low arterial PCO_2, elevated blood urea, and treatment with bicarbonate. Over-rapid delivery of fluid and insulin might be involved also. Clinicians should immediately assess children and young people with DKA for suspected cerebral oedema if they have any headache, agitation or irritability, unexpected fall in heart rate or increased blood pressure. If cerebral oedema is suspected in a child or a young person with DKA, or if there is deterioration in level of consciousness, abnormalities of breathing pattern, oculomotor palsies or pupillary inequality or dilatation, TREAT immediately with mannitol (20%, 0.5–1kg over 10–15 minutes) or hypertonic sodium chloride (2.7% or 3%, 2.5–5ml/kg over 10–15 minutes). Thereafter, seek specialist advice on further management, including deciding on the most appropriate care setting.

Type 1 diabetes has two subtypes: type 1A includes the common, immune-mediated forms of the disease, and type 1B includes the non-immune forms. The common form of type 1A diabetes is probably caused by multiple actions, and interactions, of genetic and environmental factors. Genetic

---

Box 30.2

Suspect DKA even if the blood glucose is normal in a child or young person with known T1D and any of the following:
- Nausea and vomiting
- Abdominal pain
- Hyperventilation
- Dehydration
- Reduced level of consciousness

Adapted from NICE guideline 2015 https://www.nice.org.uk/guidance/ng18?unlid=4816099252016917124749

Box 30.3

Diagnosis of DKA in children and young people is based on the following criteria:
- Acidosis (blood pH below 7.3 OR plasma bicarbonate below 18mmol/L

AND
- Presence of ketonaemia (indicated by blood beta-hydroxy-butyrate above 3mmol/L) or ketonuria (++ and above on the standard strip marking scale)
- Diagnose severe DKA in children and young person with DKA who have a blood pH below 7.1

Adapted from NICE guideline 2015 https://www.nice.org.uk/guidance/ng18?unlid=4816099252016917124749

---

linkage studies have shown significant associations between the HLA region on chromosome 6p21 and type 1A diabetes. In addition, class II genes encoding HLA-DR and HLA-DQ, as well as some other HLA foci, seem to account for most of the genetic risk for type 1A diabetes. Thus, children who carry both of the highest risk HLA haplotypes (DR3-DQ2 and DR4-DQ8) have a risk of approximately 1 in 20 for developing type 1 diabetes by the age of 15 years. Current approaches for the prediction of type 1 diabetes rely on the major genetic risk factors, genotyping for HLA-DR and HLA-DQ loci, and screening for autoantibodies directed against islet cell antigens (Figure 30.4).

Insulin regimen should be individualised for each patient according to personal and family circumstances or preferences. All children and young person with T1D should first be offered a multiple daily basal–bolus insulin regimens from diagnosis. If this regimen is not appropriate, consider continuous subcutaneous insulin infusion. Alternatively, the least preferred option of one, two or three-daily injections of short-acting or rapid acting insulin analogue mixed with intermediate-acting insulin maybe chosen. Irrespective of the insulin regimen, patients and their carers should be encouraged and supported to adjust insulin doses according to meals, blood glucose monitoring and activity levels. Patients and carers should also be explained that they may experience a partial remission phase ('honeymoon period'), lasting from a few months to up to 2 years, during which a low dose insulin (0.5units/kg body weight/day) maybe sufficient to maintain optimal Hba1c levels. This is due to a transient improvement in residual β-cell function. It is usual to maintain low-dose insulin treatment during the honeymoon period. Children and young adults with type 1 diabetes should be screened regularly for complications.

Hypoglycaemia is common in diabetic children, particularly in younger children who cannot communicate and in whom signs of hypoglycaemia (pallor, drowsiness, lethargy) are often detected by the parents. Moreover, young children are at risk of later neuropsychological impairment from severe, recurrent hypoglycaemia. Presumably, this relates to the effect of hypoglycaemia on the developing brain. Even older children are less able to detect hypoglycaemia than adults. Behavioural manifestations of hypoglycaemia include aggression, irritability, sadness, fatigue, and naughtiness (Table 30.2).

The use of Continuous subcutaneous insulin infusion (CSII, insulin pump therapy) among paediatric patients is increasing. However, Europe and many countries in the world lags behind the United States in the use of this technology. Evidence from randomised controlled study showed that compared with multiple daily insulin injection, those on CSII showed a sustained improvement in glucose control over a 5-year period. Systematic reviews and meta-analysis have reported that the use of CSII in paediatric patients with T1D was associated with better glycaemic control. When using CSII, age-appropriate structured continuous

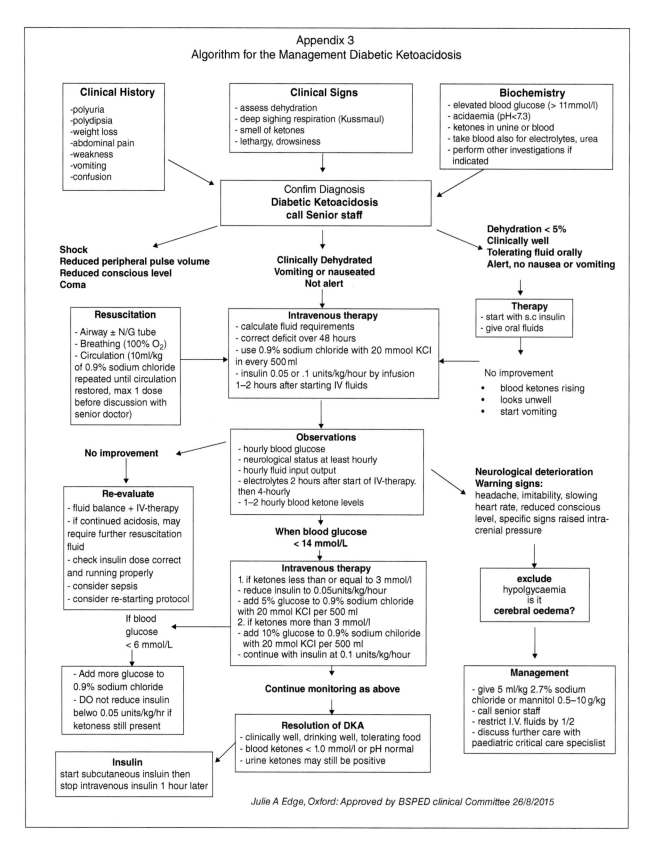

Appendix 3
Algorithm for the Management Diabetic Ketoacidosis

Clinical History

-polyuria
-polydipsia
-weight loss
-abdominal pain
-weakness
-vomiting
-confusion

Clinical Signs

- assess dehydration
- deep sighing respiration (Kussmaul)
- smell of ketones
- lethargy, drowsiness

Biochemistry

- elevated blood glucose (> 11mmol/l)
- acidaemia (pH<7.3)
- ketones in unine or blood
- take blood also for electrolytes, urea
- perform other investigations if indicated

Confim Diagnosis
**Diabetic Ketoacidosis
call Senior staff**

**Dehydration < 5%
Clinically well
Tolerating fluid orally
Alert, no nausea or vomiting**

**Shock
Reduced peripheral pulse volume
Reduced conscious level
Coma**

**Clinically Dehydrated
Vomiting or nauseated
Not alert**

Therapy
- start with s.c insulin
- give oral fluids

Resuscitation

- Airway ± N/G tube
- Breathing (100% O$_2$)
- Circulation (10ml/kg of 0.9% sodium chloride repeated until circulation restored, max 1 dose before discussion with senior doctor)

Intravenous therapy
- calculate fluid requirements
- correct deficit over 48 hours
- use 0.9% sodium chloride with 20 mmool KCl in every 500 ml
- insulin 0.05 or .1 units/kg/hour by infusion 1–2 hours after starting IV fluids

No improvement

- blood ketones rising
- looks unwell
- start vomiting

No improvement

Observations
- hourly blood glucose
- neurological status at least hourly
- hourly fluid input output
- electrolytes 2 hours after start of IV-therapy. then 4-hourly
- 1–2 hourly blood ketone levels

Re-evaluate

- fluid balance + IV-therapy
- if continued acidosis, may require further resuscitation fluid
- check insulin dose correct and running properly
- consider sepsis
- consider re-starting protocol

**When blood glucose
< 14 mmol/L**

**Neurological deterioration
Warning signs:**
headache, imitability, slowing heart rate, reduced conscious level, specific signs raised intra-crenial pressure

Intravenous therapy
1. if ketones less than or equal to 3 mmol/l
- reduce insulin to 0.05units/kg/hour
- add 5% glucose to 0.9% sodium chloride with 20 mmol KCl per 500 ml
2. if ketones more than 3 mmol/l
- add 10% glucose to 0.9% sodium chiloride with 20 mmol KCl per 500 ml
- continue with insulin at 0.1 units/kg/hour

exclude
hypolgycaemia
is it
cerebral oedema?

If blood glucose < 6 mmol/L

Continue monitoring as above

- Add more glucose to 0.9% sodium chloride
- DO not reduce insulin belwo 0.05 units/kg/hr if ketoness still present

Management
- give 5 ml/kg 2.7% sodium chloride or mannitol 0.5–10 g/kg
- call senior staff
- restrict I.V. fluids by 1/2
- discuss further care with paediatric critical care specislist

Resolution of DKA
- clinically well, drinking well, tolerating food
- blood ketones < 1.0 mmol/l or pH normal
- urine ketones may still be positive

Insulin
start subcutaneous insluin then stop intravenous insulin 1 hour later

Julie A Edge, Oxford: Approved by BSPED clinical Committee 26/8/2015

Figure 30.3 Algorithm for the management of DKA. Adapted from the updated (2015) guidelines of the British Society of Paediatric Endocrinology and Diabetes. http://www.bsped.org.uk/clinical/docs/DKAguideline.pdf)

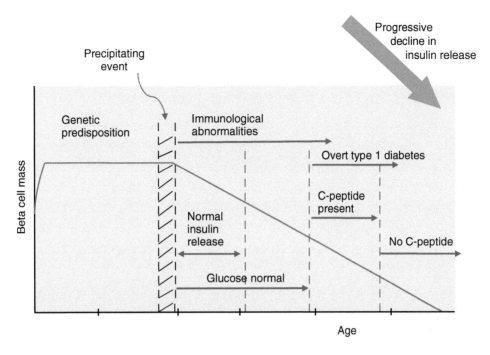

Figure 30.4 Type 1 diabetes has a preclinical phase of varying duration when autoimmune destruction of beta cells reduces beta cell mass in the pancreatic islets. This probably follows a precipitating event. Gradually, beta cell mass is reduced to a point when glucose levels can no longer be maintained within normal limits. This schematic illustrates stages in the development of type 1A diabetes. It also illustrates a potential window for therapeutic intervention during the preclinical phase to prevent the onset of overt diabetes. Trials of immunosuppressive therapies in high-risk individuals are ongoing.

education of the entire family, provided by a multidisciplinary team with a strong emphasis on psychosocial support and nutritional education, including the counting of carbohydrates is very important. The use of sensor augmented insulin pump with an automated insulin suspend function, which suspends insulin delivery at a pre-defined low glucose concentration, have been shown to reduce the time spent in hypoglycaemia, the frequency of hypoglycaemia, and the frequency of severe hypoglycaemia. Similarly, increased use

Table 30.2 Clinical features of hypoglycaemia in children.

Neuroglycopenic and autonomic	Behavioural
Reported by the children	
Weakness	Headache
Trembling	Argumentative
Dizziness	Aggressive
Poor concentration	Irritability
Hunger	Naughty
Sweating	
Confusion	
Blurred vision	
Slurred speech	Nausea
Double vision	Nightmares
Observed by the parents	
As above, plus:	
Pallor	
Sleepiness	
Convulsions	

From Mortensen et al. Diabetes Care 1997; 20: 714 – 720.

of continuous glucose monitoring (CGM) sensor technology such as Freestyle Libre@ or DEXCOM@ have improved the management of hyperglycaemia in this population and reduced risks of hypoglycaemia. Significant amount of work is also currently underway to develop an artificial pancreas system, in which CSII with Rapid Acting insulin analogue are incorporated into closed-loop insulin delivery systems. Preliminary data for the success of such systems has already been reported (Figures 30.5 and 30.6; Box 30.4).

The past three decades have seen a significant increase in the prevalence of early onset type 2 diabetes. Affected individuals are likely to be obese, have a multigenerational family history of T2DM, lead a sedentary lifestyle, be of black or minority ethnic (BME) origin and tend to come from a socially deprived group. They have a heightened risk of the premature development of microvascular and macrovascular complications, in addition to psychological morbidity, during their working life. The pathophysiology of early onset T2DM is complex, with an alteration in the balance between insulin sensitivity and insulin secretion as the most important determinant in the development of the disease. Adolescents with glucose dysregulation however are more are likely to have more impairment in insulin secretion compared with reduced insulin sensitivity (Figure 30.7).In terms of treatment for hyperglycaemia, currently, metformin and insulin are the only drugs approved for use in the paediatric population with Type 2 diabetes. However, the TODAY trial is the largest therapeutic trial to be conducted in a large cohort of

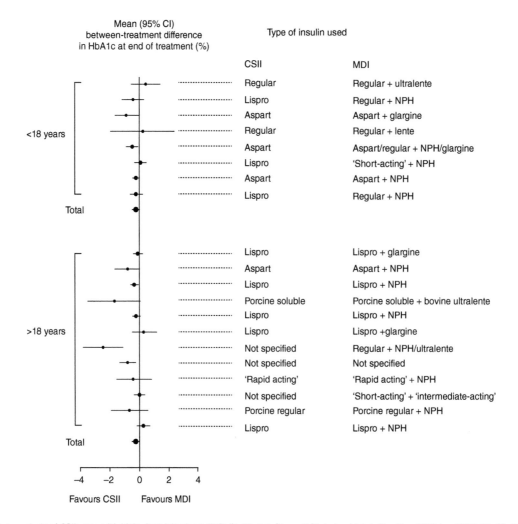

Figure 30.5 Meta-analysis of CSII versus Multiple dose injection in T1D. Pozilli et al. Figure 2 Diabetes Metab Res Rev. 2016 Jan; 32(1): 21–39. Published online 2015 Jun 22. doi: 10.1002/dmrr.2653.

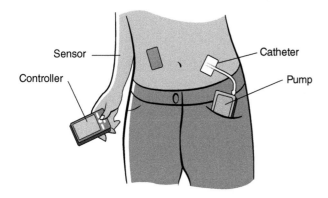

Figure 30.6 Component of a closed loop insulin delivery system. Interstitial glucose level, measured by the sensor, are transmitted to the controller, which contains a control algorithm. This modulates the pumps insulin infusion rate in real time. All communications are wireless. Pozilli et al. Figure 4 Diabetes Metab Res Rev. 2016 Jan; 32(1): 21–39. Published online 2015 Jun 22. doi: 10.1002/dmrr.2653.

Box 30.4 According to the NICE Guideline, children and young people with type 1 diabetes should be offered screening for:

- Coeliac disease – at diagnosis and every 3 years thereafter
- Thyroid disease – at diagnosis and annually thereafter
- Retinopathy – annually from age 12 years
- Microalbuminuria – annually from age 12 years
- Blood pressure – annually from age 12 years

Clinicians should also be aware of the rarer complications: juvenile cataracts and Addison's disease

adolescents with type 2 diabetes. In this 4-year follow-up randomised controlled trial, those recently diagnosed with T2DM were randomly assigned to either metformin alone, metformin and a lifestyle intervention, or metformin plus rosiglitazone. The study observed that metformin treatment failure rate was higher than is seen in older adults with type 2 diabetes, indicating that younger adults with type 2 diabetes are likely to require more aggressive polypharmacy early in the course of their disease. This trial also suggests that the benefits of lifestyle interventions in adolescents with T2DM may be limited (Figure 30.8).

There is a wide array of glucose lowering therapies currently approved for adult use, including gliptins, SGLT2 inhibitor, and glucagon-like peptide-1 (GLP-1) analogues. Such agents would, in theory, benefit those with early onset type 2 diabetes. The evidence from this however remains scarce and further studies are needed to confirm the efficacy of these commonly agents in children and young adults with type 2 diabetes. In a study in children and adolescents with type 2 diabetes, liraglutide, at a dose of up to 1.8 mg per day (added to metformin, with or without basal insulin), was shown to be efficacious in improving glycemic control over 52 weeks. However, this efficacy came at the cost of an increased frequency of gastrointestinal adverse events, which may be intolerable to children.

Modifiable

- Obesity
- Low physical activity
- High sedentary behaviour
- Socioeconomic status

NonModifiable

- Ethnicity (Pima Indian, Hispanic, Asian and Afro-Caribbean)
- Family history of type 2 diabetes mellitus
- Puberty
- Low birth weight
- Exposure to diabetes mellitus in the uterus
- Female sex
- Previous gestational diabetes

Figure 30.7 Risk factors for type 2 diabetes in youth – adapted from Wilmott et al. Early onset type 2 diabetes: risk factors, clinical impact and management. Ther. Adv. Chronic Disease 2014; 5: 234–44.

Intervention	Failure rate
Metformin alone	51.7%
Metformin + lifestyle	46.6%
Metformin + rosiglitazone	38.6%
Pairwise test	*p* value
Metformin + lifestyle versus metformin	0.015
Metformin versus metformin + rosiglitazone	0.006
Metformin versus metformin + lifestyle	0.17

The study compared the efficacy of three treatment regimens (metformin 1000mg twice daily alone, a metformin + lifestyle intervention programme focusing on weight loss through eating and activity behaviours, and metformin + rosiglitazone 4 mg twice daily) to achieve durable glycaemic control in children and adolescents with early-onset type 2 diabetes. The primary outcome was loss of glycaemic control, defined as a glycated haemoglobin level of at least 8% for 6 months or sustained metabolic decompensation requiring insulin. Results are described in the text.

Figure 30.8 Result from the TODAY Trial.

CASE HISTORY

A 13-year-old boy has a 7-year history of type 1 diabetes treated with basal bolus insulin therapy. He experiences frequent hypoglycaemic events and has had two hospital admissions with diabetic ketoacidosis over the last 12 months. These complications have become more common during his puberty. His glycaemic control is suboptimal (HbA1c ranges from 8.6–10.1%). In addition, there have been frequent episodes of severe hypoglycaemia requiring third party assistance. These have been more frequent during puberty. At his last retinal screening visit, there were signs of background retinopathy in both eyes. Increasingly, he has become angry with having diabetes, has missed a lot of extra-curricular school activities, and recently has taken to missing his insulin injections and/or missing meals.

Comment: This case history illustrates the multifactorial challenges that healthcare professionals, parents, and carers might face when managing a young person with T1D. There is clear evidence from a large scale randomised controlled trial that early tight glycaemic control has long-lasting benefits in terms of fewer complications, but balancing insulin therapy with the lifestyle of a teenager and motivating them to self-manage their disease can be extremely difficult. Assessment of the emotional and psychological wellbeing of this individual is crucial. Provision of a structured education for the patient and family is important to ensure that the patient remains on tract with self-management of this T1D. If appropriate, CSII therapy should be discussed in order to reduce the frequency of disabling hypoglycaemia and to achieve optimal glucose control.

LANDMARK TRIALS

Lind M et al. Glycemic control and excess mortality in type 1 diabetes. N Engl J Med. 2014 Nov 20; 371(21): 1972–82.

Writing Group for the DCCT/EDIC Research Group, Orchard TJ et al. Association between 7 years of intensive treatment of type 1 diabetes and long-term mortality. JAMA. 2015 Jan 6; 313(1): 45–53. doi: 10.1001/jama.2014.16107.

Patterson CC, et al. Incidence trends for childhood type 1 diabetes in Europe during 1989–2003 and predicted new cases 2005–20: a multicentre prospective registration study. Lancet 2009; 373: 2027–2033.

Harjutsalo V, et al. Time trends in the incidence of type 1 diabetes in Finnish children: a cohort study. Lancet 2008; 371: 1777–1782.

SEARCH Study Group SEARCH for Diabetes in Youth: a multicenter study of the prevalence, incidence and classification of diabetes mellitus in youth. Control Clin Trials 2004; 25: 458–471

KEY WEBSITES

- https://www.nice.org.uk/guidance/ng18?unlid=4816099252016917124749
- http://www.ndei.org/ADA-diabetes-management-guidelines-children-adolescents-type-1-diabetes-type-2-diabetes.aspx.html

FURTHER READING

Moltchanova EV, et al. Seasonal variation of diagnosis of type 1 diabetes mellitus in children worldwide. Diabet. Med. 2009; 26: 673–678.

Neu A, et al. Ketoacidosis at diabetes onset is still frequent in children and adolescents: a multicentre analysis of 14,664 patients from 106 institutions. Diabetes Care 2009, 32: 1647–1648

Bolinder J et al. Novel glucose-sensing technology and hypoglycaemia in type 1 diabetes: a multicentre, non-masked, randomised controlled trial Lancet 2016, 388; 10057: 2254–2263

Pozilli et al. Continuous subcutaneous insulin infusion in diabetes: patient populations, safety, efficacy, and pharmacoeconomics Diabetes Metab Res Rev. 2016; 32(1): 21–39.

TODAY Study Group, Zeitler, P. et al. A clinical trial to maintain glycemic control in youth with type 2 diabetes. N Engl J Med 2012; 366:

Rewers et al. Environmental risk factors for type 1 diabetes. Lancet. 2016; 387(10035): 2340–8. Review.

Pociot F et al. Genetic risk factors for type 1 diabetes. Lancet. 2016 Jun 4; 387(10035): 2331–9. doi: 10.1016/S0140–6736(16)30582–7. Review

Tamborlane WV et al. Liraglutide in children and adolescents with type 2 diabetes. NEJM 2019; 381: 637–646

Breton MD et al. A randomized trial of closed-loop control in children with type 1 diabetes. NEJM 2020; 383: 836–845

Chapter
31

Diabetes in old age

People above the age of 65 years accounts for more than 35% of people with diabetes. As such, the ageing population is one of the biggest drivers to the rising prevalence of diabetes worldwide. During the next decade, the greatest increase in diabetes is anticipated to be among persons aged 75 and older. However, although studies have estimated the prevalence of diabetes in the elderly, data relating to this relies on the diagnostic criteria being used. This is because postprandial hyperglycaemia is a prominent characteristic of type 2 diabetes in older adults, and contributes to the observed differences in prevalence depending on which diagnostic test is used. Using the HbA1c or fasting plasma glucose (FPG) diagnostic criteria, one-third of older adults with diabetes are undiagnosed compared with if a Glucose Tolerance Test (GTT) are being used.

Diabetes in older adults is linked to higher mortality, reduced functional status, and increased risk of institutionalization. Older adults with diabetes also have the highest rates of major lower-extremity amputation, myocardial infarction, visual impairment, and end-stage renal disease of any age-group. Because of the heterogeneity of their clinical status and the limited evidence-based strategies for managing older people with diabetes, the management of this group of individuals represent a unique challenge to healthcare professionals involved in the management of people with diabetes (Figures 31.1 and 31.2).

The presentation of diabetes in older people is often insidious and the diagnosis is often delayed. The symptoms can be non-specific and vague, such as fatigue, urinary incontinence, or change in mental state (e.g. depression, confusion, and apathy). Many cases are detected by finding incidental hyperglycaemia during the investigation of comorbidities, such as a delayed recovery from specific illnesses, repeated infections, or cardiovascular disease; the latter may present with atypical features, such as painless myocardial infarction,

manifested as breathlessness, lassitude, or falls. Acute metabolic disturbance is a further, rarer presentation: about 25% of cases of hyperosmolar non-ketotic hyperglycaemic coma occur in people with previously undiagnosed type 2 diabetes. The tendency to hyperosmolarity may be worse in elderly people, who may not perceive thirst or drink enough to compensate for the osmotic diuresis of diabetes, and who are often taking diuretics (Figure 31.3).

Recent guidelines from the American Diabetes Association (ADA), the European Association Study of Diabetes (EASD) and the UK National Institute of Clinical Excellence (NICE) emphasises the importance of individualising the HbA1c target. While the pursuit of low HbA1c target may not always be appropriate in the elderly patients, failing to address hyperglycaemia may significantly increase the risk of acute metabolic events and potentially morbidity and mortality. Hence, various factors needs to be considered when determining treatment options as well as treatment targets in elderly people with diabetes (Figure 31.4).

Antihyperglycaemic medication in older adults

Older adults who are fit and well, who are cognitively intact, and have significant life expectancy should receive diabetes care using goals developed for younger adults. For many elderly patients with diabetes however, treatment is mainly aimed to alleviate symptoms, to reduce the risk of hyperglycaemic crises, to prevent and manage vascular and other complications and to achieve a normal life expectancy whenever possible. Strict glycaemic control may not always be appropriate.

Metformin is often considered the first-line therapy in type 2 diabetes. Its low risk for hypoglycaemia may be beneficial in older adults, but gastrointestinal intolerance and weight loss from the drug may be detrimental in frail or nutritionally challenged patients. In addition, its increased tendency

Handbook of Diabetes, Fifth Edition. Rudy Bilous, Richard Donnelly, and Iskandar Idris.
© 2021 John Wiley & Sons Ltd. Published 2021 by John Wiley & Sons Ltd.

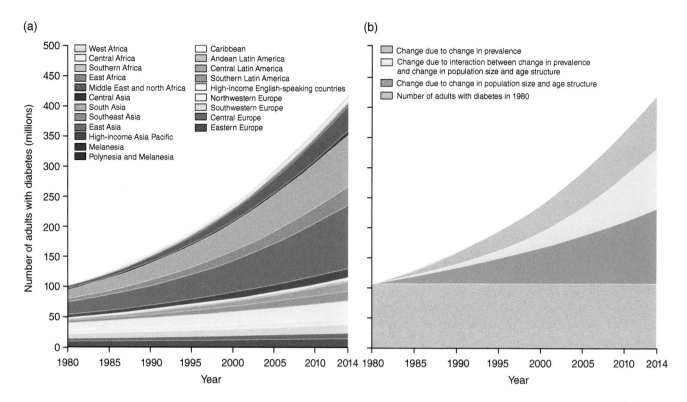

Figure 31.1 Trends in the number of adults with diabetes by region (A) and decomposed into the contributions of population growth and ageing, rise in prevalence, and interaction between the two (B). Zhou et al. *The Lancet* 2016; 387: 1513–1530. DOI: (10.1016/S0140–6736(16)00618–8).

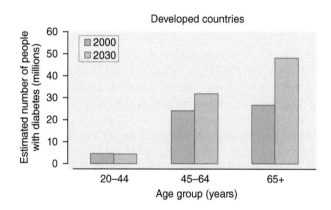

Figure 31.2 Estimated number of adults with diabetes in developed countries by age in 2030 compared with 2000. Adapted from Wild et al. *Diabetes Care* 2004; 27: 1047–1053.

- Non-specific symptoms (lassitude, confusion, incontinence, falls, etc.)
- Presentation with co-morbidity (coincidental hyperglycaemia)
  - cardiovascular disease (NB: myocardial infarction may be silent in the elderly)
  - delayed recovery from illness (e.g. stroke)
  - repeated infections
- Classic osmotic symptoms
- Acute metabolic disturbance (mostly HONK, rarely DKA)

Figure 31.3 The various ways in which diabetes may present in the elderly.

to cause lactic acidosis with renal impairment and hepatic or cardiac failure may limit its use in many older patients. Sulfonylureas (SU) are commonly used in this population, but the risk of hypoglycaemia with these agents may be problematic for older patients. Long acting SU such as Glibenclamide (Glyburide) has the highest hypoglycemia risk and should not be prescribed. Short-acting sulfonylureas such as gliclazide are therefore preferred because of the likelihood in the elderly of impaired renal function, poor nutrition, impaired counter-regulatory responses and cognition, and other factors that increase the risk of hypoglycaemia.

Dipeptidylpeptidase (DPP)-4 inhibitors are effective therapy to treat post prandial hyperglycaemia, is associated with little risk of hypoglycaemia and are well tolerated, suggesting a potential role in the elderly. However, Glucagon like peptide (GLP)-1 analogues while also effective in reducing postprandial glucose level, are associated with increased risk of nausea and vomiting, and may therefore not be suitable for the frail, older patients. Sodium glucose transporter (SGLT)-2 inhibitors are the latest class of drug for diabetes. Their role in the elderly however is currently limited due to its tendency to induced diuresis which may lead to dehydration but also its limited efficacy in patients with reduced glomerular filtration rate.

Comorbidities and geriatric syndromes

Cognitive dysfunction

Functional status

Falls and fractures

Polypharmacies

Depression

Visual and hearing impairment

Common medical conditions

Nutritional status

Physical activity, sarcopenia and fitness

Vulnerability to hypoglycaemia

Risk of undertreatment of hyperglycaemia

Life expectancy

Figure 31.4 Diabetes in the elderly: key points to consider when individualising treatment approach Adapted from Diabetes in older Adults. Kirkman MS et al. Diabetes Care 2012; 35:2650.

Insulin therapy may sometimes be required in the older patients with diabetes. Simple insulin regimens are usually the most appropriate in diabetes of old age. Twice-daily injections of premixed insulins for type 1 diabetes or NPH insulin in type 2 patients are preferred. However, the practical difficulties of administration can limit their use in some patients and once-daily insulin, though unlikely to produce good control, may be more suitable for the very old and frail. The use of once- or twice-daily injections of the long-acting insulin analogues, glargine or detemir, may be advantageous and practical. More recently, ultra-longer acting insulin such as Insulin Degludec or Toujeo are available which might benefit elderly patients who rely on others to inject their insulin once daily. The traditional multiple-dose, basal-bolus regimen for achieving near normoglycaemia is probably only suitable for the comparatively few well-motivated, mobile, and mentally alert patients who are independent in self-care and have no other medical disorders (Figure 31.5).

A framework for considering treatment goals for glycemia, blood pressure, and dyslipidemia in older adults with diabetes

Patient characteristics/ health status	Rationale	Reasonable AIC goal (A lower goal may be set for an individual if achievable without recurrent or severe hypoglycemia or undue treatment burden)	Fasting or preprandial glucose (mg/dL)	Bedtime glucose (mg/dL)	Blood pressure (mmHg)	Lipids
Healthy (Few coexisting chronic illnesses, intact cognitive and functional status)	Longer remaining life expectancy	<7.5%	90–130	90–150	<140/80	Statin unless contraindicated or not tolerated
Complex/intermediate (Multiple coexisting chronic illnesses* or 2+ instrumental ADL impairments or mild to moderate cognitive impairment)	Intermediate remaining life expectancy, high treatment burden, hypoglycemia vulnerability, fall risk	<8.0%	90–150	100–180	<140/80	Statin unless contraindicated or not tolerated
Very complex/poor health (Long-term care or end-stage chronic illnesses** or moderate to severe cognitive impairment or 2+ ADL dependencies)	Limited remaining life expectancy makes benefit uncertain	<8.5% †	100–180	110–200	<150/90	Consider likelihood of benefit with statin (secondary prevention moreso than primary)

This represents a consensus framework for considering treatment goals for glycemia, blood pressure, and dyslipidemia in older adults with diabetes. The patient characteristic categories are general concepts. Not every patient will clearly fall into particular category. Consideration of patient/caregiver preferences is an important aspect of treatment individualization. Additionally, a patient's health status and preferences may change over time. ADL, activities of daily living. *Coexisting chronic illnesses are conditions serious enough to require medications or lifestyle management and may include arthritis, cancer, congestive heart failure, depression, emphysema, falls, hypertension, incontinence, stage III or worse chronic kidney disease, MI, and stroke. By multiple we mean at least three, but many patients may have five or more (132).**The presence of a single end-stage chronic illness such as stage III-IV congestive heart failure or oxygen-dependent lung disease, chronic kidney disease requiring dialysis, or uncontrolled metastatic cancer may cause significant symptoms or impairment of functional status and significantly reduce life expectancy. †AIC of 8.5% equates to an estimated average glucose of ~ 200 mg/dL. Looser glycemic targets than this may expose patients to acute risks from glycosuria, dehydration, hyperglycemic hyperosmolar syndrome, and poor wound healing.

Figure 31.5 Proposed framework when considering treatment goals for glycaemia, blood pressure, and dyslipidaemia in older adults with diabetes.

CASE HISTORY

A family doctor was asked to review an 86-year-old lady living in a nursing home. She was confused, febrile, and incontinent of urine. Normally, she mobilises with a frame and has short-term memory difficulties, but for several days she has been unwell, more confused, and off her feet. The GP notes an episode of left leg cellulitis, treated with antibiotics, one month ago. On examination, she is obese, febrile, confused, and clinically dehydrated. The GP suspects a urinary tract infection. It has been impossible to dipstick her urine; blood tests are sent off. These confirm a raised white cell count (neutrophilia), impaired renal function, and elevated random serum glucose (23 mmol/L). HbA1c 9.1%.

Comment: Infections, dehydration, and urinary incontinence can often reflect undiagnosed diabetes in the elderly. In turn, these metabolic disturbances can affect cognitive function. The emphasis should be on symptom control. This lady needs rehydration, and treatment. With renal impairment, a glitazone or a DPP4 inhibitor may be preferred or, for practical reasons, it may be easier to start once daily basal insulin therapy instead of an oral agent, especially if her intake is limited.

LANDMARK CLINICAL TRIALS

Wild S, et al. Global prevalence of diabetes. Diabetes Care 2004; 27: 1047–1053.

Mozaffarian D, et al. Lifestyle risk factors and new-onset diabetes mellitus in older adults. Arch. Intern. Med. 2009; 169: 798–807.

Whitmer RA, et al. Hypoglycaemic episodes and risk of dementia in older patients with type 2 diabetes mellitus. JAMA 2009; 301: 1565–1572.

Biessels GJ, et al. Risk of dementia in diabetes mellitus: a systematic review. Lancet Neurol. 2006; 5: 64–74.

Cukierman T, et al. Cognitive decline and dementia in diabetes – systematic overview of prospective observational studies. Diabetologia 2005; 48: 2460–2469.

KEY WEBSITES

- http://www.diabetes.co.uk/diabetes-and-the-elderly.html
- http://www.diabetes-healthnet.ac.uk/HandBook/DiabetesSpecialCircumstancesElderly.aspx

FURTHER READING

Kirkman SM, Briscoe VJ, Clark N, Florez H, Hass, LB, Halter JB et al. Diabetes in Older Adults. Diabetes Care 2012; 35(12): 2650–2664

Sinclair A, Morley JE. How to manage diabetes mellitus in older persons in the 21st century: applying these principles to long term diabetes care. J Am Med Dir Assoc. 2013; 14(11): 777–780.

Feldman SM, et al. Status of diabetes management in the nursing home setting in 2008: a retrospective chart review and epidemiology study of diabetic nursing home residents and nursing home initiatives in diabetes management. J. Am. Med. Dir. Assoc. 2009; 10: 354–360.

Miller ME et al. Effect of randomization to intensive glucose control on adverse events, cardiovascular disease, and mortality in older versus younger adults in the ACCORD trial Diabetes Care 2014; 37: 634–643 | DOI: 10.2337/dc13–1545

Kim TN, Park MS, Yang SJ, et al. Prevalence and determinant factors of sarcopenia in patients with type 2 diabetes: the Korean Sarcopenic Obesity Study (KSOS). Diabetes Care 2010; 33: 1497–1499

LeRoith D et al. Treatment of diabetes in older adults: An Endocrine Society Clinical Practice Guideline. J Clin Endocrinol Metab. 2019; 104: 1520–1574

Diabetes and lifestyle

KEY POINTS

- Smoking confers a risk both for the development of diabetes and for its complications.
- Alcohol use is associated with hypoglycaemia in people on insulin therapy.
- Alcohol and substance abuse is associated with increased mortality and morbidity in people with diabetes.
- Most European countries issue driving guidance for people with diabetes, particularly for those on insulin or other therapies with a risk of hypoglycaemia.
- The guidance is broadly similar but needs checking in each country.

- There is no longer a blanket ban for driving commercial vehicles for people taking insulin.
- Disability discrimination legislation makes it illegal to impose restrictions on people with diabetes with regard to employment, but there are a few exceptions which vary between and within countries.
- Diabetes is not a bar to long distance travel, but planning is necessary beforehand and individual identification is essential, particularly if transporting insulin, syringes, pens and needles and devices such as glucose monitors and insulin pumps.

Introduction

Exercise has been covered in Chapter 28, and dietary issues and obesity in the sections on type 1 and type 2 diabetes. This chapter will focus on smoking, alcohol and drug abuse, employment, driving, and travel.

Smoking

People who smoke are 30–40% more likely to develop type 2 diabetes. This increased risk persists after quitting for at least 5 years, possibly because of associated weight gain. Smoking increases insulin resistance and diminishes pancreatic insulin release. Nicotine itself increases blood glucose concentrations.

People with diabetes who smoke have increased rates of both macrovascular and microvascular complications. There is an approximate 50% increase in relative risk for both all cause and cardiovascular mortality in people with diabetes who smoke compared to those who don't (Figure 32.1). Smoking increases the risk of development of diabetic nephropathy and retinopathy and also increases the rate of progression of nephropathy, especially in type 1 diabetes.

All cause mortality in people with diabetes who stopped smoking was reduced by 30% in the ADVANCE study and the benefits in terms of reductions in cardiovascular disease were seen >10 years after quitting. However, there seems to be no significant impact of stopping smoking on nephropathy or retinopathy progression, although the quality of the data is not strong.

There are no specific studies of smoking cessation interventions in people with diabetes, but the evidence suggests that the rates of success are similar to the general population. Nicotine replacement therapy, bupropion, and varenicline all seem to be well tolerated with no negative effects on glycaemia. A particular concern of patients is the potential for weight gain after stopping and this needs to be addressed with dietetic advice from the outset.

Despite the negative effects of smoking in people with diabetes, prevalence rates mirror those in the background population. Part of the reason may lie with a lack of structured advice, as a recent Diabetes UK survey revealed that 64% of people with diabetes never received advice on smoking cessation during their clinic visits.

Handbook of Diabetes, Fifth Edition. Rudy Bilous, Richard Donnelly, and Iskandar Idris.
© 2021 John Wiley & Sons Ltd. Published 2021 by John Wiley & Sons Ltd.

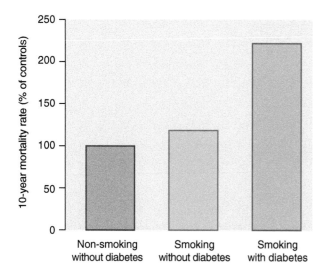

Figure 32.1 Deleterious effects of smoking and disease on 10-year mortality. Death rate is expressed as a percentage of age- and sex-matched, non-smoking populations without diabetes. From Suarez & Barrett-Connor. Am J Epidemiol 1984;120:670–675.

Alcohol

Both diabetes (mortality 10.7%) and alcohol (mortality 2.2% women, 6.8% men) contributed significantly to all cause global mortality in 2017, There is an apparent U-shaped curve for the development of type 2 diabetes in people who consume alcohol, with a nadir at 5–20g consumption per day. However, there are multiple confounders in this association and any putative protection of alcohol in terms of diabetes prevention is hotly debated.

The rates of alcohol consumption in people with type 1 diabetes seem no different to the background population, whereas for type 2 diabetes the amount of alcohol consumption may be less. However, the prevalence of alcohol abuse disorders seems greater than in the matched background population, and this is particularly so in those who have undergone bariatric surgery (with the exception of adjustable banding). The reasons are unclear but may be related to altered alcohol metabolism post surgery. People with type 2 diabetes are over-represented in the US population referred for addiction treatment.

Heavy alcohol consumption is associated with an increased all cause mortality (OR 1.35) and this seems to be related to hypoglycaemia and DKA in type 1 patients, and cardiovascular, stroke, kidney, and neuropathy related causes in type 2. In Finland, the standardised mortality ratio for alcohol related deaths in people with type 1 diabetes is 1.5 (95% CI 1.1,1.9), and 39% of deaths in the 20 year period post diabetes onset in those diagnosed between the ages of 15–29 years were alcohol or drug related. Also in Finland, the mortality rate ratio for an alcohol related death in people with type 2 diabetes was 1.71 for men and 2.10 for women compared

to matched controls without diabetes, and this increased to 6.92 and 10.60 respectively for those taking insulin. Much of this increase was related to liver cirrhosis.

Alcohol is detectable in at least 17% of hospital presentations for hypoglycaemia in people with type 1 diabetes. Alcohol itself does not lower blood glucose (a common misconception among patients), but its metabolism through acetaldehyde to acetate results in an increase in NADH and a reduction in NAD+ resulting in diminished gluconeogenesis. This, together with a relative insulin excess and reduced carbohydrate intake results in delayed hypoglycaemia often 6–8 hours after drinking. In type 2 diabetes, there is another U-shaped relationship between alcohol intake and complications. Modest white wine consumption lowers fasting blood glucose by around 1 mmol/L whilst red wine increases HDL cholesterol by 0.05 mmol/L. These benefits are also the subject of hot debate and are not thought to provide the basis for a recommendation for regular alcohol. For people with alcohol abuse disorders and type 2 diabetes, the ORs for cardiovascular disease, neuropathy and myocardial infarction are all raised at 1.35, 1.27, and 1.62 respectively, compared to those without diabetes. There appear to be no consistent links between heavy alcohol intake and microvascular complications.

The management of alcohol abuse disorders is the same for people with diabetes as for the general population, and with equal effectiveness. Routine enquiry into alcohol consumption and episodes of binge drinking during annual diabetes review is recommended. Brief (< 15 minute) counselling interventions have been shown to be effective in those identified with a problem. It should be remembered that alcohol abuse may be a manifestation of diabetes distress and/or depression (Chapter 27). Alcohol and drug abuse should be explored in people with type 1 diabetes who have recurrent admissions with hypoglycaemia and/or DKA. Education of the risks is important. Regrettably, although surveys have shown reasonable knowledge of the risks of alcohol consumption in young people with diabetes, in a recent study only 62% said they took action in terms of ensuring adequate carbohydrate intake. Apart from a consensus recommendation from professional bodies that taking carbohydrate with alcohol is advisable, there is little research on how to prevent serious hypoglycaemia. The role of technologies such as CGM or flash glucose monitoring in preventing alcohol related hypoglycaemia has yet to be established.

Drug and substance abuse

There is no conclusive evidence that cannabis and drug abuse increases the risk of developing type 2 diabetes, even though there are experimental data showing a hyperglycaemic effect with stimulants such as amphetamines, and increased appetite with cannabis. Drug use disorders are more common in those with type 2 diabetes in the USA, perhaps secondary to the widespread prescription of opioids for neuropathy.

As with alcohol, drug abuse is associated with increased mortality in people with both type 1(hypoglycaemia and DKA predominate) and type 2 diabetes. The ORs for all-cause mortality associated with cocaine, opioid, and cannabis abuse in the USA are 1.61; 1.35 and 1.49 respectively. In terms of morbidity, cocaine and cannabis use is associated with increased admissions with DKA, but whether this is due to a metabolic effect of the drugs, or secondary to treatment neglect and insulin omission, is not clear. Stroke and myocardial infarction are more common in people with type 2 diabetes who abuse opioids, and these agents commonly lead to hypogonadism which can exacerbate diabetes related erectile dysfunction. The ORs for acute stroke and myocardial infarction are 2.67 and 2.68 respectively in people with type 2 diabetes who use cocaine, and these complications often occur in younger patients who do not have the conventional risk factors for cardiovascular disease. The impact of opioids and stimulants on glycaemic control is inconsistent and the increased morbidity and mortality does not appear to be related to metabolic control.

There are no studies of management of drug abuse disorders specifically in diabetes. Methadone replacement may worsen glycaemia, and buprenorphine has some theoretical advantages for opioid withdrawal strategies.

Driving

Driving poses complex metabolic demands which increase brain glucose consumption. Because of this, there is an increased risk of hypoglycaemia, and 15–66% of people with diabetes who drive report having experienced a hypoglycaemic episode when driving. Attention, reaction times and hand/eye co-ordination are all impaired during hypoglycaemia, and visual perception is also affected, which is particularly noticeable in low light. Even modest hypoglycaemia of 3–4 mmol/L impairs responses. Subjects with induced hypoglycaemia while using a driving simulator exhibited inappropriate speeding and braking, ignored road signs and traffic signals, and had poor lane discipline. Worryingly, awareness of these potentially dangerous behaviours was also impaired. Despite this, the data on the relationship of type 1 diabetes and road traffic accident risk is conflicting and confounded by many variables. People with type 1 diabetes involved in a road traffic accident compared to those who have not, are four times more likely to have experienced a severe hypoglycaemic attack in the previous two years, and this has guided current licensing policy. There are no data on the impact of hyperglycaemia on driving ability. Regrettably, despite the theoretical risks and current regulations, 40–60% of UK drivers who take insulin never test their blood glucose before driving and 77% never test during a long journey.

In many countries, drivers with diabetes are legally required to declare the diagnosis to the national licensing authority and to the vehicle insurer. In the UK and EU, the situation has changed recently (see below and Box 32.1). Apart from hypoglycaemia, other problems that people with diabetes may have that might impact on driving are visual impairment from cataract or retinopathy, and disability from severe neuropathy, peripheral vascular disease, or leg amputation; although these disabilities can be overcome by adapting the vehicle or using automatic transmission. These problems apply equally to those without diabetes, and for details see: http://www.assets.publishing.service.gov.uk/government/uploads/system/uploads/attachment_data/file/866655/assessing-fitness-to-drive-a-guide-for-medical-professionals.pdf

Different countries apply different restrictions on the type of vehicle that can be driven by people with diabetes who are on insulin treatment. In the UK and most of the EU, vehicles are divided into Group 1 (cars and vehicles carrying up to 9 passengers, and motorcycles) and Group 2 (Buses and coaches carrying > 9 passengers, and goods vehicles). However, the regulations vary according to when the driving test was passed, and in the UK there are differences between the mainland and Northern Ireland. There is a somewhat bewildering classification of the different road traffic vehicles, and the individual eligibility for driving them now appears on the reverse of the UK card licence. For details please see www.gov.uk/old-driving-licence-categories.

Although the category nomenclature is complex, the regulations regarding eligibility of people with diabetes to drive has become simpler. Individuals in England, Wales, and Scotland have to inform the Driving and Vehicle Licensing

---

Box 32.1 UK Regulations on requirements for people with diabetes to inform DVLA (or DVA in Northern Ireland).

Cars (< 9 seats) and Motorcycles (Group 1 Licence)
1. Insulin therapy for > 3 months
2. Gestational diabetes with need for insulin 3 months after birth of baby
3. Episode of disabling hypoglycaemia and/or informed by diabetes care team that you are at risk
4. Those on tablets or non-insulin injection therapy if at risk or experience disabling hypoglycaemia (in practice those on sulfonylureas or glinides)

Buses, Coaches and Commercial Vehicles (Group 2 Licence)
1. Must inform of <u>any</u> regular medication

Those on diet therapy alone, or women with Gestational Diabetes on insulin for < 3 months, do not need to inform DVLA/DVA

Authority (DVLA) or the Driving and Vehicle Agency (DVA) in Northern Ireland if they are taking insulin for > 3 months; or if they had gestational diabetes and have to continue insulin for > 3 months after delivery; or if they have experienced (or have been told by their diabetes team that they are at increased risk of) disabling (severe) hypoglycaemia. People with type 2 diabetes with a group 1 licence only need to notify if they are treated with sulfonylureas or glinides, or any other therapy that may cause, or has caused, severe hypoglycaemia. For Group 2 licences, the DVLA and DVA need to be informed of any treatment for diabetes, except diet alone (Box 32.1).

Group 1 licences for people with diabetes who have to notify are valid for 1, 2, or 3 years, and in the UK a medical report is required for renewal. A single episode of severe hypoglycaemia while awake(defined as requiring the assistance of another person, episodes during sleep are not deemed to be relevant unless associated with impaired hypoglycaemic awareness) leads to an immediate revocation, but the individual can apply for reinstatement 3 months later with medical support from their care team. Awareness of hypoglycaemia is defined in the DVLA regulations on Medical Fitness to Drive as 'whether the licence holder or applicant is capable of bringing their vehicle to a safe controlled stop', and impaired awareness as 'an inability to detect the onset of hypoglycaemia because of a total lack of warning symptoms'. Blood glucose levels should be checked within 2 hours (preferably <1 hour) of driving and at least every 2 hours on a long journey. People should not drive with a blood glucose ≤ 5 mmol/L, the catch phrase is '5 to Drive', and are recommended to take some quick acting carbohydrate to raise their blood glucose level above this before setting off. Recently, CGM and Flash monitor readings have been approved for monitoring before and during driving, but total reliance on audible CGM alarms only has not. Readings ≤4 mmol/L and/or the driver has hypoglycaemic symptoms irrespective of the CGM reading, have to be checked with a capillary blood test. Drivers have been successfully prosecuted for failing to adhere to these rules, and non-compliance could lead insurers to limit their cover in the event of an accident. Car insurance premiums in the UK are not normally higher for people with diabetes with no previous claims history.

Group 2 licences have to be renewed every five years or at the age of 45. In addition, holders have to attend for an independent medical exam every year where they need to demonstrate that they are performing blood glucose tests at least twice a day (even when not driving). They also have to show that they test before and at least every two hours when driving, and they must show three months of uninterrupted blood glucose meter readings that are downloadable. CGM and flash monitoring is not acceptable at the time of writing.

Commercial minibus drivers should contact the DVLA for guidance as to the type of licence they require. Taxi drivers in the UK have to be authorised by the local authority, there are no national regulations, but most authorities adopt restrictions similar to those for Group 2 licence holders.

In the EU, the 3rd Directive of the European Parliament on driving licences (2006 amended 2016) has regulations very similar to those in the UK, but the definition of inadequate awareness of hypoglycaemia is left to individual member states. In Denmark, the numbers of patients reporting episodes of severe hypoglycaemia fell by 55% in the years after the Directive was introduced, presumably to avoid the risk of losing their driving licence.

Canada has regulations similar to Europe; the situation in the USA is more complicated. There are federal regulations for interstate commercial vehicle licence holders, but for car drivers each State has its own rules. The ADA offers information on its website. Australia and New Zealand have their own regulations which share elements with those in Europe.

There is general advice for people with diabetes who drive and the recommended course of action if the driver experiences hypoglycaemia when driving (Table 32.1). It is important to realise that if someone is sitting in the driving seat then they are deemed in law to be in charge of the vehicle,

Table 32.1 Recommendations for safe driving in people with diabetes taking insulin or other agents that carry a risk for hypoglycaemia.

- Always carry your glucose meter and blood glucose strips with you
- Check your blood glucose no more than 1 h before the start of the first journey and every two hours whilst you are driving
- If driving multiple short journeys, it is not necessary to test before each additional journey as long as you test every 2 h while driving. More frequent testing may be required in a circumstances where a greater risk of hypoglycemia is present e.g., after physical activity or altered meal routine
- Try to ensure that blood glucose is kept above 5.0 mmol/l (90 mg/dl) while driving. If your blood glucose is 5.0 mmol/l or less, have a snack. Do not drive if blood glucose is less than 4.0 mmol/l (72 mg/dl) or you feel hypoglycaemic
- If hypoglycaemia develops while driving, stop the vehicle in a safe location as soon as possible
- Always keep an emergency supply of fast-acting carbohydrate such as glucose tablets or sweets within easy reach inside the vehicle
- Do not start driving until 45 min after blood glucose has returned to normal (confirmed by measuring blood glucose). It takes time for the brain to recover fully from hypoglycaemia
- Carry personal identification to indicate that you have diabetes in case of injury
- Particular care should be taken during changes of insulin regimen, change in lifestyle, following exercise, during travel and during pregnancy
- Take regular meals, snacks and periods of rest on longer journeys. Do not drink alcohol before, or while driving

Reproduced from Graveling and Frier; Clin Diabetes & Endocrinol; 2015 DOI 10.1166/s40642-015-0007-3.

so it is important to switch off the engine and move to a passenger seat while correcting hypoglycaemia.

Employment

People with diabetes can and should be encouraged to undertake the widest range of employment. In the UK, diabetes is covered by the Disability Discrimination Act (1995) and the Equality Act (2010) which means that it is now possible for individuals to work in almost any area (except the Armed Forces). The Equality and Human Rights Commission offers guidance to employers about their need to provide 'reasonable adjustments' in the workplace in order to enable workers to manage their medical condition. This might involve breaks for blood glucose testing, or provision of a private area to give insulin injections for example. People with diabetes should be able to have time off to attend medical check-ups. It is not a requirement that people with diabetes have to declare their condition to their employer, but it is generally thought advisable to do so by Diabetes UK. Previous occupations such as the Emergency Services, Commercial Flying, and Air Traffic Controllers are all now open to people with diabetes, although there may be specific requirements in terms of glucose monitoring.

Travel and leisure activities.

Diabetes is not a bar to travelling, but planning is needed for extra supplies, insurance, medical identification, changes in meals, fluid intake, physical activity, and diabetes treatment en route and after arrival. It is not necessary to store insulin in a refrigerator in hot countries provided supplies are kept cool and out of direct sunlight (Box 32.2). Ensure vaccinations are up to date and check the need for malarial prophylaxis.

During long flights, blood glucose should be monitored frequently (every 2–3 hours) and glycaemic control may need to be relaxed to avoid hypoglycaemia: a few hours of moderate hyperglycaemia, say 10–13 mmol/L (180–234 mg/dL), is acceptable. Time changes of less than 4 hours in either direction require no major adjustments to the usual insulin schedule – simply give the next insulin at its usual clock time, using the destination's time zone. Westward flights effectively extend the day, and if this delay is long (>6–8 hours), extra insulin may be needed such as small doses of rapid-acting insulin injected 3–4 hourly. Long-acting insulin doses before eastward flights, which shorten the day, may need to be reduced if the day is shortened by > 6 hours (Figure 32.2).

Medical devices such as pumps and CGM can cause problems with airport security. A Medical Devices Awareness

> **Box 32.2** Recommendations for people with diabetes undertaking foreign travel.
>
> **Documentation**
> 1. Letter from health care professional confirming diabetes and listing medication (make several copies)
> 2. Personal identification such as diabetes ID card or alert bracelet
> 3. Travel insurance certificate and contacts
> 4. European Health Insurance Card (EHIC) NB ensure it is still in date (for UK nationals the EHIC card is still valid in the EU post Brexit. A new Global Health Insurance Card (GHIC) is planned)
> 5. Medical Devices Awareness Card from the Civil Aviation Authority (CAA) for insulin pump and CGM users
>
> **Medication and Equipment**
> 1. Adequate supplies of insulin, medication and testing equipment (take extra)
> 2. Carry adequate supplies in hand baggage in case any stowed bags go missing
> 3. If on an insulin pump take some long and short acting insulin in case of device failure
> 4. Check local availability of insulin and medication at destination in case of emergency
> 5. Spare batteries for devices
> 6. Small flask or cool bag to carry insulin
>
> **Security**
> 1. Letter from health care professional confirming diabetes and listing medication
> 2. If using an insulin pump or CGM do NOT pass through X ray scanners
> 3. Maximum volume is 100ml - carry quick acting carbohydrate as tablets or gels
>
> **Prevention**
> 1. Ensure vaccinations up to date
> 2. Check need for malarial prophylaxis
> 3. Use sunscreens and insect repellent
> 4. Eat what can be peeled or what is cooked
> 5. Avoid dehydration
> 6. Avoid walking barefoot

Card is available (see website below) and it is advisable to check regulations with airlines before travel.

Flying and diving are now permissible for people with diabetes taking insulin, although there are country specific regulations. The Professional Association of Diving Instructors (PADI) recommends not diving with a blood glucose <8.3 mmol/L and provides useful guidance on its website www.pros-blog.padi.com/2019/10/02/diving-and-diabetes.

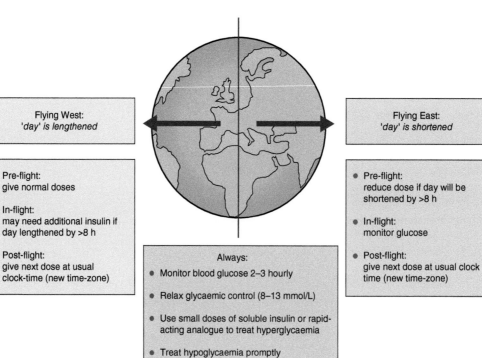

Flying West:
'day' is lengthened

- Pre-flight:
  give normal doses

- In-flight:
  may need additional insulin if
  day lengthened by >8 h

- Post-flight:
  give next dose at usual
  clock-time (new time-zone)

Flying East:
'day' is shortened

- Pre-flight:
  reduce dose if day will be
  shortened by >8 h

- In-flight:
  monitor glucose

- Post-flight:
  give next dose at usual clock
  time (new time-zone)

Always:
- Monitor blood glucose 2–3 hourly
- Relax glycaemic control (8–13 mmol/L)
- Use small doses of soluble insulin or rapid-acting analogue to treat hyperglycaemia
- Treat hypoglycaemia promptly

Figure 32.2 Scheme for adjusting insulin doses during flights that cross time zones.

CASE HISTORY

A 19-year-old with a 10-year history of type 1 diabetes experienced a severe hypoglycaemic episode in his first term at a UK University. He was living in shared accommodation and came home late one night after socialising with his flatmates. He had drunk at least eight pints of beer with spirit chasers and attended a disco. He vomited on his way home. His friends were unaware of his diabetes and left him undisturbed until late the following day. He was found deeply unconscious with signs that he had experienced a seizure (urinary incontinence and bitten tongue). He was rushed to the emergency room where his blood glucose was 2.9 mmol/L. Unfortunately, he had suffered significant brain injury and was left with major cognitive disability.

This tragic case illustrates several important points. It is important for people with type 1 diabetes to inform associates and friends if socialising in situations that increase the risk of hypoglycaemia, and they need to know what to do. The combination of vigorous exercise (dancing) and significant alcohol intake greatly increases the risk of delayed hypoglycaemia, and flatmates need to be aware of this possibility. Binge drinking games should be avoided as they increase the likelihood of serious intoxication and vomiting, in this case any carbohydrate that he had taken was almost certainly not absorbed. The modestly hypoglycaemic blood glucose concentration in the emergency department probably represented a counter-regulatory response, and he had almost certainly had much lower levels during the night and morning.

KEY WEBSITES

- Each country has its own driving regulations (these are fairly standard across the European Union) and most have their own websites.
- Information on Group 1 and 2 licences: www.gov.uk/old-driving-licence-categories
- The full fitness to drive regulations for health care professionals: https://assets.publishing.service.gov.uk/government/uploads/system/uploads/attachment_data/file/866655/assessing-fitness-to-drive-a-guide-for-medical-professionals.pdf
- Diabetes UK Guidance for Health Care Professionals: https://www.diabetes.org.uk/driving-and-diabetes--what-healthcare-professionals-should-know
- Diabetes UK Guidance for People with Diabetes: https://www.diabetes.org.uk/guide-to-diabetes/life-with-diabetes/driving
- American Diabetes Association: https://www.diabetes.org/resources/know-your-rights/discrimination/drivers-licenses/commercial-drivers-license
- Diabetes UK advice for travel: www.diabetes.org.uk/guide-to-diabetes/life-with-diabetes/travel
- Diving advice: www.pros-blog.padi.com/2019/02/diving-and-diabetes
- Diving advice : DAN.org/Health
- Cochrane library of systematic reviews on smoking cessation www.cochranelibrary.com
- Medical Devices Awareness Card : www.caa.co.uk/uploadedFiles/CAA/Content/Standard_Content/Passengers/Before_you_fly/Health/CAA_AOA_MedicalDeviceAwarenessCard.pdf
- HM Government advice on health insurance cards: www.gov.uk/european-health-insurance-card

FURTHER READING

Campagna D, Alamo A, Di Pino a et al. Smoking and diabetes: dangerous liaisons and confusing relationships. Diabetes Metab Syndr 2019; 11: 85–97

Graveling AJ, Frier BM. Driving and diabetes: problems, licensing restrictions, and recommendations for safe driving. Clinical Diabetes and Endocrinology 2015 doi:10.1186/s40842-015-0007-03

Pastor A, Conn J, MacIsaac RJ et al. Alcohol and illicit drug use in people with diabetes. Lancet Diabetes Endocrinol 2020; 8: 239–48

Tetzschner R, Norgaard K, Ranjan A. Effects of alcohol on plasma glucose and prevention of alcohol-induced hypoglycaemia in type 1 diabetes. Diabetes Metabolism Research and Reviews 2017; 34: e2965 doi.org/10.1002/dmrr.2965

Chapter 33

Organisation of diabetes care: integrating diabetes service

Providing effective high-quality diabetes care requires a co-ordinated, multi-professional team of specialists, as well as patients who are well informed and empowered (Figure 33.1). Patient-centred care is a priority in all healthcare systems, but the organisational and logistical challenges should not be underestimated. Unlike many other diseases, the management of a person with diabetes should encompass not only the provision of pharmacological therapy where appropriate to treat metabolic and cardiovascular risk factors, but also coordination of screening strategies to prevent and to detect early complications of diabetes, structured education programme to patients and carers, support with managing injectable therapies, and assessibility to health care professionals such as dietitian, podiatrist, psychologist, diabetes nurse specialist, and specialist clinicians, as well as accessibility to novel therapeutics and technologies to better manage patients diabetes. While many models of care for patients with diabetes are fairly effective in managing the acute complication or problems of diabetes, there is insufficient attention and flexibility towards the chronic nature of this condition, where patients should be placed in the centre of disease control solutions, when designs for patient education, service delivery, and payment systems should all focus on supporting patients' efforts and building the capacity of individuals and families to manage their disease effectively.

The traditional care model involves a pyramid system, between primary, secondary, and tertiary care. Patients are seen at primary care and are referred to secondary, or thereafter, to tertiary care according to clinical needs. A financial transaction and a formal referral process follows each transition of care as patients move from one health care provider to another and are seen at different tiers of health services, independent and without integration between each other. However, when this care is delivered in a fragmented

manner, it results in duplication, inefficiency and, worst of all, a poorer health experience and outcome. In the UK for example, despite the introduction of the National Service Framework (NSF) for Diabetes in 2001 which sets out a vision for diabetes services in England to be delivered by 2013, this vision is far from being achieved. While there have been some demonstrable improvements in services since the start of the delivery plan in 2003, with some good practice and effective interventions in place in some areas of the country. However, services are geographically very variable and there are still significant numbers of people with diabetes who do not have access to the agreed essential standards of care. Therefore, the integration of diabetes services is crucial to (i) improve patient experience, (ii) ensure that all healthcare organisations involved in providing diabetes care, through partnership, clearly own the responsibility for delivering excellent care to their local population, (iii) provide clearly defined terms of accountability and responsibility for each health care professional /provider and iv) reduce duplication of time, tests and information (Table 33.1).

What is integrated diabetes care?

Integrated diabetes care is both integration of a health care system **and** co-ordination of services around a patient.

"An approach that seeks to improve the quality of care for individual patients, service users and carers by ensuring that services are well co-ordinated around their needs"
- King's Fund and Nuffield Trust 2011.

In essence, diabetes integration is the whole health community joining in partnership to own the health outcomes of patients with diabetes in their local area.

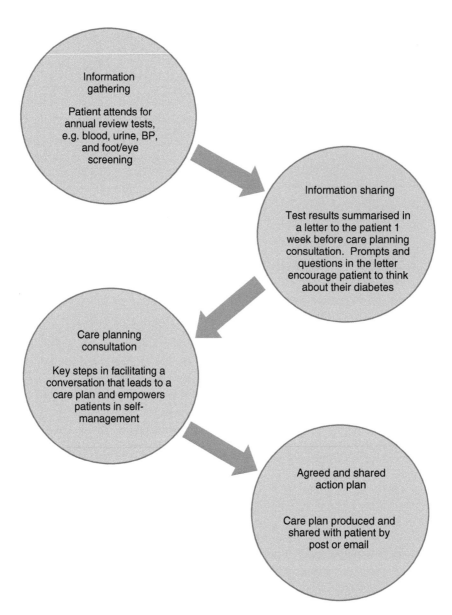

Figure 33.1 There are many different dimensions to effective diabetes services.

Table 33.1 National Institute of Clinical Excellence (NICE) for diabetes in Adults.

- Preventing type 2 diabetes in Adults (18 years and older).
- Structured education programmes for adults with diabetes.
- Care and treatment for adults with diabetes.
- Preventing and managing foot problems in adults with diabetes.

The recommendation therefore is for all local commissioners to fully and properly explore the potential benefits of joint commissioning and pooled budgets in health and social care for key populations requiring integrated approaches. Local health and well-being boards are at the centre of this approach.

What are the essential components to an integrated diabetes service?

With the development of a proposed model of care, it is important to measure both care processes and clinical outcomes. These should be used to set the priorities for commissioners and providers, ensuring all are committed to the success of the integrated service (Figure 33.2 and Table 33.2).

In the UK, proposed outcome measurements specific to diabetes would include (Table 33.3):

- Patient experience of their care, including moving between different parts of the healthcare community.
- Nine key care processes for type 1 and type 2 diabetes.
- Compliance against NICE Quality Standards for Diabetes in Adults.

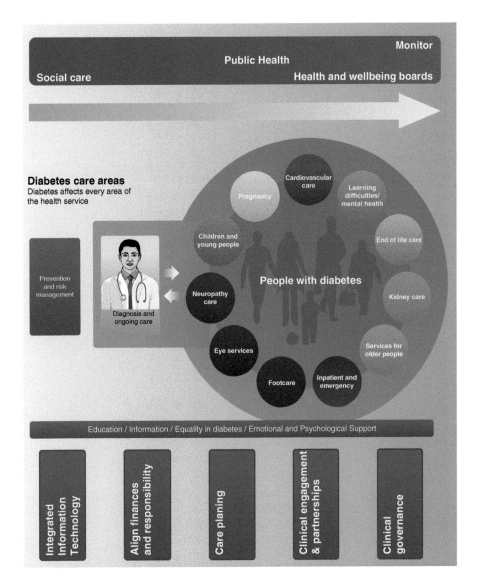

Figure 33.2 This diagram summarises the key components of integration. In particular it highlights the need to have five essential pillars of integration in place in order to facilitate the provision of different elements of diabetes care.

Table 33.2 Pillars of integration.

1. Integrated Information technology systems.
2. Aligned finances and responsibility.
3. Care planning.
4. Clinical engagement and partnership.
5. Robust shared clinical governance.

- Admissions and use of inpatient services for patients with a primary code of diabetes.
- Complications from diabetes.
- Compliance and outcomes associated with Paediatric Best Practice Tariff.

The ethos of integrated diabetes service facilitates greater involvement of people with long-term conditions

Table 33.3 The 9 Key Care process. Every person with diabetes is supposed to receive a planned programme of nationally recommended checks each year. This should be part of personalised care planning that enables them and their healthcare professionals to jointly agree actions for managing their diabetes, and to meet their individual needs. Derived from both the NSF and NICE guidance on diabetes.

1. Blood glucose level measurement
2. Blood pressure measurement
3. Cholesterol level measurement
4. Retinal screening
5. Foot and leg check
6. Kidney function testing (urine)
7. Kidney function testing (blood)
8. Weight check
9. Smoking status check.

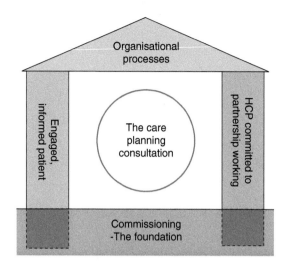

Figure 33.3 The Care Planning house model. This model was developed to illustrate the bigger picture: an engaged, informed patient and a healthcare professional committed to partnership working can achieve the best results if they are brought together in an appropriate environment with good organisational processes to facilitate their effective interaction. Robust commissioning therefore underpins the care planning 'house'.

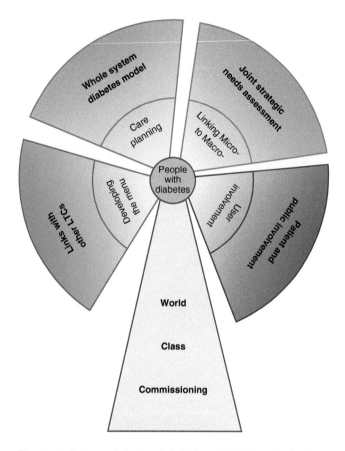

Figure 33.4 The 'commissioning windmill'. A model that illustrates key elements of service organisation to underpin care planning and the 'year of care' approach.

in planning their own care and choosing how to manage their own condition. This is in line with the emphasis placed on 'care planning' and commissioning of services to enable patients to be more informed and engaged with their treatment (Figure 33.3).

The 'Year of Care' approach has been developed in the UK in order to put the person with diabetes at the centre of decision-making and to support them in self-management. It represents care planning in action. The rationale is that each individual will have different priorities and goals, and greater opportunity to select from a range of services those that will best support and empower them in making decisions and achieving their desired outcomes. The challenge is to link each individual's needs and goals, choices, and service use into the commissioning decisions that take place at a population level. In the Year of Care Programme Evaluation people have reported an improved experience of care and real changes in self-care behaviour; professionals reported improved knowledge and skills, and greater job satisfaction, and practices reported better organisation and team-work (Figure 33.4).

The traditional annual review for patients with diabetes has sometimes become little more than a tick box exercise. Increasingly, this may be replaced by the care planning consultation in which the patient's priorities, goals, needs, and expectations contribute to a conversation leading to an action plan. There is true partnership working to develop a set of goals and action points of which the patient feels ownership. Instead of imposing management decisions and expectations, the health professional seeks to facilitate

greater ownership and engagement by the patient in setting their own aims and targets. Care planning for the year ahead will increasingly replace the current model of annual review. Beyond this, with advent of continuous glucose monitoring systems, it is increasingly feasible for patients' glucose levels to be monitored remotely by patients log on into systems, and advice can be given by diabetes specialist by phone or video links. Nonetheless, it is crucial to recognised that such strategy may only be effective when patients main issue relates to glycaemia and that assessment of vascular complications of diabetes needs to be pursued aggressively (Figure 33.5).

In order that an individual can self-manage their diabetes effectively and participate fully in decision-making, they need a good understanding of their condition and an awareness of how to access information (Figure 33.6). Thus, structured education courses have become a key component of diabetes services. An engaged, informed patient is the key to successful self-management, but it requires an individualised approach by the health professional team. As part of the NSF, many centres in the UK (>100) are now running DAFNE (Dose Adjustment for Normal Eating) courses

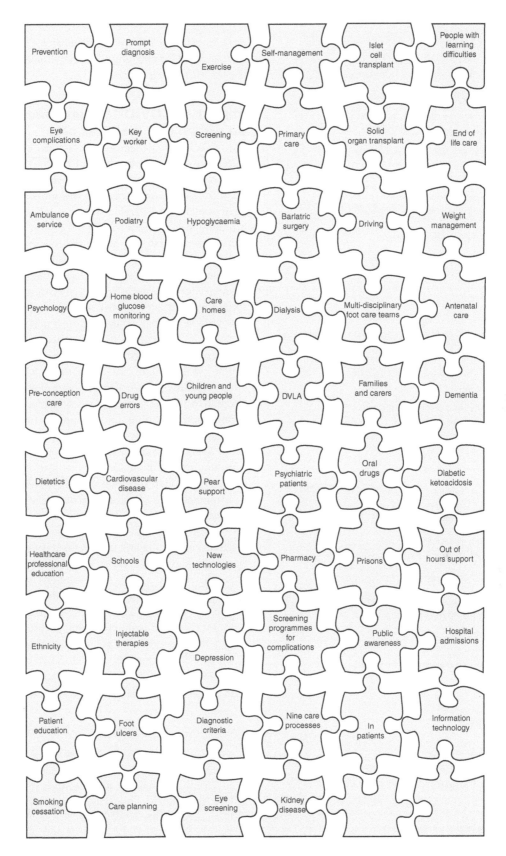

Figure 33.5 What needs to be commissioned?

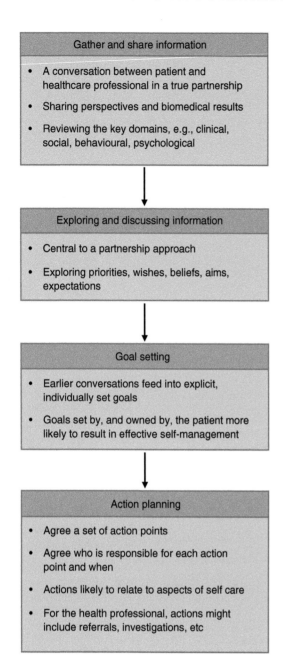

Figure 33.6 A framework for increasing the effectiveness of self-management.

for people with type 1 diabetes, and a similar number have established DESMOND (Diabetes Education and Self Management for Ongoing and Newly Diagnosed) courses for people with type 2 diabetes.

Impact of COVID-19 pandemic: lessons on organizing diabetes care

The COVID-19 pandemic started in Wuhan China in December 2019 and by the end of June 2020, there have been more than 9 million confirmed cases worldwide and around 475 000 deaths due to this virus. Various countries have implemented varying strategies to curb infectivity rate, including lockdown measures, where non key workers individuals are requested by law to self-isolate at home. This has clearly compromised the effective delivery of care for people with diabetes. As the world recover from COVID-19, a new norm needs to be established, and there is no guarantee that a second wave of infection will not occur, nor can we predict a new virus strain that would produce a new similar pandemic.

As such, innovative strategies need to be in place to ensure ongoing effective management and monitoring of people with diabetes, including those who are unable to attend routine face-to-face appointments. This requires alternative remote consultations which will require careful organisation, planning, and IT support to be able to facilitate the transformation from face-to-face to virtual consultations. Modalities may include telephone consultation, video consultation, email advice. Various platforms have become available for video consultation to be undertake effectively.

Commissioning of future diabetes services should therefore include strategies to facilitate effective collaborative care between primary and specialist teams without the need for the time-consuming and unnecessary pattern of referral, triage, and standard outpatient consultation for ongoing care. This will require effective IT solutions which enable full access to real-time patient records so that patient information can be accessed and shared seamlessly between primary and specialist teams. In addition, novel glucose monitoring technology, with cloud-based access to glucose and insulin data is required to support effective virtual consultations. It also allows services to identify those at highest risk and provide targeted care, as well as enhancing the quality of interaction.

CASE HISTORY

A 74-year-old man with type 2 diabetes, poor glucose control, foot ulcer, coronary heart disease, and frailty is reviewed by the diabetes team. An integrated diabetes care and care planning approach is implemented, replacing the traditional 'annual review' by individual healthcare professionals who focuses only on one aspect of this patient's care. Instead, a conversation about his priorities, fears, wishes, and goals was initiated. A multidisciplinary approach was used to target his multiple comorbidities including involvement of specialist foot care services to prevent the progression of his diabetic foot ulceration, assessment by a Diabetologist, dietitian, and diabetes specialist nurses to address his glucose control and coronary heart disease. These discussions and subsequent specialist interventions were conducted in the community near where this patient lives, rather than in hospital. From discussion with his GP, it became apparent that he does not want to take more than five medications, he is fearful of hypoglycaemia, and symptom-control is more of a priority. He also thinks it would be helpful to get his wife (who does the cooking) to see the dietician. He does not want to pursue aggressive HbA1c or BP targets if this means an excessive number of tablets and/or a risk of side effects. These discussions are shared within a common (ICT) computer system, so that all clinicians involved in the management of this patient would work towards the same simple goals, action points and targets.

LANDMARK CLINICAL TRIALS

Wilson A et al. on behalf of the ICCD trial Group. Evaluation of the Clinical and Cost Effectiveness of Intermediate Care Clinics for Diabetes (*ICCD*): A Multicentre Cluster Randomised Controlled *Trial*. PLoS One. 2014; 9(4): e93964

Renders CM eta I. Interventions to improve the management of diabetes mellitus in primary care, outpatient and community settings (Review). The Cochrane library 2000. Issue 4.

Davies MJ, et al. Effectiveness of the diabetes education and self management for ongoing and newly diagnosed (DESMOND) programme for people with newly diagnosed type 2 diabetes: cluster randomised controlled trial. *Br. Med. J.* 2008; 336: 491-495.

Beaglehole R, et al. Improving the prevention and management of chronic disease in low-income and middle-income countries: a priority for primary health care. Lancet 2008; 372: 940-949.

Gaziano TA, et al. Scaling up interventions for chronic disease prevention: the evidence. *Lancet* 2007; 370: 1939-1946.

Hex N et al. Estimating the current and future costs of Type 1 and Type 2 diabetes in the United Kingdom, including direct health costs and indirect societal and productivity costs. Diabetic Medicine, 2012; 29:855-62

KEY WEBSITES

- http://www.diabetes.org.uk/Professionals/Publications-reports-and-resources/Reports-statistics-and-case-studies/Reports/Diabetes-in-the-UK-2011
- http://www.diabetes.nhs.uk/work-areas/year-of-care
- https://www.diabetes.org.uk/Documents/Position%20statements/best-practice-commissioning-diabetes-services-integrated-framework-0313.pdf
- http://www.dh.gov.uk/en/Publicationsandstatistics/Publications/PublicationsPolicyAndGuidance/DH_4140284

FURTHER READING

Skills for Health / Skills for Care, Common Core Principles to Support Self Care: A Guide to support implementation (http://www.dh.gov.uk/en/publicationsandstatistics/publications/publicationspolicyandguidance/DH_084505)

Department of Health, Raising the Profile of Long Term Conditions Care: A compendium of information (http://www.dh.gov.uk/en/publicationsand statistics/publications/publicationspolicyandguidance/DH_082069)

Department of Health, Care Planning in Diabetes (http://www.dh.gov.uk/en/publicationsandstatistics/publications/publicationspolicyandguidance/DH_063081)

Department of Health, Supporting People with Long Term Conditions to Self Care: A guide to developing local strategies and good practice (www.dh.gov.uk/en/publicationsandstatistics/publications/publicationspolicyandguidance/DH_4130725)

National Diabetes Support Team, Partners in Care: A guide to implementing a care planning approach to diabetes care (www.diabetes.nhs.uk/news-1/partners%20in%20care.pdf)

Best practice for commissioning diabetes services: An integrated care framework

The management of adult diabetes services in the NHS – A progressive review. https://publications.parliament.uk/pa/cm201516/cmselect/cmpubacc/563/563.pdf

Improving integration of services – The Health and Social Care Act 2012

Integrated Care in the Reforming NHS Joint Position Statement - Diabetes UK, 2007

Integrated care for patients and populations: Improving outcomes by working together - A report to the Department of Health and the NHS Future Forum – The King's Fund, 5 January 2012

Improving the delivery of adult diabetes care through integration, Diabetes UK. https://www.diabetes.org.uk/resources-s3/2017-11/integrated%20diabetes%20care%20%28pdf%2C%20648kb%29.pdf

The NHS Atlas of Variation in Healthcare for People with Diabetes – May 2012

NHS Outcomes Framework 2012-13, Department of Health, 2011

Diabetes UK; State of the nation 2016 https://www.diabetes.org.uk/professionals/position-statements-reports/statistics/state-of-the-nation-2016-time-to-take-control-of-diabetes

Transplantation and stem cell therapy

Pancreas transplantation

Until recent advances in islet cell transplantation, whole or segmental pancreas transplantation was the only treatment for type 1 diabetes able to restore endogenous insulin secretion. Currently, about 1400 whole-pancreas transplants take place every year worldwide (Figure 34.1), with an average of 180 annually in the UK from 2016–2019. Numbers in the USA have declined from a peak of around 1400 to just under 1000 per year in the period from 2006–2017, possibly because of the increasing use of donor organs for islet cell transplants (see below). Functioning graft survival is generally better with simultaneous pancreas–kidney (SPK) grafts than with a pancreas alone transplant, probably because it is easier to detect early rejection by monitoring kidney function using serum creatinine. Around 80% of pancreas transplants in 2016/17 in the US were SPK, but the most recent reports from the Pancreas Transplant Registry do not provide graft survival rates. In the UK from 2009–2019, 1938 pancreas transplants were registered, and 5-year graft survival was 81% for SPK, but only 49% for pancreas transplant alone (PTA).

One of the problems of whole-organ transplantation is how to deal with the exocrine secretions. Many different techniques have been developed, including enteric exocrine drainage by graft-duodenojejunal anastomosis or drainage into the bladder (Figure 34.2). Enteral drainage is now the preferred technique. Venous drainage of endocrine secretions into the peripheral circulation via the internal iliac vein or by primary portal venous drainage are other options. Although some of these innovations offer theoretical advantages, there are few survival data to suggest that any specific procedure gives better long-term results. Newer immunosuppressive regimens have helped improve graft survival. The progression of diabetic complications can be halted or even reversed by pancreas transplantation if there is a sufficient period of post-transplant normoglycaemia, although up to 10 years is necessary in the case of glomerular pathology.

No controlled trials of whole organ pancreas transplant have been undertaken. Survival benefit has not been proven conclusively, but there appears to be better 10 year kidney graft survival in those undergoing SPK compared to those receiving a kidney transplant alone (KTA) (66 vs 47%), although these data are subject to patient selection bias. Patients receiving SPK may have more hospitalisations, more infections and possibly more haematological malignancies, than those

Handbook of Diabetes, Fifth Edition. Rudy Bilous, Richard Donnelly, and Iskandar Idris.
© 2021 John Wiley & Sons Ltd. Published 2021 by John Wiley & Sons Ltd.

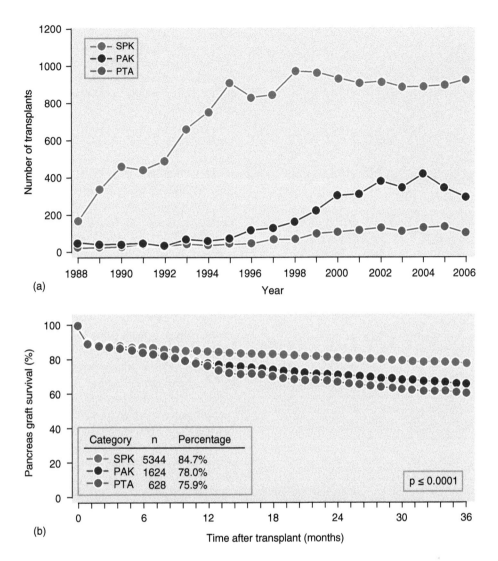

Figure 34.1 (a) Numbers of simultaneous pancreas kidney (SPK), pancreas after kidney (PAK) and pancreas alone (PTA) transplants worldwide from 1988 to 2006. (b) Percentage graft survival for the SPK, PAK, and PTA over 36 months. From White et al. Lancet 2009; 373: 1808–1801.

with KTA. No prospective evaluation of cost effectiveness has been undertaken, one retrospective analysis suggested that SPK was more cost effective than KTA or haemodialysis over 5 years. There is a compelling need for properly conducted, prospective clinical trials of whole organ pancreas transplantation along the lines of those being performed in islet cell transplantation. Currently, NICE suggests consideration of pancreas transplantation in those with sub-optimal glycaemic control who have or require a kidney transplant.

Islet cell transplantation

The clinical outcome for islet cell transplantation was transformed from the year 2000, with the introduction of the Edmonton protocol (named for the group at the University of Edmonton, Canada). The protocol is based on transplanting an adequate mass of freshly isolated islet cells, providing a potent, steroid-free and less diabetogenic immunosuppression regimen, and careful selection of patients without renal impairment. The immunosuppression involved pre- and post-transplant daclizumab (anti-interleukin 2 receptor monoclonal antibody), maintenance sirolimus and low-dose tacrolimus. Unfortunately, this combination is potentially nephrotoxic, and only patients with well-preserved renal function can tolerate it. There is research into encapsulating the islets in material that would resist both rejection and autoimmune attack in order to get around this problem. Xenotransplantation using porcine islets is a potential solution to the shortage of human tissue, but there remain potential problems with inadvertent transfer of donor animal viral pathogens.

The procedure for islet isolation is labour intensive and involves enzymatic fragmentation of the pancreas in a

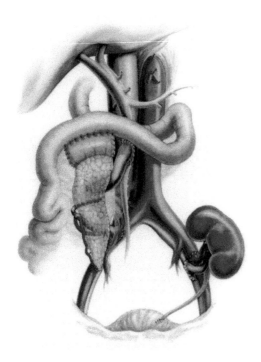

Figure 34.2 Simultaneous kidney and whole-organ pancreas transplantation showing exocrine drainage via a duodenojejunal anastomosis and venous drainage via the portal vein. The kidney transplant is shown with anastomosis to the internal iliac vessels and with ureteric implantation into the bladder. Courtesy of Dr S Bartlett, University of Maryland, MD, USA.

semi-automatic dissociation chamber. Islets are injected or infused through the percutaneous intraportal route with embolisation into the liver. An alternative approach involves direct infusion into a mesenteric vein at mini laparotomy or laparoscopy. In most cases, two sequential donors are used – approximately 850,000 islet equivalents per recipient. In the initial report of 32 consecutive type 1 diabetic patients treated in Edmonton, there was 85% sustained insulin independence and return to normoglycaemia at 1 year.

The latest report from the Collaborative Islet Transplant Registry (CITR) records data from 1086 recipients by 2015, and these individuals required 2150 islet infusions from 2619 donors. 209 of the recipients had also had a kidney transplant, 80% had severe hypoglycaemia with unawareness prior to transplantation. Over 98% were white, around 60% women, the average duration of diabetes was 29 years, and mean baseline HbA1c was 63 mmol/mol (7.9%). Full insulin independence was achieved in 50% at one year, but <30% at 5 years. However, also at 5 years, over 90% had no further recorded severe hypoglycaemic episodes, over 70% had a fasting plasma glucose <8 mmol/L and around 50% had an achieved HbA1c of <48 mmol/mol (6.5%) or a reduction from baseline of >22 mmol/mol (>2%).

In direct contrast to the situation in whole organ transplantation, more than 30 trials have been registered on ClinicalTrials.gov. Two-year data from one of them were reported in 2016. In 48 recipients with severe hypoglycaemia at baseline, and with clinical characteristics almost identical to those reported from the CITR, 52.1% were insulin independent at 1 year and 42% at 2 years. The primary endpoint of an HbA1c <53 mol/mol (<7.0%) was achieved by 87.5% and 71% at one and two years respectively. 22 procedure-specific, serious adverse events were recorded in the first year in 21 recipients, including five portal venous haemorrhages requiring transfusion, and the development of donor specific antibodies in two which will likely preclude future transplantation. Moreover, measured glomerular filtration rate declined by around 20 ml/min/1.73 m² over two years. A randomised trial of islet transplantation vs intensive insulin therapy using pumps was carried out in 50 patients in Europe with severe hypoglycaemia. At six months, glycaemic control was significantly better in the transplanted group and number of episodes of severe hypoglycaemia was reduced. Bleeding complications occurred in 7% and there was a clinically significant reduction in GFR of 20 ml/min/1.73 m² at one year, although this was less in those who had a functioning kidney transplant at baseline.

NICE originally approved islet transplantation for the indication of severe hypoglycaemia with unawareness but this has since been withdrawn. The latest type 1 guidance suggests referral of patients with hypoglycaemic unawareness that has not responded to other approaches to centres that can offer islet cell or whole organ pancreas transplantation. Further comparisons between transplantation and newer technologies such as closed-loop infusion devices should be performed in people with severe hypoglycaemic unawareness, and some are currently ongoing.

Xenotransplantation

Because of the shortage of human islets for transplantation, the use of tissue from other animals is actively undergoing research. Porcine insulin is almost homologous to human and the ready availability of animals has led to the study of transplantation into non-human primate recipients with reported long-term success for up to 804 days. There remain formidable obstacles however, notably the optimum immunosuppressive regimen and the prevention of viral transmission from donor animal to recipient. Several approaches are being tried to overcome these problems including methods of islet encapsulation and using genetically engineered pig breeds in order to reduce immunogenicity, but there remain considerable ethical and regulatory concerns that need to be resolved.

Stem cell therapy

The aim of stem cell research in diabetes is to provide a source of cells nearly identical to the pancreatic β cell for treatment

Table 34.1 Types of stem cell and their relative advantages and disadvantages as a potential β cell replacement.

Cell Type	Advantages	Disadvantages
Embryonic stem cells (ESCs)	Pluripotent Unlimited ability to multiply	Ethical constraints Teratoma risk Autoimmune response
Induced pluripotent stem cells	Easily accessible No ethical concerns	Tumour potential Problems with long-term function and viability
Nuclear transfer ESCs	ESC like potential	Limited availability
Female embryonic stem-like cells	No ethical concerns	Limited data on differentiation to functional β cells
Human testis derived embryonic-like	ESC like potential No ethical concerns	Pluripotency Male only
Mesenchymal stem cells	β cell function improved by immunomodulation Low autoimmunity Low tumour risk	Temporary efficacy requiring repeated treatments

Adapted from Lilly et al. *Am J Stem Cells* 2016; 5: 87–98.

of type 1 diabetes by transplantation. Stem cells are self-renewing cells that produce large numbers of differentiated progeny, and there are several potential sources (Table 34.1 and Figure 34.3). Embryonic stem cells are derived from the inner cell mass of mammalian blastocysts; they can be cultured *in vitro;* and when allowed to aggregate (as an 'embryoid body'), they can differentiate into all of the tissues of the embryo, including β cells. The numerous growth and transcription factors that guide embryonic stem cells to transform into endoderm and β cells are being discovered. One of the key signals is pancreatic and duodenal homeobox factor 1 (PDX-1, also known as IPF-1) and its deficiency in humans leads to pancreatic agenesis and diabetes.

Unfortunately, there is no complete road map of the the process of differentiation from stem cell to functional β cell, and this has resulted in significant biochemical and biological differences in cultured cell lines making functional reproducibility very difficult. Despite these drawbacks, engineered cell lines have been licensed for experimental use in people with type 1 diabetes and Phase 1 and 2 trials are currently ongoing.

There have been many reports of the use of undifferentiated stem cell therapy in people with type 1 and type 2 diabetes. A meta-analysis published in 2016 reported data from 22 studies involving 524 patients (300 with type 1 and 224 with type 2 diabetes) with varying results. The most promising used CD34+ haematopoietic stem cells harvested

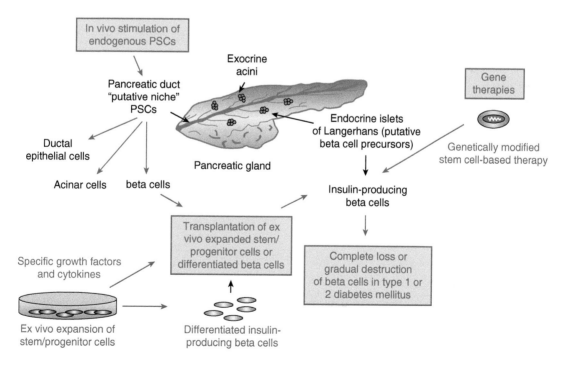

Figure 34.3 Schematic representation of the pancreas gland showing the anatomical localisation of pancreatic stem/progenitor cells (PSCs) and β cell precursors, together with potential stem cell-based therapies for diabetes mellitus. Pancreatic stem/progenitor cells exist within the ductal structure and exocrine acini; putative β cell precursors are found near or within the islets of Langerhans. From Mimeault & Batra. Gut 2008; 57: 1456–1468.

after granulocyte-colony stimulating factor therapy and leukophoresis, with a reported rate of insulin independence of 58.9% for a mean period of 16 months. Results in people with type 2 diabetes were less clear cut. However, there remain major unresolved concerns and problems with this approach. Most of the data were from uncontrolled case series not randomised controlled trials. It is unclear where the stem cells end up, in animals most cells infused peripherally seem to reside in the pulmonary and hepatic circulation. The best results in man follow direct pancreatic artery infusion, but this is obviously invasive and impractical for wider use. Finally, patients require immunosuppression, with over 20% reporting significant side effects including serious infections, although there were no reported deaths in the 22 studies.

Stem cell therapy is often marketed directly to patients and frequently delivered in unregulated facilities. It remains a highly experimental approach and patients should be advised accordingly.

Gene therapy

Gene therapy for diabetes is still at the stage of animal experimentation, but the aim is to transfer DNA to somatic cells to treat or prevent diabetes or its complications. Several strategies are envisaged, including prevention of β cell destruction through autoimmune attack by manipulating β cells to produce a survival factor (e.g. interleukin-1 receptor antagonist or anti-apoptotic factors). This requires a vector to transform the remaining β cells *in vivo* in newly diagnosed type 1 diabetic patients. Immunomodulation might be achieved by DNA vaccination in high-risk individuals, such as vaccination with glutamic acid decarboxylase (GAD) DNA to induce tolerance to this key auto-antigen. The first randomised controlled trial in 70 type 1 adolescent patients found that there was a small but statistically significantly increased C peptide concentration in the treated subjects, but no effect on insulin dose requirement. Stimulation of β cell differentiation and regeneration might involve gene therapy with transcription factors that control development (e.g. PDX-1). Other approaches have used islets which have had genes inserted that will express proteins (such as IL-10) that help resist immune attack when transplanted and avoid the need for immunosuppression. Ectopic production of insulin by several substitute cells has already been achieved, including in fibroblasts, hepatocytes, intestinal K cells, and pituitary cells. Hepatocytes have the advantages of being readily available and expressing GLUT 2 transporters and glucokinase, both of which are essential components of a glucose responsive system. However, they cannot store or secrete insulin in a regulated fashion. To overcome this, glucose responsive gene transcription controls have been employed such as glucose-6-phosphate and carbohydrate responsive element binding protein. There still remain the problems of the delivery of the modified genes and their sustainability. Viral vectors have the potential to overcome the problem of sustainability but are immunogenic and have potential

long-term safety concerns. Other approaches have used GLP-1 and fibroblast growth factor 21 genes with successful correction of hyperglycaemia and obesity in rodent models. Perhaps the most promising study to date showed correction of hyperglycaemia in diabetic dogs for four years by insertion of both the insulin and glucokinase genes into skeletal muscle cells. Gene therapy trials in other (mainly monogenic) diseases have had serious complications and there remain daunting problems to solve before they become practicable and safe for people with diabetes. Currently there are no trials registered on the Clinical Trials.gov website

---

CASE HISTORY

A 48-year-old man with longstanding type 1 diabetes of 35 years duration gradually progressed to end stage renal failure 15 years after developing severe proteinuria. He had troublesome autonomic neuropathy with postural hypotension that was hard to manage, and gustatory sweating. He underwent combined whole organ pancreas and kidney transplantation in 2015. Five years later, he had a normal HbA1c of 40 mmol/mol (5.8%) and good renal function (eGFR 48 ml/min/1.73m2). His autonomic symptoms had improved and he no longer experienced gustatory sweating or symptomatic hypotension.

Autonomic symptoms were shown to improve post pancreas transplantation in early studies from the USA. This is probably a reflection of functional improvements rather than structural changes in the nerves which would require a much longer period of normoglycemia.

LANDMARK STUDY

Shapiro AMJ, Lakey JRT, Ryan EA et al. Islet transplantation in seven patients with type 1 diabetes mellitus using a glucocorticoid-free immunosuppressive regimen. N Engl J Med 2000; 343: 230–38

After many years of unsuccessful attempts at islet transplantation, the Edmonton group were able to show prolonged survival of isles infused into the portal vein in a small number of people with type 1 diabetes using an immunosuppression protocol that avoided steroids. The results were greeted by a standing ovation when presented at the American Diabetes Association. This study paved the way for islet transplantation to become a viable option for patients with incapacitating hypoglycaemia. It led to the establishment of international collaboration in the field and of the Collaborative Islet Transplant Registry

---

KEY WEBSITES

- NICE (2015 updated 2016). Type 1 diabetes in adults: diagnosis and management. www.nice.org.uk/guidance/ng17
- Collaborative Islet Transplant Registry: 10th Annual report. Accessed through www.CITRegistry.org
- NHS Blood and Transplant. https://www.odt.nhs.uk/statistics-and-reports/organ-specific-reports/

FURTHER READING

Alam T, Wai P, Held D, Vakili STT, Forsberg E, Sollinger H. Correction of diabetic hyperglycaemia and amelioration of metabolic anomalies by mini circle DNA mediated glucose-dependent hepatic insulin production. PLoS ONE 2013; 8(6): e67515 doi: 10.1371/journal.pone.0067515

Cheng SK, Park EY, Pehar A, Rooney AC, Gallicano GI. Current progress of human trials using stem cell therapy as a treatment for diabetes mellitus. Am J Stem Cells 2016; 5: 74–86

El-Badawy A & El-Badri N. Clinical efficacy of stem cell therapy for diabetes mellitus: a meta-analysis. PLos ONE 2016; 11(4): e0151938 doi 10.1371/journal.pone.0151938

Harlan DM. Gene-altered islets for transplant: giant leap or small step? Endocrinology 2004; 145: 463–466.

Hayek K & King CC. Brief review: cell replacement therapies to treat type 1 diabetes mellitus. Clinical Diabetes Endocrinol 2016; 2: 4 doi 10.1186/s40842-016-0023-y

Hering BE, Cozzi E, Spizzo T, Cowan PJ, Rayat GR, Cooper DKC, Denner J. First update of the International Xenotransplantation Association consensus statement on conditions for undertaking clinical trials of porcine islet products in type 1 diabetes – executive summary. Xenotransplantation 2016; 23: 3–13 doi 10.1111/xen.12231

Hering BJ, Clarke WR, Bridges ND et al Phase 3 trial of transplantation of human islets in type 1 diabetes complicated with severe hypoglycaemia. Diabetes Care 2016; 39: 1230–40

Jacobsen EF & Tzanakakis ES. Human pluripotent stem cell differentiation to functional pancreatic cells for diabetes therapies: innovations, challenges and future directions. J Biol Engineering 2017; 11: 21 doi 10.1186/s13036-017-0066-3

Johnson JD. The quest to make fully functional human pancreatic beta cells from embryonic stem cells: climbing a mountain in the clouds. Diabetologia 2016; 59: 2047–57 doi 10.1007/s00125-016-4059-4

Kandaswamy R, Stock PG, Gustafson SK et al. OPTN/SRTR 2017 Annual data report: pancreas. Am J Transplant 2019; 19: Suppl 2: 124–83. doi: 10.1111/ajt.15275

Lablanche S, Vantyghem MC, Kessler L et al. Islet transplantation versus insulin therapy in patients with type 1 diabetes with severe hypoglycaemia or poorly controlled glycaemia after kidney transplantation (TRIMECO): a multi-centre, randomised controlled trial. Lancet Diabetes Endocrinol 2018; 6: 527–37

Lilly MA, Davis MF, Fabie JE, Terhune EB, Gallicano GI. Current stem-cell-based therapies in diabetes. Am J Stem Cells 2016; 5: 87–98

Park C-G, Bottino R, Hawthorne WJ. Current status of islet xenotransplantation. Int J Surgery 2015; 23: 261–66. http://dx.doi.org/10.1016/j.ijsu.2015.07.703

Prud'homme GJ, Draghia-Akli R, Wang Q. Plasmid-based gene therapy of diabetes mellitus. Gene Ther 2008; 14: 553–564.

White SA, Shaw JA, Sutherlend DER. Pancreas transplantation. Lancet 2009; 373: 1808–1817.

Vantyghem M-C, de Koning EJP, Pattou F, Mickels MR. Advances in B-cell replacement therapy for the treatment of type 1 diabetes. Lancet 2019; doi.org/10.1016/S0140-6736(19)31334-0

Index

Page locators in **bold** indicate tables. Page locators in *italics* indicate figures. This index uses letter-by-letter alphabetization.

Handbook of Diabetes, Fifth Edition. Rudy Bilous, Richard Donnelly, and Iskandar Idris.
© 2021 John Wiley & Sons Ltd. Published 2021 by John Wiley & Sons Ltd.